Comfort in Caring

Comfort in Caring
Nursing the Person With HIV Infection

Janice Bell Meisenhelder, D.N.Sc., R.N.
Director, Center for Nursing Research
New England Deaconess Hospital

Christopher L. LaCharite, B.S.N., R.N.
HIV Coordinator
Brigham and Women's Hospital

Scott, Foresman/Little, Brown College Division
Scott, Foresman and Company
Glenview, Illinois   Boston   London

Library of Congress Cataloging-in-Publication Data

Comfort in caring.
  1. AIDS (Disease)—Nursing. I. Meisenhelder, Janice Bell. II. LaCharite, Christopher L.
[DNLM: 1. Acquired Immunodeficiency Syndrome—nursing. WY 150 C732]
RC607.A26C66 1989   610.73'699   88-31914
ISBN 0–673–52004–8

Copyright © 1989 by Janice Bell Meisenhelder and Christopher L. LaCharite

All rights reserved. No part of this book may be reproduced in any form or by any electronic or mechanical means including information storage and retrieval systems without permission in writing from the publisher, except by a reviewer who may quote brief passages in a review.

2 3 4 5 6 7 8 9 10 — MVN — 94 93 92 91 90 89

Printed in the United States of America

Dedication: To Those Who Have Suffered

I see an invisible fire raging,
consuming humanity.

People,
Who have always felt outside the mainstream,
Who have been told before
they do not matter as much as the rest,
Who have felt the footprint of society
on their backs,
Now burning in an epidemic.

I feel the stabbing pain of human suffering.

At the same time,
I ache with amazement,
Awed by the resilience of the soul.

Eyes which reflect determination,
conviction,
perseverance.
Words which show me an inner strength.
untouchable by disease,
Unconquerable,
even by death.
An inner strength
augmented, matured, perfected,
by the heat of disaster.

I see the human spirit
like a Phoenix
Rising from the ashes of a wasting disease,
Soaring to heights of courage,
hope,
and faith
only imagined by us below.

And I stand with pride,
Among those who care.

J. B. Meisenhelder
1988

Contributing Authors

Margaret Benak, B.S., R.D.
Dietetics/Nutrition Department
Brigham and Women's Hospital
Boston, MA

Tara Coghlin, B.S., R.D.
Dietetics/Nutrition Department
Brigham and Women's Hospital
Boston, MA

Jeanne Watson Driscoll, M.S., R.N.
Psychiatric/Mental Health Clinical
  Nurse Specialist
Brigham and Women's Hospital
Boston, MA

David J. Hannabury, M.S., R.N.
Head Nurse
AIDS Special Care Unit
Lemuel Shattuck Hospital
Boston, MA

Jeff Huyett, B.S., R.N.
Health Care Provider Educator
AIDS Action Committee
Boston, MA

Nancy P. Karthas, B.S., R.N.
Clinical AIDS Coordinator
Children's Hospital
Boston, MA

Wm. Michael Keane, Ph.D.
Co-Director, Next Step Counseling
Newton, MA

Christopher L. LaCharite, B.S., R.N.
HIV Coordinator
Brigham and Women's Hospital
Boston, MA

Ann M. Locke, M.S., R.N.
Certified Psychiatric Mental Health
  Clinical Nurse Specialist
Massachusetts General Hospital
Boston, MA

Janice Bell Meisenhelder, D.N.S., R.N.
Director, Center for Nursing Research
New England Deaconess Hospital
Boston, MA

Martha Moon, M.S., R.N.
Clinical Director and Family Nurse
  Practitioner
Fenway Community Health Center
Boston, MA

Ruth Muller, M.S., R.N.
Staff Education Instructor
Brigham & Women's Hospital
Boston, MA

Rev. Jennifer Phillips, D. Min.
Rector, Church of St. John the
  Evangelist, Boston, MA
Chair, Ecumenical Task Force on
  AIDS
Boston, MA

Kattie Portis
Founder of Women Incorporated
Coordinator of Women AIDS Risk
 Network
Boston, MA

Berit Pratt, M.P.H., R.N.
AIDS Coordinator
Visiting Nurses Association of Boston
Boston, MA

Richard A. Rasi, D.Min
Bloom and Rasi Psychological
 Associates
Brookline, MA

Julie M. Sniffen, M.S.
Infection Control Practitioner
Brigham and Women's Hospital
Boston, MA

Jill Meredith Strawn, M.S.N., R.N.
Assistant Clinical Professor, Yale
 University School of Nursing
Certified Psychiatric/Mental Health
 Clinical Nurse Specialist
Project Director
AIDS Outreach, Prevention and
 Demonstration Project
The APT Foundation
New Haven, CT

Ann B. Williams, M.S., R.N.-C.
Assistant Professor, Yale University
 School of Nursing
Co-Director and Family Nurse
 Practitioner
Central Medical Substance Abuse
 Treatment Unit
Connecticut Mental Health Center
New Haven, CT

Preface

This book is designed to help nurses become comfortable caring for people with HIV infection. The physical care of persons with HIV infection is like the physical care of any other clients. We administer their IV medications, dress their skin ulcers, and position them in bed in the exact same manner as we do for people with other medical diagnoses who need IV medications, dressing changes, and positioning in bed. The difference in caring for people with HIV infection is not the physical care, but the emotional issues that surround and pervade the very suggestion of this disease. It's our ability to deal effectively with these issues that distinguishes acceptable nursing care from exceptional nursing care. The material in this book is specific to HIV infection. It includes all the intangible elements that make working with this population such a challenge to nurses.

The idea for this book came from seeing the unique kind of stress nurses feel in working with a stigmatized and terminal illness. We wanted to reassure nurses that everything would be all right: They had the skills they needed to care for these people well. Hence, the theme of comfort evolved for this book. In order to give comfort, nurses must first feel comfortable themselves with all the myriad of emotions and values that surround HIV infection. This book is organized around the developmental progression that nurses follow becoming comfortable with HIV infection. First, nurses deal with the threats to themselves, the causes of discomfort: fear, viral transmission, hopelessness, and lack of clear solutions to clinical dilemmas. Since this disease often brings nurses into contact with diverse groups for the first time, the second section of the book gives nurses a feel for the cultural variations found among people with HIV infection. The third section provides knowledge about the disease and nursing care of this client population: disease process, opportunistic infections, client assessment, nutritional interventions, discharge planning, needs of children, and sexual needs. The last section equips nurses with different ways of giving comfort for intangible needs: alternate care, spiritual care, psychological care, and patient teaching. Thus, the first two sections try to prepare nurses affectively, the last two sections equip nurses cognitively for working with people with HIV infection.

Throughout the book, we refer primarily to HIV infection, rather than AIDS. Although AIDS is the more common and familiar term, HIV infection better describes the clients portrayed in this book. At the onset of this epidemic, people were diagnosed with AIDS after they had become quite ill. Now, we have identified HIV infection in a range of people, from asymptomatic to critically ill. People all along this continuum of HIV infection are receiving treatment, both traditional and nontraditional. Thus, rather than distinguishing AIDS, ARC, or nonsymptomatic seropositive status, we chose to be inclusive, if not cumbersome, with the term HIV infection.

Our authors not only write about the communities and cultures that coexist with AIDS, they are a part of them. They have lived the struggles, pain, and victories of HIV infection beside their clients. In presenting these chapters, the authors have seasoned the factual information with a tender understanding of the people they serve. Our goal is to help you identify with these clients, too, for this is the key to becoming comfortable with HIV infection and being able to comfort those who suffer.

Janice Bell Meisenhelder
Christopher L. LaCharite

Contents

Part I	Comfort When Giving Care	1
1	*Overcoming the Fear*	3

    The Real Danger   4
    The Real Risk of Exposure   4
    Fear of Contagion: Manifestatons   6
    The Roots of Fear   7
    Caring Without Fear   8
    References   9

2	*Protecting Oneself: Infection Control*	13

    Transmission of HIV   14
    Risk to the Health Care Worker   15
    Universal Precautions   17
    Other Precautions   18
    Conclusion   21
    References   21

3	*Making Tough Decisions in HIV Care*	23

    Mandatory Testing Versus Informed Consent   23

xii   Contents

         Duty To Warn Versus Confidentiality   25
         Right To Treatment Versus Right To Die   26
         Duty To Care Versus Personal Risk Taking   27
         Conclusion   28
         References   29

4   Sustaining Our Hope   31

         The Meaning and Need for Hope   31
         The Process of Involvement With HIV-Infected People   31
         Spiritual Dimensions of Care Givers' Fears   32
         Befriending Our Mortality   34
         Grief, Hope, and Burnout   35
         Helplessness and Hope   36
         Self-care   37
         Finding Hope   38

Part II   Comfort With Cultural Differences   41

5   Interacting With Gay Families   43

         Understanding the Gay Family   43
         Understanding the Emotional Issues   46
         The Nurse's Interaction With the Gay Family   49
         References   51
         Recommended Videos and Readings   51

6   Managing Addictive Behavior   53

         Key Attitudes   54
         Psychosocial Profile   54
         Nursing Approach   56
         Specific Drugs of Abuse   56
         Treatment for Heroin Addiction   59
         Cocaine Treatment   62
         Referral for Drug Abuse   63
         Intravenous Drug Abuse and AIDS   63
         The Intravenous Drug Abuser as a Person With
            HIV Infection   65
         References   65

7	***Breaking Down Barriers: HIV Infection and Communities of Color***	67
	My Experience With Breaking Down Barriers 68	
	Barriers for Communities of Color 69	
	AIDS and Communities of Color 70	
	Communities of Color and the Health Care System 71	
8	***Counseling Women With HIV Infection***	75
	Epidemiology of AIDS in Women 76	
	HIV Transmission in Women 76	
	Reproductive Concerns 78	
	Risk-Reduction Strategies for Women 80	
	Psychosocial Issues for Women With AIDS 82	
	Conclusion 84	
	References 85	
Part III	**Comfort With Physical Needs**	**87**
9	***Understanding the Disease***	89
	Human Immunodeficiency Virus (HIV) 89	
	Clinical Spectrum of HIV Infection 90	
	HIV Testing 91	
	Asymptomatic HIV Infection 93	
	HIV and Its Effects on the Body 93	
	Effects on the Immune System 93	
	HIV Effects on the Central Nervous System 94	
	Peripheral Nervous System Effects 96	
	HIV Effects on Lymphocytes and Platelets 97	
	HIV-Associated Malignancy 97	
	Zidovudine (AZT) 98	
	Summary 99	
	References 99	
	Appendix 9.1: Opportunistic Infections Associated With HIV Infection 102	
10	***Assessing the Client's Needs***	109
	Functional Health Patterns 111	

Physical Assessment 117
Compiling the Data 118
References 119
Appendix 10.1: Nursing Care Plan for Person
With AIDS 120

11 *Nutrition: Controlling the "Slims"* 129

How AIDS Undermines Nutrition 129
Assessing the Client at Nutritional Risk 131
Unproven Nutritional Regimes 132
Meal Plans 135
Appendix 11.1: Difficulties Meeting Nutrition
Requirements: Some Solutions 136
Appendix 11.2: Daily Meal Plans 143
Appendix 11.3: Supplements 148

12 *Getting Them Home: Discharge Planning* 149

The Need for Home Care 149
The Discharge Process 150
Summary 155
References 155

13 *Identifying Special Needs: Children With HIV Infection* 157

The HIV-Infected Family 158
The Clincal Picture 159
The Nursing Role 161
The HIV-Infected Child in the Community 163
References 164

14 *Teaching Safer Sex* 167

Gaining Comfort in Teaching and Counseling 168
Conducting a Sexual Assessment 168
Teaching Safer Sex 172
Barriers to Safer Sex Practices 176
Summary 177
References 177

Part IV	**Different Ways of Comforting**	**179**
15	*Complementary Therapies: Maximizing the Mind-Body Connection*	181

        Mind-Body Connections   182
        Long-Term Survivors of AIDS   183
        Cancer as a Rehearsal for AIDS   184
        Common Complementary Therapies   184
        The Underground Network   190
        Responsibility Versus Blame   191
        The Nurse's Role in Complementary Therapies   191
        The Bottom Line: Keeping Hope Alive   194
        Resources   194
        References   196

16	*Nurturing the Spirit*	199

        Loss and Change as Spiritual Stressors   199
        Building Community in the Face of Fear   204
        Emerging Spiritual Questions   207

17	*The Psychosocial Impact of HIV Infection: Minimizing the Losses*	213

        The Expressed Concerns   213
        The Family's Experience   221
        References   223

18	*Patient Teaching: Empowering for Self-Care*	225

        Individualize for Effective Teaching   225
        Maximizing the Teaching Time   226
        The Content: What Clients Need to Know   227
        Developing Additional Learning Tools   234
        Appendix 18.1: Definition: Pneumocystis Carinii Pneumonia   236
        Appendix 18.2: Definition: Kaposi's Sarcoma   237
        Appendix 18.3: Medication: Trimethoprim/Sulfamethoxazole (Bactrim, Bactrim DS, Septra)   238
        Appendix 18.4: Medication: Ketoconazole (Nizoral)   239

Appendix 18.5: Medication: Acyclovir (Zovirax) 240
Appendix 18.6: Medication: Nystatin Suspension (Mycostatin, Nilstat, Nadostine) 242
Appendix 18.7: Medication: Pentamidine Isethionate (Pentam 300) 243
Appendix 18.8: Zidovudine (Retrovir, formerly AZT) 245
Appendix 18.9: Home Care Guidelines for People With AIDS, ARC, and HIV Infection 247
Appendix 18.10: Checklist for PWAs: Items To Have on Hand 252
Appendix 18.11: "To Do List": Suggestions for PWA or PWARC to Consider 253

Appendix A.1   **255**

Appendix A.2   **271**

Appendix B   **278**

Glossary   291

Index   299

Comfort in Caring

Notice

The authors and publisher have made every effort to ensure the accuracy and appropriateness of the drug dosages presented in this textbook. The medications described do not necessarily have specific approval by the Food and Drug Administration for use in the diseases and dosages for which they are recommended. The package insert for each drug should be consulted for use and dosage as approved by the FDA. Because standards for usage change, it is advisable to keep abreast of revised recommendations, particularly those concerning new drugs. We urge you to check the dosage information on the manufacturer's package insert before you administer any drug.

Part I

Comfort When Giving Care

Chapter 1

Overcoming the Fear

Janice Bell Meisenhelder

A fearful epidemic spreads throughout society: Acquired Immunodeficiency Syndrome (AIDS). It strikes the young, the healthy. It lies dormant for years, waiting to emerge into the deadly syndrome at an unknown time. It passes innocently, silently, undetected, from person to person. It evolves into a devastating, wasting disease. The very hint of its symptoms guarantees a gruesome, inevitable death.

As nurses working with clients who suffer from AIDS, we suffer too. We feel helpless and afraid. We see the devastating end result, the last final stages of physical and emotional pain. We feel the most exposed, the most vulnerable, not only to the agony of watching people die, but vulnerable to the virus itself. We are the front line. How can we be comfortable giving compassionate care when we are confronted with such an intangible threat to our own safety?

Fear of contagion, an anxious response to the perceived threat of contracting AIDS, grips all of us at one time or another. Our society's characteristic response to this infection has been widespread, extreme fear that evokes irrational behavior. As nurses, we need to face the realistic fears, take reasonable precautions, and overcome the exaggerated fears through a better understanding of ourselves. This chapter focuses on fear of contagion, the irrational anxiety of catching a disease. Both the real and the imagined threats are examined. We will discuss how to prevent our fears from compromising our care.

The Real Danger

Acquired immunodeficiency syndrome (AIDS) and AIDS related complex (ARC) result from an infection caused by a retrovirus, the human immunodeficiency virus (HIV). Unlike other viruses that reproduce themselves independently, a retrovirus uses the host's own cells to reproduce. HIV invades predominantly white blood cells and takes over the protein (DNA and RNA) production. Under the virus's control, the white blood cell makes the virus's DNA rather than its own. Thus, the cell reproduces the virus, not the cell. An active HIV infection results in a decrease in the number of white blood cells and a production of more virus, which continues to invade other healthy cells in order to reproduce (Kunkel & Warner, 1987).

Three characteristics make this infection particularly threatening. First, since most of the viral activity is inside the cell rather than in the bloodstream, the immune system does not detect the viral invasion immediately. There is a time lag between the initial invasion and the formation of antibodies that can last up to several months (Simmonds et al., 1988). Thus, identifying noninfected persons with absolute certainty by laboratory tests is impossible. Second, the virus may lie dormant in the initial cell for years before it begins to reproduce. Thus, the incubation period, the time between initial infection to onset of symptoms, could be six years or longer in some cases (Moss et al., 1988). Since this is a relatively new disease, with such a long potential incubation period, it is impossible to know what percentage of people currently infected actually will be afflicted with the illness. Estimates range up to 75 percent, but such figures remain educated guesses based on an insufficient amount of evidence (Barbour, 1987; German Study, 1987; Health & Public Policy Committee, 1988; Kunkel & Warner, 1987; Moss et al., 1988).

Third, this virus mutates and produces a variety of related strains. This virus could produce a strain that differs from the current strain in antibody formation, response to medication, and incubation period. Because HIV has this capacity to be evolving and changing constantly, we can never be certain that what we know to be true today will be true tomorrow, especially in regard to treatment and vaccine. We may never know all we want to know about this infection.

These three characteristics of HIV infection portray the doomsday foreboding of a science-fiction thriller. Fear of acquiring this virus is understandable. Fortunately, HIV infection is relatively difficult to acquire. The properties of HIV outlined above make vaccine, treatment, and cure very difficult, but not prevention! Scientists *do* know how the virus transmits from person to person. Although HIV infection should be avoided at all times, avoiding exposure to this virus is relatively easy to do.

The Real Risk of Exposure

HIV is a fragile virus that needs blood-to-blood, semen-to-blood, or vaginal-secretions-to-blood contact to be transmitted. Thus, a limited, defined set of conditions must exist to contract this microbe. There must be mucus membrane contact or a break in the skin to allow the virus to reach the bloodstream. There must also be sufficient virus in the body fluid to infect. HIV infection spreads by infusion of contaminated blood, through sexual activity, and from mother to fetus or newborn. With the exception of vertical transmission from mother to unborn child, some degree of consent takes place with adult exposure to this virus. The majority of infections result from sexual activity and intravenous drug use with blood-contaminated needles (CDC, 1987; Friedland & Klein, 1987; Sande, 1986).

Because of the unknown elements of this disease, multiple rigorous studies have been conducted on how HIV spreads. In order to rule out the possibility of infection through saliva, tears, or other body fluids, people living with persons with HIV infection have been closely watched. Under all family living conditions, including displaying affection and sharing meals and lavatories, no one has contracted the virus through close contact. The only family members to be exposed to the virus were the sexual partners of the infected. This was true in three separate studies of household members (Graaf & Diepersloot, 1986). These studies provide conclusive evidence that HIV cannot be transmitted through casual contact, such as hugging, kissing, shaking hands, or sharing drinking cups.

The risk to health care workers from exposure to blood continues to be a major focus of AIDS research. However, even an inoculation of infected blood from an accidental needlestick is usually insufficient exposure to transmit the virus. Multiple studies from around the United States and Great Britain have together evaluated over 3,500 health care workers who have intensive exposure to HIV. These studies first establish the negative-antibody status of the health care workers, and then follow them for one year or longer to see if they develop the antibody for HIV. Most of the subjects of these studies have had exposure to the virus through needlesticks with infected blood or other skin, or parenteral contact with infected body fluids. From all of these studies, scientists calculate a risk of transmission of HIV in the occupational setting to be less than one in a thousand (<0.1%) per year of exposure. The risk of developing antibodies after accidental needlestick exposure is less than five in a thousand (<0.5%). These calculations of risk include health care workers who were not using recommended precautions. Compared to all other infectious diseases, HIV is the hardest to contract in the health care setting (CDC, 1987; Gerbering et al., 1987; Gerbering & Henderson, 1987; Henderson et al., 1986).

These studies say that for every 1,000 nurses who stick themselves with needles containing HIV-infected blood, 999 nurses will remain free of infection. HIV infection *can* and has been spread by blood on infected needles, or exposure of infected blood to the oral mucus membrane or eye. These cases are rare and occur primarily when the appropriate precautions are ignored. When the recommended precautions are followed, this risk becomes almost nonexistent (CDC, 1985; CDC, 1987; Friedland & Klein, 1987).

Although HIV is never contagious by casual contact and rarely contagious by health care contact with precautions, this virus does readily transmit sexually and through blood-to-blood contact. The above studies of health care workers eliminated those people who contracted the virus sexually, through intravenous drug use, or through receiving contaminated blood. Although people rarely acquired the virus from exposure at their jobs, there are probably hundreds of health care workers who have been exposed to HIV through activities in their personal, rather than professional, lives.

Fear of Contagion: Manifestations

If the risk of acquiring the virus through casual touch or health care is almost nonexistent, why then is there so much fear among health care workers and the public in general? Repeatedly, people behave as if this virus could be acquired through public rest rooms or cafeterias, rather than through deliberate, intimate contact. The contagiousness of this virus becomes largely exaggerated by fear.

Examples of irrational, fearful overreactions to this epidemic include public proposals that call for mandatory blood testing of everyone, or compulsory identification cards for persons with AIDS or ARC. One proposal even suggested HIV-infected individuals be tattooed (Ballard, 1987; Kirby, 1986). Some government proposals include quarantine of all homosexuals who are HIV-positive, an impossible suggestion of lifetime imprisonment of over a million people. These proposals strive to identify and isolate the virus in order to contain it. In an attempt to separate uncontaminated people from those contaminated, they seek to set up a system similar to the lepers of ancient times who had to warn those near them of their untouchable condition. However, HIV is not contagious by casual or public contact. These suggestions for identification serve only to impose a social isolation on those infected with no consideration for their well-being.

Persons with HIV infection repeatedly encounter rejection and ostracism due to their disease. They have been refused services by welfare staff, funeral directors, and sanitation workers (Cecchi, 1986; Deuchar, 1984). They have been fired from their jobs, evicted from their homes, suspended from their schools, and abandoned by their families (Ballard, 1987; Cassens, 1985; Deuchar, 1984; Krapfl, 1986).

Such rejection occurs even among health care workers. Persons with HIV infection have been denied admission to intensive care units, recovery rooms, and hospitals due to their diagnosis (Loewy, 1986; Rosendorf & Hatfield, 1984). Some health care personnel have refused to give basic hygiene, deliver meal trays, give treatments, or even step into the room of a person with HIV infection (Banning, 1985; Cecchi, 1986; Deuchar, 1984). Nurses have left their jobs to avoid contact with these clients (Brock, 1986). Four studies of attitudes of hospital workers show misinformation and anxiety over catching HIV infection among both professional and paraprofessional staff (M.A. Cummings, Rapaport & K.L. Cummings, 1986; L. O'Donnell & C.R. O'Donnell, 1987; L. O'Donnell,

C.R. O'Donnell, Pleck, Snarey, & Rose, 1986; Polan, Hellerstein, & Amchin, 1985). In addition to outright rejection, fear of contagion causes health care workers to take unnecessary and extreme precautions against exposure to the disease (Cecchi, 1986; Lillard, Lotspeich, Gurich, & Hesse, 1984). Elaborate gowns, gloves, and goggles for each entrance into the room only intensifies the client's feeling of isolation and loneliness. Nurses exhibit approach-avoidance behavior by their willingness to give care, while avoiding any verbal or physical contact that is not absolutely necessary. Such reluctant interaction only heightens the psychic agony of living with this disease (Rosendorf & Hatfield, 1984; Wolcott, Fawzy, & Pasnau, 1985).

These fearful public health and health care reactions to persons with HIV infection fall into four behavior patterns: 1) avoidance of exposure, 2) attempting extreme precautions, 3) displaying a lack of regard for the afflicted, and 4) expressing fear of catching the disease (Meisenhelder & LaCharite, 1988). These behaviors comprise the result of fear of contagion, but what is the cause? If HIV infection is relatively difficult to contract, why are people so afraid of even seeing those afflicted? Some explanation for this fear comes from our cultural and social values.

The Roots of Fear

Our fear of AIDS becomes exaggerated by our social and cultural values, which attach a symbolic meaning to illness. Dreaded diseases surrounded in mystery become perceived and treated as contagious. For example, people used to respond to cancer as if they could "catch" it from visiting those afflicted. The unknown cause of cancer, its ability to strike without warning, its association with certain death, all heighten its image as contagious. Illnesses that have no cure, that are poorly understood, whose cause is unknown, summon the most fear. Regardless of the type of disease, such fear leads to an assumption of contagion (Sontag, 1977).

Just as mystery feeds into the fear of an illness, so does its connotation with death and punishment. Our society has always hidden death, packed it away in hospitals or funeral parlors, separated it from the mainstream of life. Death is the ultimate insult, the final loss of control. As such, death is denied, concealed, shunned. Any illness associated with death takes on the same meaning, the same stigma of repulsion, the same response of avoidance. Death by disease often becomes interpreted as punishment of those afflicted. The illness then takes on a moral purpose, a judgmental meaning (Sontag, 1977).

People tend to assign meaning to that which they do not understand. Persons sitting quietly in a room, startled by an unrecognized sound outside, will investigate until they can conjure some reasonable explanation for the sound, regardless of its accuracy. People need to attribute meaning to the events around them. Thus, the less understood the illness, the more meaning we attach to it. For a disease associated with death, the meaning becomes punishment, corruption, moral wrong-doing. The disease becomes a metaphor of all that is feared: evil, destruction, ruin.

If the associations of mystery and death can produce such fears of contracting the disease, how much more so the stigma of a sexually transmitted disease. Human sexuality in our society represents a misunderstood, repressed, and feared taboo. A disease transmitted by sexual relations, much less homosexual relations, becomes contemptible. The association of punishment cements in a sexually transmitted disease. Any illness contracted through sexual actions incriminates its victim. Society views persons with HIV infection, not as helpless prey of a deadly microbe, but as having caused their own fate. An unspoken accusation of irresponsible, if not offensive, behavior fastens to the label AIDS. The sexual transmission of this disease renders it that much more reproachable, unacceptable within the context of cultural values (Brandt, 1986; Sontag, 1977).

We dread AIDS not only because it is deadly, but because it is despised. The diagnosis becomes a social verdict of guilty, the punishment justified. As a mysterious, deadly, sexually transmitted disease, AIDS represents the ultimate metaphor for sin, pollution, decay. Since HIV is such a feared entity, its contagion becomes exaggerated. The horror of possibly contracting this shameful and lethal illness augments our perception of how exposed we may be. We may not be able to control that fleeting feeling of panic as we step into a client's room, but we can remind ourselves that the fear of getting the disease does not change the facts about its transmission. Our fears evolve from complex socio-cultural values that influence us even without our awareness.

Caring Without Fear

Those of us who work with persons with HIV infection have already dealt with many of our fears in order to fulfill our role. However, the destructive nature of this retrovirus and the high anxiety of those around us often rekindle the feelings of threat. To some extent, we can recondition ourselves to respond more reasonably and less emotionally to this disease.

We take the first step in decreasing our fears by grounding ourselves in accurate information on the transmission of HIV. Misinformation adds to the AIDS hysteria, a catching anxiety (L. O'Donnell & C.R. O'Donnell, 1987). Reviewing the ways that HIV infects and the efficiency of the recommended precautions helps to lower the feelings of vulnerability to a more accurate level. Likewise, feeding accurate information to those around us, colleagues, friends, and family, defuses much of their anxiety, which tends to fuel our own.

Second, the more we can identify with persons with HIV infection, the less we will fear them. Research shows social interaction as decreasing fear of contagion, probably because it increases sensitivity to the plight of those infected, thus removing the cultural associations of disgrace (L. O'Donnell & C. R. O'Donnell,

1987; O'Donnell et al., 1987). Symbolic meaning melts as our clients become individuals in our eyes, rather than diagnoses. The more we understand our clients' feelings, empathize with them, recognize the sameness of their humanity, the less fear and reproach we will feel for the disease, the less contagious it will seem.

Third, we need to recognize the fears of our loved ones as the response to the threat of death, sexuality, homophobia, or lack of control, rather than an accurate reflection of our risk. The more we can separate our thinking from that of fearful people around us, the more we can control our own emotions and behavior. We need to share our experiences, feelings, and needs with other professionals within the AIDS community who have also conquered their fear. A person's educational level may not be the most accurate indicator of his or her helpfulness in overcoming fear. Rather, the best role models are those people who have eliminated their prejudice and stereotypes of persons associated with high-risk behavior. We can overcome fear by seeking not only information but emotional support from those who are already comfortable with giving care.

Human Immunodeficiency Virus is clearly a deadly and legitimately frightening disease. Our fear will help us take logical action to prevent exposure. Our understanding of the facts of transmission and the pain of persons with HIV infection will help us care with increasing comfort and compassion.

References

Ballard, K.A. (1987) Public and private sector responses to AIDS. In J.D. Durham & F.L. Cohen (Eds.), *The person with AIDS: Nursing perspectives* (pp. 253-267). New York: Springer.

Banning. J. (1985). Education blitz necessary to reduce fear of AIDS. *The Canadian Nurse, 81*(10), 10.

Barbour, S.D. (1987). Acquired immunodeficiency syndrome of childhood. *Pediatric Clinics of North America, 34*(1), 247-268.

Brandt, S.D. (1986). Historical analogies to the AIDS epidemic. In M.D. Witt (Ed.), *AIDS and patient management: Legal, ethical and social issues, 159-163*, Owings Mills, MD: National Health.

Brock, R. B. (1986). On a nursing AIDS task force: The battle for confident care. *Nursing Management, 17*(3), 67-68.

Cassens, B.J. (1985). Social consequences of the acquired immunodeficiency syndrome. *Annals of Internal Medicine, 103*, 768-771.

Cecchi, R. (1986). Living with AIDS: When the system fails. *American Journal of Nursing, 86*(1), 45-47.

Centers for Disease Control. (1985, November 15). Recommendations for preventing transmission of infection with human T-lymphotropic virus III/lymphadenopathy-associated virus in the workplace. *Morbidity & Mortality Weekly Report, 34*(45), 681-686+.

Centers for Disease Control. (1987, May 22). Update: Human immunodeficiency virus infections in health care workers exposed to blood of infected patients. *Morbidity & Mortality Weekly Report, 36*(19), 285-289.

Cummings, M.A., Rapaport, M., & Cummings, K.L. (1986). A psychiatric staff response to acquired immunodeficiency syndrome. *American Journal of Psychiatry, 143*(5), 682.

Deuchar, N. (1984). AIDS in New York City with particular reference to the psychosocial aspects. *British Journal of Psychiatry, 145*, 612-619.

Friedland, G.H., & Klein, R.S. (1987). Transmission of the human immunodeficiency virus. *New England Journal of Medicine, 317*, 1125-1135.

Gerberding, J.L., Bryant-LeBlanc, C.E., Nelson, K., Moss, A.R., Osmond, D., & Chambers, H.F. (1987). Risk of transmitting the human immunodeficiency virus, cytomegalovirus, & hepatitis B virus to health care workers exposed to patients with AIDS and AIDS-related conditions. *Journal of Infectious Diseases, 156*(1), 1-8.

Gerbering, J.L., & Henderson, D.K. (1987). Design of rational infection control policies for human immunodeficiency virus infection. *Journal of Infectious Diseases, 156*, 861-864.

German study: 75% will get AIDS within seven years. (1987, Jan.). *AIDS Alert,* p. 19.

Graaf, M. van der, & Diepersloot, R.J.A. (1986). Transmission of human immunodeficiency virus (HIV/HTLV-III/LAV): A review. *Infection, 14,*(5), 203-211.

Health and Public Policy Committee. (1988). The acquired immunodeficiency syndrome (AIDS) and infection with the human immunodeficiency virus (HIV). *Annals of Internal Medicine, 108*, 460-469.

Henderson, D.K., Saah, A.M., Zak, B.J., Kaslow, R.A., Lane, H.C., & Folks, T. (1986). Risk of nosocomial infection with human T-cell lymphotropic virus type II/lymphadenopathy-associated virus in a large cohort of intensively exposed health care workers. *Annals of Internal Medicine, 104*, 644-647.

Kirby, M.D. (1986). AIDS legislation—turning up the heat? *Journal of Medical Ethics, 12,* 187-194.

Krapfl, M. (1986). As AIDS hysteria spreads, so does the need for cool-headed education. *Occupational Health Nurse,* 20-26.

Kunkel, S.E., & Warner, M.A. (1987). Human T-cell lymphotropic virus type III (HTLV-III) infection: How it can affect you, your patients, and your anesthesia practice. *Anesthesiology, 66*(2), 195-207.

Lillard, J., Lotspeich, P., Gurich, J., & Hesse, J. (1984). Acquired immunodeficiency syndrome in home care: Maximizing helpfulness and minimizing hysteria. *Home Healthcare Nurse, 2*(5), 11+.

Loewy, E.H. (1986). AIDS and the physician's fear of contagion. *Chest, 89*(3), 325-326.

Meisenhelder, J.B., & LaCharite, C.L. (1988). Fear of contagion: A stress response to AIDS. *Advances in Nursing Science, 11*(2) (in press).

Moss, A.R., Bacchetti, P., Osmond, D., Krampf, W., Chaisson, R.E., Stites, D., Wilber, J., Allain, J.P., & Carlson, J. (1988). Seropositivity for HIV and the development of AIDS or AIDS-related conditions: Three-year follow-up of the San Francisco General Hospital cohort. *British Medical Journal, 296* (March 12), 745-750.

O'Donnell, L., O'Donnell, C.R., Pleck, J.H., Snarey, J. & Rose, R.M. (1987). Psychosocial responses of hospital workers to acquired immune deficiency syndrome (AIDS). *Journal of Applied Social Psychology, 17,* 269-285.

O'Donnell, L.& O'Donnell, C.R. (1987). Hospital workers and AIDS: Effect of in-service education on knowledge and perceived risks and stresses. *New York State Journal of Medicine, 87,* 278-280.

Polan, H.J., Hellerstein, D., & Amchin, J. (1985). Impact of AIDS-related cases on an inpatient therapeutic milieu. *Hospital and Community Psychiatry, 36*(2), 173-176.

Rosendorf, L.L. & Hatfield, S. (1984). Acquired immunodeficiency syndrome: Rules for pestilential contagion revisited. *American Journal of Infection Control, 12*(1), 31-33.

Sande, M.A. (1986). Transmission of AIDS: The case against casual contagion. *New England Journal of Medicine, 314*(6), 380-382.

Simmonds, P., Lainson, F.A.L., Cuthbert, R., Steel, C.M., Peutherer, J.F., & Ludlam, C.A. (1988). HIV antigen and antibody detection: Variable responses to infection in Edinburgh hemophiliac cohort. *British Medical Journal, 296*(February 27), 593-598.

Sontag, S. (1977). *Illness as a metaphor.* New York: Farrar, Straus & Giroux.

Wolcott, D.L., Fawzy, F.I., Pasnau, R.O. (1985). Acquired immune deficiency syndrome (AIDS) and consultation-liaison psychiatry.*General Hospital Psychiatry, 7,* 280-293.

Chapter 2

Protecting Oneself: Infection Control

Julie Sniffen, Christopher L. LaCharite, Janice Bell Meisenhelder, and Jeff Huyett

Human immunodeficiency virus (HIV), the AIDS virus, HTLV-III—all are synonyms of a well-known infectious disease. No other disease has sparked such fear of contagion among health care workers, although many diseases with which we have contact in the health care setting are much more readily transmissible. Recently, these have taken a back seat in people's minds since most are treatable and few are fatal. This chapter explains this virus's transmission and reproduction, with clear guidelines on how to protect yourself from exposure to HIV infection.

The causative agent of acquired immune deficiency syndrome has been epidemiologically linked to a family of viruses known as retrovirus. Retroviruses characteristically induce a variety of neoplastic diseases among humans and animals and were the first infectious agents found to be oncogenic. In contrast to most viruses, which kill the cells they infect, retroviruses establish a chronic infection in their host cells that allows them to survive indefinitely. Once introduced into the bloodstream of its host, HIV establishes itself mainly in lymphocytes, macrophages, and parts of the central nervous system. The virus integrates into the DNA of the host cell where it can remain as part of the cell or produce thousands of new viruses. New viruses leave the host cell and are free to infect other susceptible cells within the system.

Since the virus has the capability of surviving in the host without causing disease, persons infected with HIV may *not* exhibit symptoms or feel ill. Once infected with the virus, however, a person potentially may transmit the virus through blood or other body fluids in which lymphocytes, macrophages, etc., may be found.

HIV has been isolated from blood, semen, vaginal secretions, cerebrospinal fluid, breast milk, amniotic fluid, urine, saliva, tears, and alveolar fluid of infected individuals (Friedland & Klein, 1987). The Centers for Disease Control, however, recently advised that, for health care workers, blood is the single most important source of both HIV and hepatitis B virus in the occupational setting (Centers for Disease Control, June 24, 1988).

In addition, other body fluids such as semen, vaginal secretions, peritoneal fluid, cerebrospinal fluid, synovial fluid, pleural fluid, pericardial fluid, and amniotic fluid should be considered infectious as well. However, body fluids such as feces, nasal secretions, sweat, tears, vomitus, and urine, unless they contain visible blood, have not been shown to play a role in the transmission of HIV or hepatitis B (CDC, June 24, 1988). (See Appendix A.2 at the back of this book.)

Transmission of HIV

Transmission of HIV occurs through sexual contact, parenteral exposure to blood and blood products, and from mother to infant during the perinatal period. No other routes of transmission have been shown to exist (Friedland & Klein, 1987).

Parenteral Exposure

In the health care setting, exposure is usually through direct blood-to-blood contact with a person infected with HIV by way of a needlestick injury. Blood exposure to nonintact skin (chapped, broken, or cut) or mucous membranes (eyes, mouth) has also been implicated in transmission of virus among health care workers (CDC, May 22, 1987).

IV Drug Abuse

Twenty-five percent of AIDS cases are present in those who have used intravenous drugs; 17 percent are those for whom IV drug use is their only risk factor (CDC, August 22, 1988). Transmission can occur through contaminated needles, syringes, and other drug paraphernalia.

Blood Transfusions

Three percent of all cases of AIDS have occurred as a result of delivery of contaminated blood products (CDC, August 22, 1988). This route has virtually been eliminated with the advent of donor screening, voluntary referral, and testing for HIV antibodies. Other possible sources of infection include artificial insemination with infected semen and organ donation from an infected source.

Sexual Transmission

In the United States, sexual transmission has occurred mostly in homosexual men. Risk of infection increases with the number of partners and the frequency of receptive anal intercourse (Winkelstein et al., 1987). Nationally, heterosexual transmission accounts for 4 percent of the AIDS cases (CDC, August 22, 1988). Vaginal and anal intercourse probably play the major role in heterosexual transmission.

Perinatal Transmission

Transmission of HIV from mother to infant can occur through three possible routes: during pregnancy, at delivery, and during breast feeding (Friedland & Klein, 1987). Preliminary short-term studies have suggested that transmission from mother to child occurs in about 20-50 percent of births (Minkoff, 1987).

Risk to the Health Care Worker

Multiple studies indicate that the risk of contracting HIV infection from delivering health care to infected individuals is very low. Of the thousands of health care workers who are in daily contact with persons with AIDS, as of April 1987, only six health care workers had been known to have developed HIV antibodies through health care exposure. Four of these were the result of needlesticks obviously contaminated with infected blood, while the other two involved extensive exposure to infected blood and body fluids. These last two individuals were not observing routinely recommended barrier precautions (CDC, May 22, 1987).

In May of 1987, the Centers for Disease Control reported the seroconversion of three additional health care workers who had nonneedlestick exposure to HIV-infected blood. This report has generated a great deal of anxiety among the health-care-providing community. However, *none* of these three individuals was *following infection control recommendations* for the handling of blood and body fluids. Although the antibody status of clients was unknown to the providers, it has been recommended by the CDC that all blood and body fluids be handled as if they were infected. If appropriate precautions were being taken, it is unlikely that these three providers would have seroconverted (CDC, May 22, 1987).

One of the problems with anecdotal reports such as those above is the possibility of nonoccupational exposure to HIV, which may be unknown to the individual. The best measure of occupational risk is through studies that follow seronegative health care workers for a period of time to see if they convert after known occupational exposure, such as needlesticks with infected blood. Four such longitudinal studies of health care workers in a variety of settings provide strong evidence for the low risk of contracting HIV infection through a health occupation.

First, in a study at San Francisco General Hospital, 175 health care workers were followed for seroconversion of HIV antibody. The participants had a wide variety of exposure to patients with HIV infection. Exposures ranged from casual, infrequent contact to extensive exposure including needlestick. No health care worker developed HIV antibodies during the study period, an average of ten months. All participants who were at high risk for developing HIV infection through other exposures were excluded from this study, as well as workers who were HIV antibody positive at the start of the study (Gerberding et al., 1987). Further testing on more health care workers in this hospital has confirmed one seroconversion after a needlestick injury (Gerberding & Henderson, 1987).

In Britain, 150 health care workers were followed for nine to twelve months after an accidental exposure to HIV-infected blood: needlestick or other sharp injuries, splashes to mucous membranes or broken skin, inhalation of aerosols, and injuries sustained during postmortem examination. The sample was composed mainly of nurses (61 percent), but also included physicians (21 percent), laboratory workers, and others. All subjects were seronegative at the time of injury and had no history of high-risk activity. No one seroconverted. There was no evidence of transmission of HIV regardless of the method of exposure (McEvoy et al., 1987).

The third study of risk to health care workers consisted of a prospective study of 531 health care workers at the National Institute of Health. One hundred and fifty of these workers had reported percutaneous or mucous membrane exposures to blood or blood products in caring for 238 persons with AIDS over four years. Six to forty-six months after exposure to the virus, no one had seroconverted. Of the initial 531 employees tested, 3 were found seropositive. These three people had engaged in high-risk behavior in their personal life. This study provides more evidence that the risk to health care workers is sexually and IV-drug-related, rather than occupational (Henderson et al., 1986).

Fourth, a Los Angeles study followed 246 female health care workers, primarily nurses, for nine to twelve months. As in all the studies, all subjects were seronegative upon entry into the study. These employees were divided into three groups depending on the intensity and frequency of contact with blood or body secretions of clients with AIDS: high exposure (102), low exposure (43), and no exposure (101). No employee showed serologic evidence of HIV infection at the end of the year (Kuhls et al., 1987).

On a national scale, the Centers for Disease Control has organized a cooperative surveillance project following health care workers with parenteral or mucous-membrane contact with HIV-infected blood. As of June 30, 1987, 883 health care workers were being followed. Of the 425 participants who had serum samples tested for the presence of HIV antibodies both at the time of injury and more than three months later, only 3 participants had seroconverted (CDC, August 21, 1987).

A study of 1,309 dentists, hygienists, and dental assistants did one-time testing of serum samples for HIV. Most of these people worked in geographic areas with reported AIDS cases, and many failed to use barrier precautions when giving care and experienced frequent accidental puncturing of skin with instruments. Only one dentist who denied high-risk behavior was found seropositive for HIV (Klein et al., 1988).

The case for low risk to health care workers is further supported by the studies on family members of persons with AIDS. In three separate studies of household members of persons with AIDS (total n = 153), none of the household members had contracted the virus by contact through bathrooms, kitchen utensils, or social kissing. Thus, all studies thus far have failed to demonstrate transmission of the virus through saliva, tears, or perspiration (Graaf & Diepersloot, 1986).

An analysis of the studies to date estimates the risk of HIV transmission is less than one in a thousand (<0.1%) per year of exposure, even when standard infection control procedures are not followed. The risk for transmission following direct inoculation with infected blood during accidental needlestick injuries is less than five in a thousand (<0.5%). In order for transmission to occur, enough blood containing sufficient virus has to be introduced directly into the host, which is rarely the case. Therefore, "HIV is one of the least transmissible nosocomial pathogens" in the hospital environment (Gerberding & Henderson, 1987).

Universal Precautions

The term *universal precautions* has been adopted to represent protection of health care workers from blood or other body fluids that may contain HIV or hepatitis B virus. The recommendation for instituting universal precautions came from the Centers for Disease Control in August 1987 and was updated in June 1988. (See Appendixes A.1 and A.2 at the back of this book.)

The philosophy behind the idea is simple: The majority of persons infected with either HIV or hepatitis will not be known. Therefore, it is wise to consider the blood and bloody body fluids from *all* patients as potentially infectious. Also, treat as infectious genital secretions and body fluids normally limited to internal cavities such as the pleural, spinal, synovial, and amniotic cavities. It has been estimated that as many as 1.5 million individuals are infected with HIV, and almost as many carry the hepatitis B surface antigen in the United States. Since most people are asymptomatic carriers of either virus, and serologic evaluation is not recommended common practice, the majority of virus carriers will remain unrecognized.

Universal precautions are meant to protect health care workers to the fullest extent from occupational exposure to HIV or hepatitis B. The most effective means of protection is through the consistent use of protective barriers: gloves, face protection (goggles, mask), and impervious gowns. See Table 2.1 for barrier technique guidelines.

Most blood exposures that occur in the health care setting are the result of needlestick accidents. Extreme care should be taken when handling any needle or sharp instrument. See Table 2.2 for needle-handling precautions.

Table 2.1. *Barrier Technique Guidelines*

1. Medical gloves (vinyl, latex) should be worn for all contact with blood, body fluids, or others fluids that may contain HIV. Gloves should be worn for procedures that may result in contact with blood, etc. Reusable rubber gloves can be worn in special instances, i.e., equipment cleaning. Hands should be washed following any exposure and after removal of gloves. Gloves should be removed after each patient contact.
2. Face protection, in the form of protective eyewear and masks, or face shields, should be worn during procedures that may aerosolize blood, such as arterial line manipulation (dialysis) or CPR.
3. Impervious gowns should be worn for situations where there might be exposure to large quantities of blood, such as emergency care to a trauma patient, or in labor/delivery area.
4. Shoe covers and hats are not required as protective clothing.

Table 2.2 *Needle Handling Precautions*

1. Needles should NOT be recapped after use. Most needlesticks are the result of missed needle recapping.
2. Do not cut, break, or bend needles after use, as this may release aerosolized blood in the needle shaft.
3. Do not leave used needles lying around and do not dispose of in ordinary trash receptacles.
4. Dispose of used needles in appropriately labeled, impermeable needle containers.

It is extremely important to report all needlestick or sharp exposures and mucous membrane splashes to the appropriate department for follow-up evaluation. All health care workers exposed need evaluation for antibodies to hepatitis B and administration of appropriate immune globulin and/or vaccine. The health care worker needs follow-up for HIV exposure, if applicable, and appropriate counseling. Recommendations for occupational exposure to HIV have been published by the CDC. (Refer to Appendixes A.1 and A.2 at the back of this book.)

Other Precautions

Most infections associated with HIV disease are not transmissible from person to person. Organisms such as candida, pneumocystis carinii, toxoplasma gondii, and mycobacterium avium-intracellulare, or Kaposi's sarcoma are referred to as opportunistic because they do not cause disease in an immunocompetent host. Most adults have already been exposed to these organisms, or actually harbor them as their own normal flora. The transmission of opportunistic infections poses no threat in the health care setting. However, bacteria or viruses that are transmissible and are capable of causing disease in immunocompetent individuals warrant appropriate isolation precautions. Good hygienic practices, especially frequent hand washing, will reduce the risks of cross-contamination in most instances. Herpes viruses usually will require specific precautions for contact with lesions or respiratory secretions. For example, herpes zoster (shingles), if disseminated, requires the addition of respiratory precautions and restricts contact of nonimmune individuals with the patient. A diagnosis of tuberculosis, causing active pulmonary disease, requires the institution of respiratory precautions. Ordinarily, however, the adoption of universal precautions by all health care workers will greatly reduce the risk of contact with most undiagnosed infectious diseases.

Tuberculosis

Tuberculosis (TB) is a respiratory disease caused by a bacteria known as (Mycobacterium Tuberculosis (MTB). Although there are many other species of bacteria in the mycobacterium genus, only MTB is capable of being readily transmitted from person to person. The organism is spread by respiratory secretions, called droplet nuclei, which are exhaled by persons with active pulmonary tuberculosis when they cough. Individuals may become infected with TB if they breathe in airborne organisms exhaled from persons with active pulmonary disease.

Other mycobacteria, such as mycobacterium avium complex (MAI), are found in the environment (soil, water) and cannot be transmitted from person to person.

TB and AIDS

Although mycobacterium avium complex is the most common cause of bacterial infections in persons with AIDS (Young, Inderlied, Berlin, & Gottlieb, 1986), mycobacterium tuberculosis is being recognized with increasing frequency (Snider, Hopewell, Mills, & Reichman, 1987). MTB infection can occur in a variety of sites throughout the body in a person with HIV infection, but it is only contagious when the site of infection is the lungs. Because TB is one of the few infectious respiratory diseases associated with HIV infections, it is important to identify in order to treat and prevent further spread. The diagnosis of tuberculosis usually precedes the diagnosis of AIDS, but may be made simultaneously or after the diagnosis of HIV infection (see Figure 2.1).

The occurrence of TB and AIDS is most striking among groups where there is a high prevalence of TB already, i.e., Haitians, Hispanics, and intravenous drug users. Studies have reported that approximately 2 to 10 percent of persons with AIDS also have tuberculosis, depending upon location and study population (Handwerger et al., 1987; CDC, July 18, 1986; November 14, 1986; December 11, 1987; January 1, 1988).

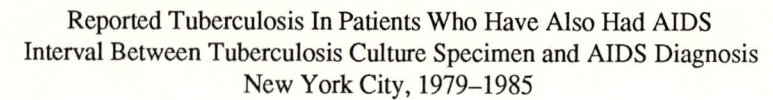

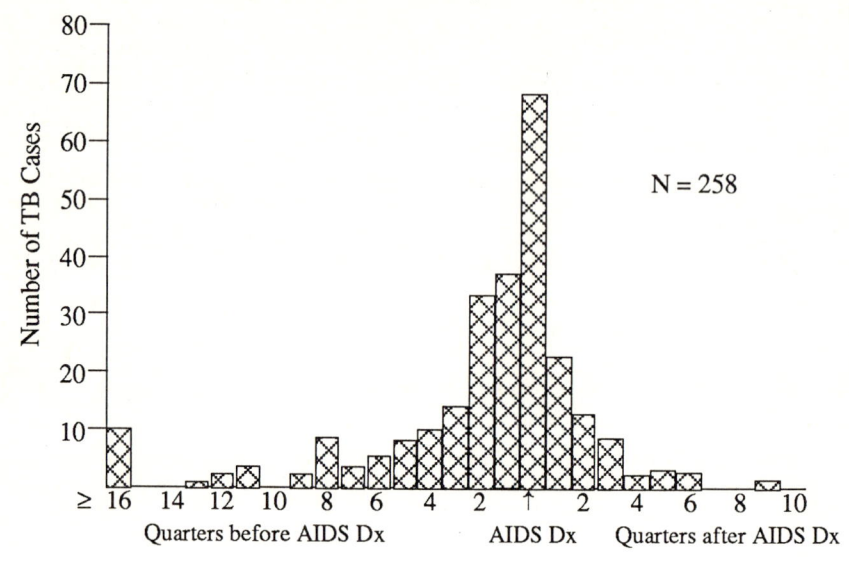

**Reported Tuberculosis In Patients Who Have Also Had AIDS
Interval Between Tuberculosis Culture Specimen and AIDS Diagnosis
New York City, 1979–1985**

Figure 2.1

SOURCE: Snider, D.E. (1987, September 29). *The Continuing Challenges in TB Control.* Paper presented at the Georgia Department of Human Resources' Community Health Section Conference, Savannah, GA.

Diagnosis of Pulmonary TB

A Mantoux tuberculin skin test (PPD) to assess MTB exposure is generally performed on patients with HIV infection and undiagnosed pulmonary infiltrates.

Sputum specimens should be obtained for both acid-fast stain and TB culture. Staining for the presence of acid-fast organisms is quick and nonspecific whereas culture is the more specific but lengthier process. A positive stain indicates the presence of acid-fast organisms, which might be TB. A culture is required to identify the specific acid-fast organism, regardless of the result of the stain. For infection control purposes, a positive acid-fast stain of sputum should be treated as tuberculosis. Generally, the client is placed on respiratory precaution and standard tuberculosis treatment is initiated. Respiratory precautions may be discontinued after about fourteen days of therapy.

Conclusion

Part of being comfortable while providing care to persons with HIV infection is being familiar with the proper infection control guidelines. This chapter has outlined the current thought regarding known modes of transmission, universal precautions, and general information about AIDS and TB. Although overuse of precautions can make a client feel dirty and shameful, the appropriate use of precautions is necessary in providing a safe environment for both you and your client.

References

Centers for Disease Control. (1986, July 18). Diagnosis and management of mycobacterial infection and disease in persons with human T-lymphotropic virus type III/lymphadenopathy associated virus infection. *Morbidity and Mortality Weekly Report, 35*(28):448-452.

Centers for Disease Control. (1986, November 14). Tuberculosis—United States, 1985. *Morbidity and Mortality Weekly Report, 35*(45):669-703.

Centers for Disease Control. (1987, May 22). Update: Human immunodeficiency virus infections in health-care workers exposed to blood of infected patients. *Morbidity and Mortality Weekly Report, 36*(19):285-9.

Centers for Disease Control. (1987, August 21). Recommendations for prevention of HIV transmission in health-care settings. *Morbidity and Mortality Weekly Report, 36*: 1S-18S.

Centers for Disease Control. (1987, December 11). Tuberculosis and acquired immune deficiency syndrome—New York City. *Morbidity and Mortality Weekly Report, 36*(48):785-795.

Centers for Disease Control. (1988, January 1). Tuberculosis: Final data United States, 1986. *Morbidity and Mortality Weekly Report, 36*(50&51):817-820.

Centers for Disease Control. (1988, June 24). Update: Universal precautions for prevention of transmission of human immunodeficiency virus, hepatitis B virus, and other bloodborne pathogens in health-care settings. *Morbidity and Mortality Weekly Report, 37*(24):337-88.

Centers for Disease Control. (1988, August 22). AIDS Weekly Surveillance Report. Department of Health and Human Services, Atlanta, Georgia.

Friedland, G.H., & Klein, R.S. (1987, October 29). Transmission of the human immunodeficiency virus. *New England Journal of Medicine, 317*(18): 1125-1135.

Gerberding, J.L., Bryant-LeBlanc, C.E., Nelson, K., Moss, A.R., Osmond, D., & Chambers, H.F. (1987). Risk of transmitting the human immunodeficiency virus, cytomegalovirus, and hepatitis B virus to health care workers exposed to patients with AIDS and AIDS related conditions. *Journal of Infectious Diseases, 156*, 1-8.

Gerberding, J.L., & Henderson, D.K. (1987). Design of rational infection control policies for human immunodeficiency virus infection. *Journal of Infectious Diseases, 156,* 861-863.

Graaf, M.V.D., & Diepersloot, R.J.A. (1986). Transmission of human immunodeficiency virus (HIV/HTLV-III/LAV): A review. *Infection, 14,* 203-211.

Handwerger, S., Mildvan, D., Erie, R., McKinley, F.W. (1987, February). Tuberculosis and the acquired immune deficiency syndrome at a New York City hospital: 1978-1985. *Chest, 91*(2): 176-80.

Henderson, D.K., Saah, A.M., Zak, B.J., Kaslow, R.A., Lane, H.C., & Folks, T. (1986). Risk of nosocomial infection with human T-cell lymphotropic virus type II/lymphadenopathy-associated virus in a large cohort of intensively exposed health care workers. *Annals of Internal Medicine, 104,* 644-647.

Klein, R.S., Phelan, J.A., Freeman, K., Schable, C., Friedland, G.H., Trieger, N., & Steigbigel, N.H. (1988). Low occupational risk of human immunodeficiency virus infection among dental professionals. *New England Journal of Medicine, 318*(2): 86-90.

Kuhls, T.L., Vider, S., Parris, N.B., Garakian, A., Sullivan-Bolyai, J., & Cherry, J.D. (1987). Occupational risk of HIV, HBV and HSV-2 infections in health care personnel caring for AIDS patients. *American Journal of Public Health, 77,* 1306-1309.

McEvoy, M., Porter, K., Mortimer, P., Simmons, N., & Shanson, D. (1987). Prospective study of clinical, laboratory, and ancillary staff with accidental exposures to blood or body fluids from patients infected with HIV. *British Medical Journal, 294,* 1595-1597.

Minkoff, H.S. (1987). Care of pregnant women infected with human immunodeficiency virus. *Journal of the American Medical Association, 258*(19): 274-7.

Snider, D.E., Hopewell, P.C., Mills, J., Reichman, L.B. (1987). Mycobacterioses and the acquired immunodeficiency syndrome. *American Review of Respiratory Diseases, 136,* 492-6.

Winkelstein, W., Jr., Padian, S.M., Padian, W.S., Wiley, J.A., Lang, W., Anderson, R.E., & Levy, J.A. (1987, June). The San Francisco men's health study: III, Reduction in human immunodeficiency virus transmission among homosexual/bisexual men, 1982-1986. *American Journal of Public Health, 77*(6):685-9.

Young, L.S., Inderlied, C.B., Berlin, O.G., & Gottlieb, M.E. (1986). Mycobacterial infections in AIDS patients, with an emphasis on the mycobacterium avium complex. *Reviews of Infectious Diseases, 8,* 1024-33.

Chapter 3

Making Tough Decisions in HIV Care

Martha Moon

Nurses working with HIV infection are often confronted with ethical dilemmas unique to this population of clients. The issues can be complex and tangled, requiring the wisdom of Solomon to resolve the conflict. We can easily feel overwhelmed by the insight needed to make fair and just decisions. This chapter presents some of the common issues that face us in AIDS care at the bedside level. The concerns are presented in a case example, with a discussion of the opposing perspectives as well as some guidelines for looking at each issue. Instead of providing right or wrong answers, we hope to equip you with the perspective to see both sides of an issue so that you can base your decisions on factual information and an empathy for everyone involved.

Before deciding on a course of action, we need to clarify our values: identify those beliefs that are most important to us. The process of values clarification entails looking at all the available options, deciding which alternative seems best, and acting on that decision. The more we crystalize our values, the more positively our decision will affect us and the people we serve (Kirschbaum, 1977). Evaluate the strengths and weaknesses of both viewpoints presented in the arguments below, choosing the decision that most clearly reflects your values. Consider which actions seem to represent the least harm for the most potential good.

Mandatory Testing Versus Informed Consent

You are the head nurse on a general medical-surgical unit. A man with a history of intravenous drug use, who has been drug-free for three years, is admitted for medical treatment of a peptic ulcer. He is married with two children, ages seven and ten, and employed by a construction firm for the past two years. He has stated that he understands his risk for HIV infection, and has used safer sex practices for the past three years. One of your nurses accidentally sticks herself with a needle that has just been used to give an intramuscular injection. The nurse wants the client to be tested for HIV antibodies. The client refuses. You are working in a state where informed consent for HIV testing is *not* required by law: You could legally test the man against his will. You consult the physician who says: "It's your nursing staff. You decide." What would you do?

The Nurse's Perspective

"The Centers for Disease Control recommends testing clients for HIV antibodies in the case of a needlestick exposure to a health care worker. This gives health care workers some idea of their risk and important information for making decisions about safer sex practices. In this case, I was stuck with a needle that came directly from the client and could contain infected blood. Since the client denies engaging in risk behavior for the past three years, an antibody status would probably be accurate. If the client tested positive, then I would need to change to condom use in sexual relations with my husband, as well as undergo HIV antibody testing myself on a repeated schedule for several years. If the client tested negative, then I would not have to use safer sex practices and could proceed with my plans to get pregnant in the coming year. I have a right to know the client's antibody status."

The Client's Perspective

"Current laws and recommendations favor the health care worker's rights, often at the expense of the client's rights. In this case, the risk to the nurse is minimal. Studies have shown a significant amount of blood needs to be introduced in order for HIV exposure to occur (Friedland & Klein, 1987). The chance that the nurse has been exposed to HIV is 1 in 200 (Gerberding & Henderson, 1987). She can determine her antibody status by being tested herself, in a relatively short period of time, without my being tested, and should do so regardless of my antibody status. The risk to the nurse is minimal, but the risk to me is tremendous. There is a high probability that I would test antibody-positive. Since my medical records can be summoned in a court of law at any time, this is not information that can really be kept confidential. My employers have fired people who are HIV antibody positive, and this is likely to happen to me. We are currently renting an apartment in a nice neighborhood that is very conservative. We could lose our housing. My family would be out on the street, with no income. I couldn't stand to see that happen. I couldn't handle knowing that I had caused my wife and kids so much pain. After years of hurting people, I've finally got my life together and have been able to be a decent father and husband. I couldn't take going back to being a failure. That's what HIV seropositive means: disgrace and shame. I'd kill myself first. At least they would have the insurance money and would be spared the humiliation. They would be better off without me. Being HIV antibody positive would ruin, if not end, my life. I have a right to withhold that information. I have a right to privacy, autonomy, and informed consent."

Discussion

The issues raised above are common ones. Many nurses caring for HIV-infected clients are of childbearing age, making safer sex a more complicated matter. Nurses are more aware of their rights with HIV clients and insist on them. The risks outlined by the client are also accurate. People have returned to drug use and committed suicide upon learning of the HIV status. Discrimination against HIV-infected people is common and widespread. These are not unrealistic fears of the client. Both sides have good arguments for what should be done. The verdict is up to you.

In deciding similar cases surrounding HIV testing, find out what will be done with the information. In this case, it would impact the nurse's sexual practices and possible childbearing plans. However, in many cases, health care workers have an emotional need to know, without a rational need to know. Since universal precautions apply to all clients, nursing practice remains the same regardless of the client's HIV status. Knowing the HIV status of all clients just for the sake of knowing could be dangerous to both clients and staff. It leads staff into a false sense of security with those clients testing negative who could still be infectious. For the HIV-labeled clients, it creates a group of people who will be treated differently, if not in physical practice, then in psychosocial needs. Testing should be done with the client's consent, with professional counseling before and after testing, and with complete confidentiality.

Duty To Warn Versus Confidentiality

You are the primary nurse for a 45-year-old man who is admitted with a fractured pelvis from being hit by a car. An unusually low white blood cell count suggests that the man might be HIV antibody positive. Upon questioning, the physician learns that the man periodically engages in homosexual activity, unknown to his wife of 22 years. The physician, a woman, feels strongly that the wife should be told of her potential risk to HIV. The social worker, a man, argues that the client's privacy should be protected. You are mediating the discussion to come to a team decision. What would you do?

The Social Worker's Perspective

"In this state, we have no legal right to disclose a client's diagnosis to anyone. For us to tell this wife that her husband might be HIV antibody positive is breaking the law. Such action violates the client's right to privacy and could seriously damage the family dynamics. He could sue us for doing so. What right do we have to interfere in other people's marriages? If this man is HIV antibody positive, the wife is already exposed. Since they are married, there is no danger of the wife's infecting others with the virus. This is not a public health problem. This is a personal, private matter that must be left up to the client. It is his family and his life."

The Physician's Perspective

"This is a public health issue. We have a duty to warn those at risk of being exposed. Here is an unsuspecting woman whom we must protect by equipping her with information. She has a right to know her risk. She could sue us for *not* telling her, if she became infected and symptomatic. Since we do not *know* her sexual activity, we cannot assume that she may not now or in the future potentially spread the virus to others. As health care professionals, we are ethically obligated to protect people from harm and prevent the spread of infection."

Discussion

Some important principles arise in this discussion. First, actions that are legal may not be ethical. In this case, the physician felt the legal action was not ethical. Since states differ in their protection of clients' rights, the legal boundaries vary depending on your location. Nevertheless, we need to know the laws of our states and be aware of when we are contemplating violating these laws and the potential consequences.

Secondly, ethical decisions are often based on the individual with whom the decision maker identifies. The woman identified with the wife, while the man identified with the husband. Trying to separate our own issues and feelings of vulnerability from our clients' is difficult. The best we can do is be aware of our biases and try to adjust for them in decision-making situations.

Lastly, health care workers tend to assume that sex with an HIV-infected person is dangerous. On the contrary, many people possibly exposed to HIV are careful and highly knowledgeable about safer sex. The first action in the above case is to find out if the client and his wife correctly use condoms, which would eliminate any reason to speak to the wife. If they are not currently practicing safer sex, then speak to the husband about initiating this, with or without divulging his bisexual behavior. If the client refuses both options, then your dilemma remains the same.

Right to Treatment Versus Right To Die

You are the primary nurse for Harry, a 27-year-old gay man with pneumocystic carinii pneumonia (PCP). He has told you that he is not ready to die. His condition suddenly worsens; he is hypoxic, restless, with difficulty breathing. Now the health care team is wondering whether or not to admit him to the ICU for aggressive therapy or just keep him comfortable. His family is supportive of the decision for minimal intervention, saying that they cannot stand to watch him suffer. What is your input to the team?

Argument for Aggressive Therapy

"Since the client has expressed his wish, he should have the determining choice. Although PCP is often fatal, many people have recovered from acute episodes to live with AIDS for years after. The will to live is a critical therapeutic factor that defies calculation. We owe it to the client to give him every chance possible."

Argument for Conservative Therapy

"We are obligated to give humane treatment, not to prolong suffering from our own inability to accept the inevitable. If the family, the people who love him, feel a conservative approach is best, then who am I to interfere?"

Discussion

The decision about how aggressively to treat occurs with many illnesses. The one difference in HIV infection is the usual assumption that AIDS is a terminal disease. Many people live for years with AIDS and have recovered from critical illness to go back to work and relationships. When the client cannot make the decision, the potential for recovery needs to be considered carefully. Given the current social prejudices against people with HIV infection, they hold a vulnerable position for having their needs pushed aside.

Duty To Care Versus Personal Risk Taking

You are the head nurse on a medical-surgical unit. Three of your nurses refuse to care for any clients with HIV infection because they are pregnant. The other staff members are willing to cover for the pregnant nurses. Should you allow staff to manipulate the assignment so that pregnant nurses can avoid caring for people with HIV infection?

Argument for Duty To Care

"The Code of Ethics of the American Nurses Association (ANA) states that nurses have a duty to care for all clients, regardless of the nature of the health problem (Code for Nurses, 1985). The ANA again addressed this issue by publishing criteria for the nurse to be obligated to provide care: when giving care does not present more than minimal risk (ANA Committee on Ethics, 1987). The Centers for Disease Control states that pregnancy is unrelated to risk in acquiring HIV infection (CDC, August 21, 1987). Pregnant nurses are no more or less vulnerable than nonpregnant nurses. Therefore, the decision to refuse to care is a violation of the professional principles of equal care for all without valid rationale. If I, as a head nurse, allow nurses to switch off HIV-related assignments, then I reinforce irrational prejudice and discrimination against a group of people entrusted to my care."

Argument for Nurse's Risk of Infection

"As a head nurse, I want to respect the feelings and needs of my staff, even if irrational. I need to keep my staff satisfied with their jobs, or they might quit. In the face of a severe nursing shortage, more staff attrition could force me to close admissions to some beds, which would compromise the care of all clients. If I require all nurses to care for HIV-infected people, what kind of care will fearful nurses give? As long as all my clients get good care, I can justify allowing some nurses some extra privileges."

Discussion

The head nurse faces very real trade-offs: supporting the professional ethical position versus respecting and keeping her staff. The most common solution is probably to allow nurses to choose to whom they give care, since it is easiest for us to identify with the concerns of other nurses. We need to be careful to avoid abusing those nurses who are comfortable giving care, providing maximum emotional support to all nurses involved with intense care issues. The best defense against this dilemma seems to be an educated staff who are free of fears of contagion and comfortable with the cultures and lifestyles associated with HIV infection.

Conclusion

One major difficulty in sorting through ethical dilemmas is the impact of our emotions on our decisions. Often we identify with one side, rendering it impossible to function as an impartial judge. Other times we harbor unconscious associations: If I support duty to care, will it increase my chance of being exposed to HIV? Does changing our values toward AIDS put us at risk of acquiring the infection? If we change our perspective on AIDS, will family, friends, or co-workers feel antagonistic toward us? In working through the above dilemmas, we are responsible to consider all the information as having equal worth, reflectively considering which ideas appear more justified, and be willing to change our opinions as new evidence arises (Steele, 1986). Our responsibility is to our profession, to our clients, and to ourselves. How this responsibility translates into our actions and practice is up to us.

References

American Nurses Association. (1985). *Code for Nurses: with Interpretive Statements.* (Publication Code No. G-141). Kansas City, MO: Author.

American Nurses Association Committee on Ethics. (1987, January 16). *Statement Regarding Risk Versus Responsibility in Providing Nursing Care.* (Available from American Nurses Association, 2420 Pershing Road, Kansas City, MO 64108.)

Centers for Disease Control. (1987, August 21). Recommendations for prevention of HIV transmission in health care settings. *Morbidity and Mortality Weekly Report, 36*(2S), 1S-18S.

Friedland, G.H., & Klein, R.S. (1987). Transmission of the human immunodeficiency virus. *New England Journal of Medicine, 317,* 1125-1135.

Gerberding, J.L., & Henderson, D.K. (1987). Design of rational infection control policies for human immunodeficiency virus infection. *Journal of Infectious Diseases, 156,* 861-864

Kirschbaum, H. (1977). *Advanced Values Clarification.* University Associates: La Jolla, CA

Steele, S.M. (1986). AIDS: Clarifying values to close in on ethical questions. *Nursing and Health Care, 7*(5), 247-248.

Chapter 4

Sustaining Our Hope

Jennifer Phillips

The Meaning and Need for Hope

As care givers to people affected by human immunodeficiency virus (HIV), we may find ourselves asking the same question: "How are we to maintain our hope in the face of so much loss and death?" We need to ask this question together with clients, recognizing our common ground with those to whom we give care. Hope is the ability to invest our energy and vision in a reality beyond our sight in the present moment, the capacity to yearn for and expect a meaning deeper and an outcome better than the circumstances seem to allow. We must first sustain our own hope in order to support the hopes of clients and loved ones. Hope cannot be based on groundless wishes. If it is to carry us through the crisis of AIDS, our hope must resonate with a truth felt within our hearts and minds. We find hope in different places. By sharing the grounds of our hope, we strengthen hope in one another. Sustaining hope is the essence of self-care.

As a hospital chaplain, I have labored with nurses and clients in their struggle to sustain their hope. The following discussion touches on some of the emotional and spiritual obstacles to hope for care givers: fears, grief, and helplessness. The chapter closes with strategies for self-care and finding hope.

The Process of Involvement With HIV-Infected People

When first confronted with HIV infection, the issues of self-care for nurses may differ substantially from those issues that arise after a long exposure to working with this disease. The resources we bring to our clients may also differ, depending on our length of experience with HIV infection.

When beginning work with HIV infection, we are faced with learning complex issues of treatment. We may encounter intravenous drug users for the first time, stirring up feelings or values about such behavior that make empathy difficult. Our comfort levels in working with gay clients may also vary. Such discomfort is heightened by the need to talk to HIV-infected clients about issues of intimacy and sexuality. A small support group may be helpful at the onset of working with HIV-infected people in order to discuss and explore our feelings and values related to HIV-affected populations.

As we gain experience working with HIV infection, loss accumulates quickly. So many clients are not only losing so many parts of their lives during their illness but will also die within months or a year. Nursing HIV-infected people presents us with a special challenge to be self-aware, to detect mounting feelings of sadness or anger, and to respond to our need for a change of pace or additional sources of support. Many care givers report that their HIV-infected clients and families draw them to open their professional boundaries of intimacy and become involved in ways that are uncommon with other groups of patients. Issues of HIV infection become more personal when they confront us, not only in the hospital but also in the community and even in our own family circles.

At first, our hope may focus on technology and new developments in research and on the stimulation of beginning to "do something" about the AIDS crisis in a practical way. As experience increases, we tend to decrease our expectations for a quick remedy from experimental medicine, making it more difficult to maintain our hope in the midst of feeling helpless or overwhelmed as the numbers of affected people, living and dead, increase.

Having a setting in which to talk through feelings and care issues on a regular basis can be helpful, though nursing shortages are making it difficult for many staffs to find time for peer support. Where there is an HIV-designated unit, the entire care team may appropriately meet for rounds and team support. When staff come from various parts of the institution, the idea of a support group may be more difficult to implement. Some staff find it easier to justify taking time from a busy schedule to attend an educational or case-study group than a self-care group. Try building supportive sharing into a variety of group formats.

Spiritual Dimensions of Care Givers' Fears

When the self feels threatened in any way, a fear response is likely to arise, producing the tendency either to run away from the perceived threat or to rally and fight. The fear response is both emotional and physiological. It is not based in reason. Reason only helps fearful individuals decide how to behave in the presence of their fear. Neither feelings of fear nor the fight or flight responses are good or bad in themselves. Fear is an adaptive behavior to protect the self. Any response may be adaptive or maladaptive, depending on the circumstances.

HIV-related fears are no different. It may be adaptive to have a level of fear of HIV infection that causes one to observe careful hand washing and universal precautions in handling body fluids, or to follow prevention recommendations in personal life. It may be maladaptive to don protective clothing from head to toe to deliver a meal tray. The need to flee the overwhelming sadness of watching the decline and death of a series of clients may result in the adaptive behavior of taking a respite break from HIV care, or the maladaptive behavior of avoiding clients who are dying by reducing time spent in their rooms. The urge to fight may lead a care giver to become a strong advocate for clients' needs, or it may be acted out in hostility and judgmental behavior toward the infected person.

Fear has a spiritual dimension. Our first impulse in managing fear may be to gain information. Information goes perhaps 50 percent of the way toward alleviating fear; but some fear remains, even when we feel fully informed about HIV infection. To acknowledge and then act despite our fear is a moral choice based in our sense of our humanity, purpose, and transcendent values, as well as professional pride and vocation. The process of moving beyond fear to give care takes time and is deserving of respect. Some care givers may be ready to work with HIV-infected clients sooner than others. For the nurse-manager, compelling care may be less helpful than modeling care. Fear, whether of HIV infection, sexual difference, ethnic difference, or addictive behavior, tends to diminish as contact and direct experience with the affected populations increases. We may choose to enter into very small but real risks in order to be compassionate professionals, consistent with our own vision of an ideal self. Our fears are transcended, though not necessarily removed.

Compounding our fear is the influence of family and friends, who may also be called upon to transcend their fears. The process of transcending fear is not so much a conquering as a befriending process. Be gentle with yourself. Give yourself inner permission to feel afraid and to experience a part of yourself as protective of the part that feels irrationally vulnerable.

Ironically, fear may arise equally when a client is perceived as being very much like oneself, or as radically different. The similar client stimulates feelings related to our own death, suffering, and loss. The client who is different by virtue of addictive behavior, ethnic origin, or sexual practice may seem alien, incomprehensible, or hostile to our own deeply held values and attitudes. With sensitivity to ourselves or with feedback from a strong support group, we can recognize the signs of overidentification with a client in time to clarify our boundaries. When we find ourselves strongly identifying with a client, we may be tempted to magnify the perceived differences in order to distance ourselves from the painful and frightening feelings. This coping mechanism can result in blaming and isolating those with HIV infection, thus adding to their suffering. We have far more in common with clients and their families than at variance; we share a common humanity and vulnerability. We both contribute at times to our own ill health as well as to our own wellness. Focusing on common ground without overidentification can be an effective way of transcending fear in order to give care.

Befriending Our Mortality

In the hospital environment, death is often regarded as the ultimate enemy, with systems and procedures set up accordingly. Nurses know, sometimes more clearly than others on the health care team, that when the body becomes uninhabitable for the desperately ill, death brings less anguish and suffering than its postponement. Death can be most difficult when both the client and the care giver are young. The death of children is particularly distressing to many. At this point in time, a diagnosis of AIDS brings with it a prognosis of death, usually within three years, and often to a relatively young person. At the heart of coping with this illness lies the process of coming to terms with mortality. This is as true for care givers as for clients and their families.

We will be most helpful to our clients when we have become acquainted with our own dying and no longer regard death as an enemy. There are a variety of ways of setting about this befriending process. It can be helpful to sit quietly and imagine step by step our dying: the deathbed (who is there, what they might say, how they look, how we feel); the actual dying (leaving the body, floating upward or traveling through a passage or tunnel into a place of light or darkness); experiencing in some way the Eternal Dimension (meeting loved ones who have died, meeting a Holy Presence, looking back over life); and watching from afar our funeral and burial. It can be helpful to write our own epitaph, make a will, or plan our funeral, and to revise these at intervals. We may think, write, or talk out our expectations of death and an afterlife. Many religious traditions encourage the believer to take stock of life on a daily basis and to live each day as though it were the last, with a minimum of unfinished business, unexpressed feelings in relationships, and unreconciled conflicts. We might choose to reflect about who it is who is actually dying: who dies, who remains, and in what fashion. Such exercises are not morbid; rather, they are ways of experiencing our full humanity as mortal and finite beings to whom death will indeed come in time. It is likely that sad and possibly frightening feelings will emerge while considering death. If we can accept these feelings, acknowledge them, and allow them to pass by, they will become resources for empathy with our clients.

Death that is run away from becomes an enemy, and the self becomes its victim. People with HIV infection are often anxious to be recognized as people, not victims. We can be most helpful to our clients if our perspective and language emphasize their individuality and humanity rather than the helplessness of their condition.

In the sixties, Elizabeth Kubler-Ross categorized stages of dying, though her work has been criticized as an oversimplified model. Rather than in discrete stages, most people coping with their own or a loved one's dying fluctuate back and forth between fear, anger, denial, bargaining, depression, grief, acceptance, and a variety of other responses to mortality. We will be seen as allies if we can empathize flexibly with the changing stances of dying persons, recognizing that our clients and their loved ones may not experience similar feelings at similar times. When the coping stances of clients and families collide, we may be able to highlight the commonality of coping beneath the differences of style and assist their empathy and humor with one another.

When care givers see many successive people die awful deaths from HIV-related illness, death may begin to overshadow the rest of life. The workplace may become a place of dread. Maintaining a balanced vision is important: recognizing that living is going on even while death is approaching.

Grief, Hope, and Burnout

The phenomenon labeled "burnout" may most often be simply grieving that has not been done, but has accumulated until it incapacitates the care giver from further work. It is the phenomenon of the closed system, like a rocket that, having expended its fuel, falls into the sea. As nurses caring for HIV-infected individuals, we will need to find ways of being an open system: nourishment, care, and refreshment coming in, and grief and other strong feelings being released out. Hoarded or repressed negative feelings will cripple us from effectively giving care over the long term.

Grief may include not only profound sorrow, but also rage. Just as sorrow unexpressed tends to settle into that numbing of feeling and energy known as depression, rage unexpressed tends to harden into cynicism and scapegoating or blaming the victim.

There is much to grieve for the care giver watching people losing their health and intact bodies, the support and esteem of friends and family, the intimacy of their sexual relationships, their jobs, insurance, housing, goals, dreams, and ultimately, their lives. HIV infection also brings grief into the wider community, especially areas that are most heavily affected by the epidemic. Members of the gay community, clients, and care givers mourn what feels like the death of their whole culture just as it was beginning to blossom and be recognized. Inner cities mourn the deaths of hundreds of needle users and their partners and babies, and the way that those deaths make the tears in the fabric of society more visible to everyone. In time, the entire world will be grieving the devastation of HIV infection. The care giver may not find respite from the grief of the workplace at home.

There is a special grief for those who tend people with HIV-related disease of the central nervous system. Nurses experience the loss of these patients from relationships long before they actually die, as their personalities change, their communication falters, and their memories fade.

Nurses, like many others in society, may tend to cope with grief by moving faster and doing more. There is always another patient needing care and another task to be done. Grief that is not given time to be felt does not go away. It accumulates under the surface and ultimately leaks out as depression or irritability or explodes in rage, despair, or a decision to quit. The ongoing work of grieving is facilitated where there is a strong nursing team. The team provides support for the times of grief, and colleagues who can fill in while a grieving nurse takes time to work through feelings. The team also may share in the grieving by exchanging stories about the client who is the focus for grief.

The individual nurse, the health care team, and society as a whole will have increasing need for rituals of mourning that facilitate grieving. A broad repertoire of personal rituals of mourning is useful. Rituals of mourning may consist of five minutes to sit and remember and cry, a conversation over a cup of tea, a walk outside the hospital walls, or holding a team quiet time of remembrance. Rituals of mourning may extend into our daily, personal lives, such as planting a flower in someone's memory, attending a funeral, recording the date of a death in a diary, soaking in a bath, writing a poem, sending a note to the family on the six-month and first-year anniversary of a death, putting a photograph in an album, or saying a prayer.

Grief is not an illness to be healed or a disability to be repaired. It is a daily, restoring, homeostatic activity. Grieving keeps people in balance and in touch with their deepest responses to the ongoing losses and changes of life. Rather than excluding the possibility of enjoyment and celebration, grieving frees the energy of sorrow for renewed investment in life and sustains our hope.

Helplessness and Hope

HIV infection lays waste the lives of clients and their loved ones. As yet, there is relatively little that we can do to change that reality. While so few treatments are available and death seems inevitable, we, as care givers, may be left feeling helpless and out of control.

Our desire for control may lead us to focus our energy on concrete outcomes, such as family unity or acceptance of death. We may encourage clients to put their affairs in order or to search for meaning in their experiences in order to achieve some level of peacefulness. Such nursing goals are helpful to some clients in some situations. However, the desire for control may prompt us to nudge clients unhelpfully toward the stereotyped image of a "good death." While some people may reach a point of folding their hands, gathering their loved ones around the bed, and departing with a prayer, others leave the world with their lives unfinished, in fear and great anger about going. Sometimes, it is uniquely fitting to individuals that they die in protest or in the midst of sadness and depression. We may feel that we have failed if a client dies before acknowledging or accepting the disease and death. Sustaining care requires relinquishing to clients the responsibility for their own living and dying that is properly theirs. Sometimes, amazing reconciliation is possible at the end of life. More often, a family network will continue in the same functional or dysfunctional patterns of relating they have always known up to and through the death of one of its members.

Helpless feelings generate the need to do something or change something. Often, our most therapeutic response is to let go of the compulsion to do and simply to focus on being: being present, being still, being available, and being calm. Our best intervention may be tolerating our own helplessness and empathizing with the helplessness of the client, family, and friends.

Away from the bedside, coping with helplessness by doing may have more value. We may find becoming a community educator or AIDS-service advocate helps to mobilize some of the energy of helplessness that HIV infection generates.

If there are only limited ways of doing something about AIDS, how do we maintain hope in the midst of helplessness? One avenue is through reflecting on metaphors of choice for our role. At different moments, we may envision this role as midwife, teacher, companion, conscience, supervisor, parent, police officer, pastor, witness, or friend. Some metaphors suggest more functional and fitting modes for professional behavior by portraying the appropriate limits of our responsibility in relating with another adult. Metaphors of shared responsibility and flexible roles may be the most useful for maintaining sustained care. Companions will be better stewards of their energy than "white knights" riding to the rescue or parents trying to enforce sexual- or addictive-behavior change in an adult. Our feelings of loss of control multiply if we try to control too much. By attending to the limits of our responsibility, we conserve our energy for sustaining a positive outlook in the midst of HIV-infection care.

Self-care

Taking the time for self-care is one of the hardest tasks for nurses to do. Yet, unless we take care of ourselves and respect our own needs, we will be unable to care for others. With deliberate concentration, we can develop sensitivity to our inner feelings and needs in order to detect the early symptoms of overload. We need to cultivate the art of taking guilt-free breaks at the first signal of needing a change: when feelings of frustration, helplessness, anger, or depression mount despite our normal ways of coping. Self-care ranges from taking a coffee or bathroom break *when needed* to getting away for a week at the beach. Stress-management techniques, such as meditation, guided imagery, and relaxation exercises, help to reduce the strain of the patient-care demands on our minds and bodies. Laughter provides a release of tension and a perspective on life. Even the dark humor of the health care setting effectively reduces stress, as long as it is not at the expense of others. We need to balance our work with HIV infection with life-affirming activities: cooking, dancing, making music, growing a garden, or raising a child.

We can help our efforts for self-pacing by developing a strong health care team. A team can provide the necessary relief from the constant involvement in close, intense relationships with dying clients. In between deaths, we all need time to withdraw and breathe, to move into less intense relationships. Although the primary nurse may take responsibility for the management of care, no one person can be expected to be the primary support for each client. Some relationships draw forth more intimacy than others. Clients themselves choose which relationships to develop. A team approach allows for: a choice of confidants for the client, a rotation of care givers in order to offset the strain on any one individual, and the camaraderie and warmth of group support for the nurses involved.

In an independent practice or ambulatory-care setting, care givers may find themselves trying to supply all the clients' needs single-handedly, since other health care professionals may simply be unavailable. Community services may provide the extra help needed to relieve some of the pressures on nursing. Local AIDS networks often supply the physical support of home care and the emotional support of companionship and comfort. Such resources are critical to the person whose network of family and friends collapses because of HIV infection. When people are abandoned due to their diagnoses, we become their main support system. The rigors of this closeness require us to pace ourselves and draw others into the support team to help us.

There may come a time when any one of us has spent long enough caring for those with HIV infection. When the work begins to sap the celebration out of the rest of life, it may be time for a change of job. This is not burnout, but normal human finitude: a sign of healthy pacing. The nurse leaving the field can pass on a legacy of information and experience to the new hands who come to take up the work.

The more we can pace and renew ourselves on a daily basis, the longer we will be effective in administering compassionate care over time. The foundation for sustaining empathy in caring over the long term is the ability to receive love and care from others, so that the wellsprings of kindness going out are replenished in order to achieve an overall balance in the whole of life.

Finding Hope

"In the face of HIV infection, where does your hope lie?" Nurses and clients may pose this question to themselves and others again and again over time. In the journey to find hope, nurses and clients often travel the same roads, at times together.

For the past few decades, technology has offered the brightest hope for many coping with illness, both clients and care givers. Technological solutions to the suffering of HIV infection seem still far off. As a society, Americans are beginning to grieve the lost myth of the omnipotence of science and medicine. Many clients and their loved ones experience the recognition of this loss of hope and the working through of the resulting disappointment. They discover that medicine is not black and white, but an art of woven hypotheses, trial and error, risk and benefit. Their first response to this realization may be one of anger and disbelief.

Faced with the lack of a miracle cure or even effective treatment, many persons with HIV infection are exploring holistic approaches to illness and wellness and insisting that these modalities be included in their regimen of care. Some health care clinicians and researchers are beginning to recognize the potential positive impact of such holistic means as diet, meditation, prayer, attitude, and stress reduction, in addition to conventional treatment. Clients may have much to teach us about the healing benefits of such practices on the immune system.

HIV infection leads some individuals to reexamine their spiritual roots, to seek hope in the Eternal Dimension, whether through their religious communities of origin or in a new fashion. Nurses and clients may enrich one another through dialogue about their differing spiritual journeys. Some place hope in a promise of heaven, some in the general beneficence of the cosmos. Some do so in explicitly religious language, and others use a more generic language of spirituality. We can communicate a supportive openness to the client's explorations by raising questions once a comfortable relationship has been established. We might ask: "Have you thought about whether there is anyone up there keeping an eye on you?"; "Do you have any expectations of what might come after you leave this life?"; or "How is your inner person doing in the midst of all this?" Ways of making meaning out of illness deserve much respect, even if they do not make sense or sound helpful to us. The content of the meaning may matter less than the fact that some meaning has been perceived. Try to hear it without trying to change it or evaluate it. Some individuals make meaning by interpreting illness as divine punishment or testing. If the concept of a severe, judgmental God conflicts with our own image, we might be tempted to debate such a statement. For the client, it may be more comforting to see God as a harsh parent than to risk thinking that there is no God at all, that all of the lifelong images of God are inadequate and wrong. Perhaps a suitable response for such a client might be: "How does that experience of God help you to find hope in the middle of your illness?"

Many people have less concern with cosmic hopes than with the small hopes of daily life. A desperately ill client may find hope in little things: a comfortable day, a sound night's sleep, a trip to the front door in a wheelchair, being able to eat a small meal, a visit from friends. Such hopes can be important and sustaining in their own way, as the small triumphs of life in the midst of dying.

Both nurses and clients may rest much hope in community, whether a small circle of friends and relatives or the larger society and world. At times, persons with HIV infection experience the loss of one community, friends and relatives of the past, only to find a new loving community in the AIDS network. This epidemic makes even more poignant the loss of the myth of the normative family, since for some, especially those who are gay, the structure of husband-wife-children-grandparents may have ceased to be a reality years before the onset of HIV infection. As we assist our clients to cope with new dimensions of the loss of family, we may find our own sense of safety in the rightful order of relationships painfully challenged. We may find ourselves grieving the lost myth also, along with embracing a new concept of social support. New structures of "family" are emerging in the lives of many people with HIV infection. We need to respond with flexibility in our policies and practices in order to facilitate our clients' community source of hope.

One of the most powerful ways to nurture hope is to tell one another the stories of relationships, particularly the stories of success, triumph, and reconciliation. The media tend to tell stories of the failure of caring: children with HIV infection whose house is burned, people who lose their jobs and housing. Stories of courage, humor, toughness, and love remind those who see so much suffering that there is more to life. Perhaps every HIV-team rounds should include updates about the clients who are doing well out of the hospital, or living well despite symptoms. Share news about families who have rallied round to help, and successful referrals to the community AIDS network that brought solutions to last week's problems. Even remembering the beloved people who have died can bring a sense of hope in the goodness of humanity and the possibilities of inner healing. The world outside the hospital walls also needs to hear some of these stories of hope.

David, newly diagnosed with AIDS, said to the chaplain on one visit, "AIDS is so terrible, I keep asking myself why it's here, why now, all over the world. And I hope that perhaps it's so that the world will finally learn to work together and be a kinder place." He speaks for many clients and care givers who place hope in the possibility of change toward a more humane world. At various points in history, nations or groups of people have created myths that envision their sense of the emerging purpose in their lives: manifest destiny, the new frontier, the lady with the lamp beside the golden door. HIV infection challenges all affected to envision a new myth with power to engender hope by embodying the compassion and inclusiveness that will sustain caring on an individual and global level.

Part II

Comfort With Cultural Differences

Chapter 5

Interacting With Gay Families

W. Michael Keane
Richard A. Rasi

A nurse working with a gay man with HIV infection is immediately involved in a complex set of emotional and social dynamics that can be overwhelming. Knowing the particular factors that are specific to gay relationships and gay families will greatly facilitate the nurse's capacity to work with these clients. Most of the material in this chapter has been drawn from the authors' work with groups composed of friends and lovers of people with HIV infection. At various times we have had friends, lovers, brothers, sisters, aunts, cousins, brothers-in-law, and roommates in the group. Everyone has been a principal caretaker. Most have been gay men. In sharing their heartache, their anxieties, their confusion, and their strength, we have been able to put together some of the essential ingredients for providing satisfying care to a person with HIV disease.

Acknowledging that nurses, particularly primary-care nurses, become an integral and pivotal part of the care and support team, what do they need to know, learn, and do to provide the best possible conditions to ride the waves that buffet the person and his family? First, we will give an overview of our conception of the gay family, then discuss the nurse's role in interacting with that family.

Understanding the Gay Family

Gay families formed out of the human need to be in a relationship with someone other than oneself. We all grow up in families and we all want to create our own.

A gay family consists of two men in a lover relationship, a group of friends, or, more likely, a combination of the two.

From an anthropologist's perspective, a family is composed of a group of people related by kinship ties. Kinship is established by being born to a set of parents or by marrying into a family. Family members are identified as mothers, fathers, brothers, sisters, cousins, aunts, uncles, grandparents, nieces, and nephews. People can also be brought into a family as godparents. So what is a gay family? How is it created? How does it exist without the kinship ties or the ritual ceremonies that are used to initiate people into a family? Clearly, the concept of a family based on same-sex intimacy forces us to broaden our concept of family.

Growing up in a culture in which a family is based on marriage and the children that arise from this union, most people do not conceive of two gay men as being a family unit. Gay men do form relationships that last over time. These relationships become the foundation of the gay family. In the book *The Gay Couple* (McWhirter & Mattison, 1984), the authors cite various types of gay couples and the stages of development through which they progress. The unit in the gay family known as the lover relationship consists of two individuals of the same sex who are romantically, sexually, and emotionally involved with each other. It is not rare to find many gay men and women who have been in a lover relationship from several weeks to years. For instance, in our Friends and Lovers support group, there is Larry who has been involved with John for eight years. They have lived together for the last five years, sharing friends and weekend co-parenting John's two children from a previous marriage. John's AIDS has caused a strain in the relationship because he will not reveal his diagnosis to his children or biological family. Then there is Bob who has been with his lover, Ed, for eight months. They have separate apartments but many mutual friends. Because of Ed's diagnosis, they have planned to move in together so that Bob can take care of Ed through the illness.

Gay families also consist of a network of friends. Within this network, a gay man may have friends with whom he is closer than with any biological relatives. As in any family, he depends upon these friends for his nurturing, support, and growth. In the crisis time that HIV infection brings, these are the friends to whom he turns for physical and emotional support. As stated by Morin and Batchelor (1984), "Because AIDS is a mysterious and stigmatized illness, the psychological issues raised for significant others may be more complicated than those for other life-threatening illnesses." For instance, in our group there are three men who are friends of Frank. Each shares in the responsibilities of taking care of Frank. Nate takes him to his appointments and the hospital when the need arises. Jim makes sure that his meals are prepared, and Steve checks in with him each night to chat. Responsibilities are interchangeable as the needs arise. There is a commitment to one another and to Frank to take care of him throughout the course of his illness. When assessing a client, it is important to note the significant other people who will be responsible for care both in and out of the hospital. This group of people can include lovers and best friends as well as biological family. Often within a friendship group, the members are called brothers or, jokingly, "sisters." The latter, when used between men, seems to refer to the special bonding and sharing of emotions that is more clearly expressed by women, or "sisters," in our culture. Knowing the network is essential for keeping the communications clear and open.

Although society does not allow lovers or friends legalizing rituals, i.e., marriage, commitment can be expressed in different ways. For example, a couple might decide to celebrate with a commitment ceremony to which friends and relatives are invited. This ceremony might even include the presence of a clergyperson to offer a blessing. For instance, in our group there is a couple who had been in a relationship for ten years and decided that they would like to celebrate their commitment. They did this by inviting all their family members and their friends to a ceremony in which they exchanged rings, shared stories of themselves as a couple, and made a vow for their continuing relationship. For other couples or even groups of friends, their commitment might be buying a house together and establishing a home. Others might assign a lover as a beneficiary of an estate or a life insurance policy. Moving in together and signing a lease is often a means to commit to a relationship.

HIV infection has a profound impact on a relationship. We have seen lovers who have been in a relationship for short periods of time break up over the diagnosis of AIDS. We have seen others develop a stronger bonding. We have been witness to couples who had been splitting up but then decided to remain together when one of the two was diagnosed with AIDS. We have seen men return to former lovers, and we have seen people take in best friends in order to care for them. In other cases, we have heard of men who have been thrown out or asked to leave their homes, because of fear or ignorance. We have heard of people shunned and disowned by their families.

Biological families vary in their involvement with the gay family according to the level of sharing that has occurred among them. Sharing the fact that you are gay (known as "coming out") is not easy, even if the gay man's family is caring and understanding. Individuals in the family react differently to the "news." One group member, Ralph, said, "When I told my father I was gay, he put his arms around me and told me that it would be OK. He would find a good psychiatrist to cure me. My mother told me, after almost three years, that she blamed herself for being such a dominant mother. I still haven't been able to tell my brother because I'm afraid that he would never talk to me again." Even in open and caring families there is ambivalence. However, "many families are not ambivalent; they are clearly rejecting" (Geis, Fuller, & Rush, 1986). For some, the diagnosis of AIDS is the first time that the family becomes aware of the gay man's sexuality. In these cases, both the family and the individual are left dealing with both the gay identity and HIV infection.

The three primary groups we have identified in the gay family are the extended-kinship family, the lovers, and the friendship network. These three groups have many overlapping issues. There is a mutual need for networking, a need to prevent social isolation, and methods to deal with the grief of multiple losses over time. In order to develop strategies for interacting with these groups, we would now like to explore how these issues and other issues manifest themselves.

Understanding the Emotional Issues

Each member of the family system is impacted upon by the diagnosis of HIV infection. Immediate shock sends emotional waves through the family system. Disbelief, anger, denial, guilt, hopelessness, fear, rage, anxiety, grief, vulnerability, and helplessness are all emotions that emerge and reemerge in various combinations. For instance, in our group, one member, a roommate of someone diagnosed with AIDS, kept saying over and over again, "It all seems like a big shock. I've known about AIDS for a long time, but I never thought anyone close would get it. I'm scared. It's too close."

As any of these emotions are experienced by a member of the family system, each of the members will be affected. For the person with HIV disease, first arises his sense of vulnerability, anxiety of death, fear of physical debilitation, and anger at the foreshortening of life. From these emotions arise such questions as: When will I die? How will I die? What can I do to feel better? Lovers and friends ask similar questions: How will I take care of him? How and when will he die? What do I do with my own feelings of vulnerability? What do I do with my feelings of loss and abandonment? What does this say about my own contamination? What can I do to make him feel better? What do I do with my anger?

As time continues, the person may feel a lack of control. He might consider that this is not the way life was supposed to be. He faces a sudden restructuring, if not dashing, of dreams, expectations, plans, goals, and careers. Life suddenly feels very tenuous. Some people are very open in dealing with their disease. Others make valiant attempts to hide the reality. The fear of rejection and abandonment can create isolation. For instance, a young doctor in the group expressed extreme frustration that his lover had forbidden him to talk to anyone. He said, "What am I supposed to do? I can't talk to him because he is sick, and he won't let me talk to anyone else. I'm scared. I'm anxious and I feel alone. No one knows how sick he has become. It's the shame. He feels so much shame. It's a web of guilt and self-hate, and I'm caught in it with him." Despite the group's encouragement to involve others, his diagnosis remains a secret.

Shock, anger, anxiety, and depression are a few of the emotions that face the lover and friends. These feelings can precede an AIDS diagnosis if a person had seropositive HIV test before becoming symptomatic (Grant & Anns, 1988). Because AIDS is opportunistically unpredictable, the lover can find himself on an emotional roller coaster. This unpredictability creates a sense of walking on eggs. Many lovers live with the fact that things could come crashing down at any moment. Many men faced with this type of uncertainty will spend every free moment with the client. This can lead to a lack of social contacts that are so needed at this time. He may have a sense that he has no personal space and that the boundaries of the relationship have become fluid. For instance, he may become preoccupied at work about his lover's daily routine. How is he eating? Is he taking his medication? How is he feeling? The pervasive sense of anxiety and worry can take its toll. It may be difficult to concentrate on his work or explain to his boss why he needs to take off so much time. Needing to take time to communicate with the physician, with the lover, with the support system, takes time away from work, which may suffer.

A good example of this dilemma is Roger. Roger began to take care of his ex-lover who lived in an apartment upstairs. When his ex-lover developed central nervous system involvement that left him disoriented, Roger began round-the-clock surveillance. He prepared all the meals, left work at noon, and checked in constantly. He couldn't concentrate on his job. As Roger said, "I couldn't stop thinking about him. I'd get so angry at his neediness. Then I'd get guilty about wanting to run away. I felt totally trapped." The group helped Roger to expand his network so that other people could take turns with the caretaking.

When the situation becomes so overwhelming, it is healthy to take time out for oneself. For many, taking time out becomes a source of anxiety and guilt for having one's own life and one's own needs. Any lover who is at this point needs to be encouraged to take time out for himself so that he can be there for himself and for the person with HIV infection. In our group, members talk about the frustration of their lives being on hold. "Sometimes I feel like my life has ended at twenty-eight. We used to go on vacations, but now John is too sick to travel. I'm too guilty to go away without him. I'm so tired and miserable." Another member who did go away for a week's vacation reported, "He looked so sad when I left. Yet, I felt relieved to be away and not always caring for him. Just to pretend to be free of this damn disease for a few days was a relief. It was hard to see him when I returned, and I had to suppress my good-time stories. I feel guilty I had such a good time, but I'm glad I went. I can be more there for him knowing I'm not trapped." The group always supports people taking time out, yet few seem to take it.

When under such pressure, the lover may turn to his biological family for support and help. For a gay man, this might be the first time that the issue of his sexual preference is disclosed to his family. Families respond differently. The worst case is when the family totally rejects and abandons the gay couple. The best is when they pitch in and form a caring network. In her book *The Screaming Room,* Barbara Peabody (1987) describes her involvement with caring for her son, Peter, during his illness. Micki Dickoff's film, *Too Little, Too Late,* documents the formation of a mothers' support group. Within these support groups, the mothers describe their individual experiences of taking care of their sons with AIDS. Sometimes they take care of the son and his lover. This can sometimes lead to a mixed emotional experience. One man described the arrival of his "mother-in-law" as a mixed blessing. "She tries to take care of both of us, and I feel like there is hardly any room for the two of us together. She does forget, or maybe doesn't want to acknowledge, the relationship between me and her son. Yet she is wonderful. She cares. She's there."

She'd do anything to make him more comfortable. I guess I can put up with a little bit of her insensitivity and possessiveness."

There have been other cases where the client's family immediately takes over. They leave the lover totally outside the decision-making process. In certain cases, the person with HIV disease has been removed from the environment with the lover and has been taken away or back home for care. In one case, the lover was totally removed from the caring process. As he lamented his feelings of powerlessness, he said, "They just swept in and scooped him. He was so sick. He wanted to go because they can make him more comfortable. They ignore me completely. I can visit, but I can't stay. I feel so angry and abandoned, and he is too sick to care. I don't know what to do. We've spent two years together."

For the couple dealing with AIDS, physical intimacy becomes an ongoing struggle. Sexual activity declines from fear of contagion, the physical disability of the client, or the lover's fear of exposing the client to new infections. To avoid creating more stress over the lack of this intimacy, the lover may refrain from discussing his needs. The lover might find himself being attracted to other men and may entertain fantasies about sexual intimacies with them. These desires can be an indication of the lover's own need for attention, caring, and physical contact. Guilt over these feelings can lead to a distancing or an overinvolvement in caretaking. The only antidote is openly talking out the dilemma. A group member described his situation as follows: "I felt so frustrated. He was too sick most of the time, and even when he was well, we were too afraid of his getting sick again. I felt so guilty wanting to go out with other men. We never talked about it, yet I had all these feelings. He'd get angry even when I had a dinner with a friend. When we finally talked, he said that he was afraid that I would have sex with someone else and leave him. He said that he felt badly not being able to make love with me anymore. I felt so much better knowing he still cared and we've actually had some safe physical contact since then."

The lover's anxiety about infection by the HIV is based on reality. This disease is spread by intimate sexual contact. Often lovers have revealed their inner fear that they will get sick and die. Because they have been involved with someone who has or had AIDS, they fear rejection. Many lovers also develop a realistic anxiety of being stigmatized by other gay men. As one group member put it, "I hate the whole disease. I want it to go away. Every time I talk on the phone, someone else has just been diagnosed. I feel like it is only a matter of time until the ax falls on me. I'm scared to meet new people. I feel that even if I don't have it, I'm contaminated for life by having a lover who has had it."

What about the friends of the person with HIV infection? They differ from the lover in the levels of commitment and intimacy. Yet, often they share many of the emotions and involvements. If the ill person does not have a lover, the responsibilities may be shared with a group of friends. There may be relationships in which the lover, through his inability to deal with the illness, might distance himself from the client, leaving the friends to take up the responsibilities. Friends can wind up in the position of attending to the person at night, watch-dogging the medication, transporting to the physician or hospital when necessary. Sometimes a friend has to clarify his boundaries in regard to his involvement. In one instance, a friend had to confront the client, saying he would no longer care for him in his home. He felt guilty yet realized that his own relationship and his own work was suffering as he tried to juggle too much. In another situation, a roommate had to confront a lover to take more responsibility for the client's care.

Often, groups of friends will make a commitment to one another about the care that they will give to the client. The client might be invited to move in with one of them to facilitate care during acute illness. Emotional involvement of friends with the client and with each other can become intense as the bonds between them are deepened during the course of the illness. One person remarked, "We've never been lovers. It's real close, this relationship with him. Like being lovers without sex. We are family, I guess." Again boundaries can be blurred. A friend can find that all his time is taken up caring for the client. Sometimes he experiences guilt over wanting to have his life back again. As one group member said with a sigh, "I made this commitment to care for him, and I'll do it. I just get so sad and tired. I love him. He's my family, yet, sometimes I wish he'd die so I could have my life back."

Like a lover, a close friend can be confronted with his own mortality and the possibility of illness. "I hate that so many people with AIDS are my age. I think: maybe I'm next. Every time I get a cold or feel sick—there it is—AIDS."

The Nurse's Interaction With the Gay Family

In the work that we have done with individuals in gay families of persons with HIV infection, you as the nurse are the single most important health care provider in the health care system. You are the liaison with physician and medical team, counselor, medicator, comforter, nurturer, teacher, and advocate. In order to be able to fulfill each role, you will need to clarify your own feelings, boundaries, and needs in an ongoing manner.

Most of us have grown up hearing negative comments about homosexuality. It is almost impossible to avoid being influenced by early childhood teaching. Our task in adulthood is to review and reconstruct our associations about gay people, basing our concepts on our own experiences. Most people begin to develop positive connotations of homosexuality as they form relationships with gay people. Until then, we may be bothered by unconscious anxiety as we walk into the room of a gay client, or see two men hugging. The more we learn about homosexuality and the closer we become to a gay person, the more comfortable we will be in these situations. As we develop friendships with gay people, we discover they are just like all people, but with a natural sexual attraction for their own gender. For many nurses, their clients become the gay people with whom they bond, grow, and understand. If you feel some discomfort working with gay men and their families, reach out to someone. Professional support groups, counselors, and AIDS community groups may offer support and comfort for understanding homosexuality. Gay hotlines or gay publications often list such resources. It's OK to have feelings of discomfort with your clients and families. Ask questions. Be open with your clients about your desire to understand. They will appreciate your concern and interest as a form of caring.

There is much written on the care of the AIDS client, less about the care and needs of friends and lovers. Almost nothing has been presented about the care of the care givers. As aptly stated by Sandi Feinblum (1987): "When the experts discuss the psychosocial problems AIDS creates for clients, they seldom address the psychosocial problems that people who care for clients with AIDS must face." For example, in a support group for nurses, one nurse said, "No one understands the stigma that comes in taking care of a person with AIDS. I actually have friends who won't talk to me or spend time with me because of their fear of contamination."

Self-care is important. You must understand your own boundaries and needs to avoid burnout. As with other chronic illnesses where there are multiple hospitalizations, there can be a tendency to get overinvolved with patient and family. Because this population is often young, open, and composed of men who are allowed by their sexual preference to be more expressive of their emotions, it is easy for the nurse to identify with them. When you work with clients for a long time, you develop relationships. No one tells you how to deal with the loss and grief when they die. As one nurse said in a support group, "I get so involved, I spend extra time. The need is so great, and so many people don't understand. I often become so exhausted that I can barely go home and take care of my own family. I can get so close, I hate to lose them. Sometimes I get to the point that I can't take care of one more patient with AIDS. Yet I know I can't stop now." Her additional statement, "If it wasn't for this support group, I know I couldn't go on," is an indication of the strong need for support groups. You will do well to establish yourself in a support network with whom you can process your own feelings.

Your understanding and sensitivity to the dynamics at play within the various relationships of the gay family as outlined above determine the way in which you will interact. Without such understanding, you may unknowingly make interventions that potentially have profound effects on individuals. If an individual feels unaccepted or judged in any way, the levels of trust are severely reduced. For any relationship to be helpful, the establishment of trust is important. When interactions and interventions are made with sensitivity and understanding, you can be healing and helpful to the individuals involved who so deeply need your help. First, get to know your gay client's family structure. Over time, the inner circle of intimate connections must be identifiable. You may be comfortable asking clarifying questions, such as if he has a lover or designated friend to communicate with the health care team.

The more you know your client's family structure, the better you can serve as his advocate. You may need to run interference with other hospital staff who might question relationships. Sometimes, the most important family members are prevented from seeing the client in an ICU because they lack a blood kinship. You may also be instrumental in referring clients and families to local AIDS organizations or professionals who are sensitive to the needs of this population. By making appropriate referrals, you provide more possibilities for intervention for the gay family members.

Just as family therapists will arrive at a point in the interaction with families where they are admitted as adjunct members of the families, so too nurses might find themselves invited into gay families. The individuals in a family often find nurses to be people who will listen to their struggle. As the individuals in the family experience the myriad of issues surrounding the illness, the nurse might be the one readily available as a listening ear. During the course of the illness, there are many questions, many unknowns. The nurse may be identified as the one to whom the questions can be addressed. It is the nurses who have direct contact with the doctor and who will be around to express concern to the doctor, long after the family might have left the hospital. The nurses give relief to the family members in caring for the client. Knowing and trusting the nursing staff allows a lover or friend to leave the client with a sense of comfort, secure that the nurses care not only with their hands, but with their hearts.

Gay families, like other families, share the crisis of their loved one's illness. As you facilitate family support and coping, you comfort both the client and family in their struggle to live with HIV infection.

References

Feinblum, S. (1987). Pinning down the psychosocial dimensions of AIDS. *Nursing and Health Care, 7*(5): 255-257.

Geis, S., Fuller, R., & Rush, J. (1986). Lovers of AIDS victims: Psychosocial stresses and counseling needs. *Death Studies, 10,* 43-53.

Grant, D., & Anns, M. (1988). Counseling AIDS antibody-positive clients: Reactions and treatment. *American Psychologist, 43,* 72-74.

McWhirter, D., & Mattison, A.M. (1984). *The male couple.* Englewood Cliffs, NJ: Prentice-Hall, Inc.

Morin, S., & Batchelor, W. (1984). Responding to the psychological crisis of AIDS. *Public Health Reports, 99,* 4-9.

Peabody, B. (1986). *The screaming room.* New York: Avon Books.

Recommended Videos and Readings

An Early Frost. (1987). RCA/Columbia Pictures Home Video, 3500 West Olive Avenue, Burbank, CA 91505. 97 min.

Overcoming Irrational Fear of AIDS, A Coping Strategy for Health Care Providers. Carle Medical Communications, 611 West Park, Urbana, IL 61801. 22 min.

Parting Glances. (1986). Key Video (a division of CBS Fox Video), 39000 Seven Mile Road, Livomia, MI 48152. 90 min.

Too Little, Too Late. Fanlight Productions, 47 Halifax Street, Boston, MA 02130. (617) 524-0980. 48 min.

Clark, D. (1987). *The New Loving Someone Gay.* Berkeley, CA: Celestial Arts.

Morin, S., Charles, K., & Malyon, A. (1984). The psychological impact of AIDS on gay men. *American Psychologist, 39,* 1288-1293.

Silverstein, C. (1981). *Man to Man.* New York: William Morrow and Company, Inc.

Chapter 6

Managing Addictive Behavior

Ann Williams

We are nurses because we value and respect individuals. We are concerned with more than the technology of modern medicine. The desire to help people help themselves is intrinsic to good nursing practice. We seek always to return as much control as possible to the client. What happens then when we are faced with clients who do not choose to help themselves or who, when given control, make choices that are self-destructive? Or when the client, instead of responding to us with gratitude, is actively hostile, perhaps even abusive?

We respond in a variety of ways. We may categorize clients as "noncompliant" and hopeless. We may unconsciously punish clients by withdrawing or by setting limits to our interactions that effectively distance both them and the challenge they represent to our view of ourselves. We punish ourselves as well. We feel guilty for not liking the client, for not helping more effectively, for not being "better" nurses.

People who use illegal drugs intravenously evoke just this set of dilemmas for nurses. It is hard for us to understand why they do what they do and why they don't respond when we try to help. In addition, most intravenous drug users are mistrustful, angry, and scared. They have had tumultuous relationships with society in general and hospitals in particular in the past and they enter the medical system prepared to do battle. We continue to look for the magic word, the special approach that will enable the client to do better (to stop using drugs) and that will restore our own image of ourselves as caring, helpful, effective nurses.

There is no "magic bullet." Science has very little understanding of addictive disease; indeed, there is no agreement that addiction is a disease. Drug use in our country is complicated by social, political, and moral attitudes that cloud the medical issues and make solutions even more difficult to see. But we are not totally helpless. By seeking to understand both ourselves and our clients and by placing each individual in a larger social and health care context, we can perhaps create a climate where help can be offered and accepted. We cannot cure addiction but often we can facilitate a more positive experience for the hospitalized person with HIV infection who uses drugs. In this way, we may be able to offer hope and the possibility of a more satisfying life.

Key Attitudes

To understand and reach patients who use drugs, we must first examine our own attitudes toward drugs and alcohol. Ask yourself these questions:

Do I drink or use drugs to an extent that others may find excessive and, as a result, deny a client's problem?

Does a member of my family or a close friend drink or use drugs? If so, how does that person's drug use affect my attitude toward my clients? Does it encourage me to deny the seriousness of their problems? Does it lead to an inability on my part to sympathize with the client?

Do I use drugs and alcohol moderately myself and therefore assume that all intelligent people can do the same if only they choose to do so?

Do I abstain from drugs and alcohol entirely and lack respect for others who don't?

It isn't necessary to change our personal beliefs or behavior about drug and alcohol use in order to care for clients who are different, but it is important to understand what our attitudes are and how they influence our feelings about clients as we give care. Being clear about ourselves will help us to see our clients more clearly as individuals. We can then respond to their needs with less interference from our own unexamined assumptions.

People who use drugs are generally quite mistrustful. They have often had negative experiences in the past that put them on guard and make them very sensitive to nuances and nonverbal behavior. It is, therefore, important to be as straight-forward and honest as possible. Try to convey genuine concern and a nonjudgmental attitude. Being nonjudgmental does not mean condoning drug use. If you are genuinely concerned about clients and value them as individuals, then you will be able to offer support and understanding without enabling self-destructive activity.

Psychosocial Profile

Stereotypes about people who use intravenous drugs abound. Such stereotypes are a great mistake. Parenteral drug abusers are a heterogeneous population who are drawn from all social and economic classes. Some common themes of personality organization, however, have been described and these may be helpful to the nurse in developing an understanding of how best to approach and care for clients who use drugs.

Most of the research has been with clients who are addicted to opiates, usually heroin, because these are the people who have been available for studies through drug treatment programs. Much less is known about cocaine or poly drug abusers. A significant finding in studies of heroin addicts has been the presence of major depressive symptoms (Rounsaville, Weissman, Crits-Cristoph, Wilber, & Kleber, 1982; Rounsaville, Weissman, Kleber, & Wilber, 1982). There is often a history of profound emotional deprivation in childhood, poor relationships with parents and family, and a significant lack of closeness to others. Many opiate addicts have a low tolerance for painful dysphoria and great difficulty with feelings of anxiety and anger.

Most opiate addicts will meet diagnostic criteria for a psychiatric disorder other than drug addiction at some time in their lives. Although there is no one "addicted personality," many opiate-dependent people exhibit features of major depressive disorders, personality disorders, and alcoholism (Rounsaville, Weissman, Kleber, & Wilber, 1982).

Drug abusers respond to painful feelings in a variety of ways. Drug use itself is a psychological defense. Heroin and sedative-hypnotics sedate and decrease anxiety through regression and withdrawal from others. The narcotic euphoria provides feelings of nurturance and safety as well as orgasmic satiety. People who take heroin find their anxiety relieved by feelings of "Everything is OK; nothing matters." In contrast, cocaine offers a surge of feelings of power and competence. People who use cocaine find anxiety relieved by feelings of "I can handle anything; I'll take care of it all."

Drugs relieve anxiety. It should not surprise us then that some intravenous drug users respond to a diagnosis of AIDS, ARC, or HIV seropositivity with increased drug use. A number of former drug users have said that they are afraid that if they were told they had AIDS, the temptation to return to drug use would be irresistible.

Other psychological defenses used by intravenous drug abusers include denial, externalization, projection, and personalization. These defenses lead to paranoia and mistrust of others, especially of professionals. The suspicion is reinforced in interactions on the street and with professionals in the social services, law enforcement agencies, and health care facilities.

Intravenous drug abusers are often overwhelmed by feelings of guilt, shame, and personal worthlessness. Neither the drug user nor society really believes that addiction is an illness, and both condemn the user for not stopping. Clients are extremely anxious about the health risks of drug use, including HIV infection, but are often unable to act on their concerns to change their behaviors effectively. They may respond to this anxiety, particularly in the hospital setting, with angry and demanding behavior.

Nursing Approach

Keeping in mind the psychosocial profile of drug users as well as one's own attitudes toward drug use, there are a number of ways to defuse the situation, decrease suspicion and frustration for both the client and the nurse, and improve communication and care.

1. Be alert to signs of anxiety that may be masked by anger and denial.
2. Try to hear what clients want and what worries them. What is the client's agenda for this hospitalization? It may be different from yours.
3. Speak directly to the client's concerns.
4. Be very clear and straightforward about who you are, and what you will be doing and why. This approach will decrease paranoia and suspicion.
5. Remember when talking with clients that many of the behaviors you are discussing are illegal and they may have good reason not to be forthcoming. This is not a reflection on you but on society.
6. Keep in mind the tendency toward personalization and avoid generalization in your discussion with the client. Choose your words carefully.
7. Be supportive and understanding without sanctioning the behavior.
8. Don't set yourself and the client up for failure by defining the success of your interventions in terms of abstention from drugs. A more realistic and helpful goal is to establish a caring relationship based on mutual respect.

People who use drugs are individuals. The first step in working with people who have this problem, as with anyone, is learning who they are as individuals. Drug users expect to be categorized as difficult or undesirable clients. This expectation often leads them to present initially in a defensive, sullen, or hostile manner. Many times you will be able to step around this anger quickly by showing your interest, concern, and respect.

When working with an angry or difficult client, threats are rarely effective. Remember that risk taking is part of drug use; intravenous drug users risk death every time they use a needle. However, it is often necessary to establish boundaries. To do this, you must know yourself and the rest of the health care team. You must be clear as to what behaviors are not acceptable and why, then firmly communicate this information to the client. Explicit limitations presented in an objective, matter-of-fact way communicate a genuine concern for the individual. The key to setting limitations is to do so consistently with all members of the health care team at all times, while still maintaining a continual, attentive concern for the person's felt needs. Try to hear what is behind the anger. For most clients, it will be overwhelming fear and anxiety, which can be defused with careful, repeated assurances of your concern and attention.

Specific Drugs of Abuse

Caffeine, tobacco, alcohol, barbiturates, sedatives, tranquilizers—all are abused. But only the opiates and the stimulant drugs are used intravenously. Most people who "shoot" drugs in the United States use either heroin or cocaine. An understanding of the physiological and psychic effects of these drugs is essential in caring for clients who have used them.

Heroin

Heroin is a short-acting narcotic that is metabolized to morphine in the body. It is the primary narcotic drug used to the point of dependence. Recently, a number of synthetic narcotics have been produced and marketed. They are known by a variety of "street" names such as "P-dope" or "Blue Thunder." Their effects are similar to that of heroin; users will tell you that these new drugs are more powerful and more addicting than heroin. Some users believe that the synthetic drugs are responsible for the HIV epidemic.

Heroin may be administered intranasally by inhalation ("snorting"), injected intravenously ("shooting"), or injected intradermally ("skin popping"). It produces an acute brief period of euphoria—the "high"—followed by sedation—"nodding." Users describe the high as unlike any other physical sensation, "better than sex." Heroin and other narcotics have many acute and chronic effects, which are listed in Table 6.1 (Jaffe, 1970b).

Table 6.1 *Heroin*

Psychic Effects

Euphoria
Sedation

Physiological Effects

Respiratory depression	Pupillary constriction
Lowered temperature	Peripheral vasodilatation
Hives	Pruritis
Decreased GI motility	Urinary retention
Pulmonary edema	Respiratory arrest

Tolerance to the effects of heroin develops at different rates for each effect (Jaffe, 1980). Tolerance to euphoria, for example, develops much more rapidly than tolerance to respiratory depression. One tragic result may occur when a user attempts to recapture euphoria by increasing the amount of the drug injected; the discrepancy in tolerance may lead to death from respiratory failure.

Heroin is very short-acting. The total duration of action is only three to five hours. The peak effect and euphoria are felt immediately; within thirty to sixty minutes, the euphoria has disappeared, to be replaced with feelings of sedation. Withdrawal symptoms in the dependent person will begin in three to six hours if additional drugs are not administered. Withdrawal symptoms are listed in Table 6.2 (Jaffe, 1980a).

Table 6.2 *Narcotic Withdrawal*

Signs and Symptoms	
Lacrimation	Nausea
Rhinorrhea	Vomiting
Yawning	Diarrhea
Piloerection	Abdominal pain
Shivering	Tachycardia
Diaphoresis	Hypertension
Restlessness	Myalgias
Insomnia	Muscle spasm

Heroin and Pregnancy

Opiate dependence in a pregnant woman results in fetal opiate dependence. Prior to the advent of methadone maintenance as a treatment for heroin addiction and the development of sophisticated neonatal technology, the morbidity and mortality associated with maternal narcotic dependence were extremely high. By 1979, straightforward, effective, safe protocols for the medical management of drug dependence in pregnancy and the neonatal period had been developed (Finnegan, 1979). In the absence of methadone treatment, pregnant women who are opiate-dependent suffer a high rate of spontaneous abortions, miscarriages, premature labor, and fetal stress (Finnegan, 1979).

Cocaine

The United States is in the midst of a cocaine epidemic as the result of the increasing supply and decreasing price of this very powerful drug. The National Institute of Drug Abuse estimated that, by 1986, more than 10 million people abused cocaine regularly (Adams, Gfroerer, Rouse, & Kozel, 1986). After a period of believing that cocaine was a relatively "safe" drug, experts now agree that it is extremely addictive and an abstinence syndrome has been described (Gavin & Ellinwood, 1988).

Cocaine is a central nervous system stimulant that produces euphoria, hyperstimulation, alertness, and feelings of power. The euphoric effect of cocaine is very short-lived, generally less than forty-five minutes, and is followed by a debilitating "crash" that includes feelings of negativism and irritability (Gavin & Ellinwood, 1988; Van Dyke & Bych, 1983). (See Table 6.3).

Table 6.3 *Cocaine*

Psychic Effects

Euphoria	Alertness
Hyperstimulation	Feelings of power

Physiological Effects

CNS stimulation	Myocardial infarction	Elevated temperatures
Blood pressure elevation	Seizures	Cardiac arrhythmias
Rapid respirations	Vasoconstriction	Cerebral hemorrhage
Palpitations	Rapid pulse	Status epilepticus

Cocaine can be administered in a variety of ways. The water-soluble hydrochloride salt can be inhaled or injected intravenously. When cocaine is altered to form cocaine base, or "free base," it can be smoked. In the past two years, large inexpensive quantities of free-base cocaine, also known as "crack," have been available in many urban areas, leading to a significant increase in cocaine abuse. Many heroin users combine cocaine hydrochloride with heroin in a mixture known as a "speedball" that prolongs heroin's euphoric effect and lessens the subsequent feelings of sedation.

Treatment for Heroin Addiction

Medicating a physiological opiate dependence, although not complicated, is not the same as treating the addiction and is rarely successful without a complete drug treatment plan. Options for drug treatment include detoxification, psychotherapy, and methadone maintenance (Table 6.4). Methadone, a synthetic, long-acting narcotic (Jaffe, 1970a), and clonidine hydrochloride (Gold, Redmon, & Kleber, 1979), an alpha andrenergic agonist, are both effective agents for treating narcotic abstinence syndrome and can be used in either an outpatient or in-hospital setting. Many addicts will become drug-free during a hospitalization. The challenge then is to help them remain drug-free after discharge.

Table 6.4 *Treatment Options for Opiate Addiction*

Drug-free treatment	Individual
	Group
	Residential/therapeutic community
Narcotic antagonist treatment	Naltrexone
Methadone Maintenance Treatment	

Methadone Maintenance

For many heroin addicts, methadone maintenance has proved to be the only treatment modality that allows them to lead a normal life. Nurses in acute care hospitals are caring for increasing numbers of persons with HIV infection who are taking daily methadone. It is useful to have a basic understanding of what the drug provides, the framework in which it is used, and its physiological effects.

Methadone is a semisynthetic, long-acting narcotic that can be administered orally as well as parenterally (Jaffe, 1970b). The half life is between twenty-four and forty-eight hours. Because of the drug's stable plasma level, a client who is taking methadone regularly at a fairly high dose (70 mg) will not experience euphoria, will be freed from the highs and lows of the heroin cycle, and thus will be able to change behavior patterns. An individual's drug-seeking behavior decreases as the craving for heroin is reduced. (See Table 6.5.)

Table 6.5 *Differences Between Heroin and Methadone*

	Heroin	*Methadone*
Administration	IV (usually)	PO (usually)
Onset	Immediate	30 minutes
Duration	3 - 6 hours	24 - 36 hours
Euphoria	1st 1 - 2 hours	None
Withdrawal	After 3 hours	After 24 hours

Methadone is a very safe drug. In the first six months of treatment, a client may present with a number of side effects (see Table 6.6) that are common to all narcotics (Kreek, 1983). Most side effects resolve as the person develops tolerance. Constipation may be a persistent problem and should be addressed in the hospitalized client.

Pain Management

Clients who are on methadone maintenance therapy are often afraid that when they are admitted to the hospital, they will not receive adequate pain medication. Often, their fears are well-founded. They are tolerant to the analgesic effects of methadone and their pain threshold is the same as if they were not taking a narcotic. They will require as much or more analgesic medication as a nondrug-dependent person (Kreek, 1983). Nurses and physicians are often concerned about contributing to the individual's drug problem or about "readdicting" the patient. These fears are unnecessary. Occasionally, clients will try to increase the amount of pain medication they are receiving or prolong the duration of prescription, but, more often, inadequate doses of analgesics are prescribed for too short a time.

Table 6.6 *Methadone Side Effects*

Central Nervous System	Depressed cerebral functioning:	Analgesia Sedation Mood changes Difficulty concentrating
	Depressed respiratory center:	Shallow breathing Decreased respiratory rate
	Stimulated chemotrigger zone:	Nausea Vomiting
Gastrointestinal Tract	Decreased motility: Increased muscle tone: Biliary tract spasm	Constipation Abdominal cramps Abdominal pain
Urinary Tract	Increased tone of urinary bladder: Increased tone of urethral sphincter:	Urgency Hesitancy
Peripheral Vasculature	Dilation of cutaneous vessels:	Flushing Hypotension Diaphoresis
Allergic Reactions	Histamine release:	Rash Hives Pruritis
Hormonal System	Antidiuretic hormone release: Decreased FSH and LH: Altered prolactin release	Edema Menstrual irregularities

Drug Interactions With Methadone

Drug	Effect	Solution
Rifampin	Increased hepatic metabolizing of methadone, abrupt onset of withdrawal symptoms	Choose another antitubercular agent
Phenytoin	Enhanced methadone metabolism, mild narcotic withdrawal 2 - 4 days after beginning phenytoin	Observe and increase methadone dose, if necessary

Methadone itself should not be used for analgesia when the patient is on methadone maintenance. First, its effectiveness is quite limited in the tolerant individual. Second, the methadone dose was established as part of the therapeutic plan developed by the drug treatment team and should not be altered without their participation. Other drugs not to be used are mixed agonist-antagonists such as pentazocine (Talwin) and nalbuphine (Nubain) because they will precipitate withdrawal in an opiate-dependent person (Kreek, 1983). Normal or slightly higher than normal doses of drugs such as meperidine (Demerol) and codeine are appropriate.

Clients with a drug addiction are often placed on methadone at the time of admission to a hospital. The amount of methadone needed must be carefully established according to (a) reported daily intake of addictive drugs and (b) signs and symptoms of withdrawal (see Table 6.2).

Drug-seeking behavior can also occur when additional pain medication is unavailable to clients. Some of these problems can be avoided by consulting both nursing and medical experts in drug addiction early in the client's admission in order to develop a solid care plan for the whole health team.

Narcotic Antagonist Therapy

Another, newer pharmacologic approach to the treatment of opiate dependence is based on the use of a long-acting narcotic antagonist, naltrexone (Trexan). Naltrexone blocks the effects of opiates by competing for opiate receptor sites. When a client who is taking naltrexone uses narcotics, the antagonist blocks the narcotic and the client fails to experience the euphoric effects of the drug (Anonymous, 1985).

Naltrexone has a long duration of action and is often taken only two or three times a week (Anonymous, 1985). It has few side effects, little or no "street" value, and no addictive potential. Naltrexone will precipitate withdrawal if given to an individual who is currently opiate-dependent. The client who has been using short-acting narcotics such as heroin, morphine, or dilaudid will need to be drug-free for one week before beginning naltrexone therapy (Anonymous, 1985). Clients taking naltrexone must be given only nonnarcotic pain relievers.

Naltrexone is particularly useful for highly motivated clients who are able to maintain the initial drug-free state required to begin naltrexone therapy and who are motivated to continue to take the medication. For these individuals, naltrexone can prevent impulsive use of narcotics and readdiction. Naltrexone is attractive because it is a nonaddictive treatment for opiate dependence, but it has not been well accepted by the majority of heroin addicts, and methadone maintenance remains the treatment of choice for many.

Cocaine Treatment

Treatment protocols for severe cocaine abuse are not well-established. Most psychotherapeutic approaches have been tried and some pharmacotherapies are being studied. One group has used desipramine hydrochloride with some success (Gavin & Kleber, 1986). Treatment for this problem is probably most effective in a program designed specifically for cocaine abusers; unfortunately, there are few such programs. Many methadone maintenance programs offer special groups for cocaine abusers in the context of a full-service drug treatment program.

Referral for Drug Abuse

Nurses are frequently frustrated in their attempts to help people with HIV infection who also have drug problems. Substance abuse is a complex psychological, physiological, and social problem that can rarely be "cured" in the context of an acute care admission. Helping the client make contact with the appropriate drug treatment agency is often the most valuable service the nurse can provide.

Community resources vary tremendously in the types of services available as well as in the number of "treatment slots." Methadone programs in particular are limited by federal and state regulations in the number of clients they are allowed to serve. Many urban areas have waiting lists for methadone treatment. However, methadone programs may also have special slots for "medical emergencies" or be able to refer the patient to another treatment modality such as a drug-free residential program, detoxification, or naltrexone treatment.

It makes sense to contact community agencies early in the client's hospitalization and to include agency staff in discharge planning. With the client's consent, information can be shared and care coordinated. Case conferences can be of immense help in difficult management problems such as that of the methadone client who continues to use cocaine intravenously, is homeless, and is about to be discharged.

Frequent communication is essential when the client is already enrolled in a drug treatment program. In these cases, clients will most likely already have a primary drug abuse counselor who will know them, their family, and their social situation well. When the client declines referral, drug treatment staff can still be a valuable resource in developing a care plan and understanding the client's behavior. Consultation requests can be made without violating the client's confidentiality by discussing the situation without divulging the client's identity.

Intravenous Drug Abuse and AIDS

Throughout the course of the AIDS epidemic, a steady 16 to 17 percent of the cases of AIDS reported to the Centers for Disease Control have been in persons who used drugs intravenously. An additional 8 percent have been among men who were gay or bisexual and also used drugs. Pediatric AIDS and heterosexually acquired AIDS are also closely tied to intravenous drug abuse. In some parts of the urban Northeast, intravenous drug abuse is emerging as the major risk behavior associated with HIV transmission.

Prevention Education—Needle Use

HIV is presumed to be transmitted from one intravenous user to another through shared needles, syringes, and other paraphernalia containing infected blood. A number of studies have shown that HIV infection among intravenous drug users is associated with shooting gallery use (Schoenbaum et al., 1986). Shooting galleries are often abandoned buildings or back rooms of apartments or stores where needles, syringes, and other equipment are rented. Such equipment may be used sequentially by multiple anonymous individuals.

In order to interrupt transmission, users must be cautioned not to use the equipment in shooting galleries. Needles either should not be shared or should be cleaned effectively. Studies have demonstrated that the majority of drug abusers are aware of the way HIV is transmitted and what they must do to protect themselves (Selwyn, Feiner, Cox, Lipschultz, & Cohen, 1987). Since the anxiety associated with hospitalization may provide an additional motivation for changing behaviors, nurses should take every opportunity to reinforce this information.

Needle sharing is associated with a lack of access to individual needles and with the overwhelming need to use drugs to ward off withdrawal symptoms or to satisfy cocaine craving. Most intravenous drug users do clean their needles but they often clean with water (A.B. Williams, D'Aquila, & A.E. Williams, 1987). To be effective, education about needle cleaning should take into account the realities of daily life for addicts. Methods that require boiling, long periods of soaking, or unusual disinfectants are not likely to be used. Liquid household bleach, either full strength or diluted with water in a 1:10 solution, is effective. Equipment should be soaked for thirty minutes if possible; if soaking is not possible, full-strength bleach is preferred.

Many nurses are uncomfortable providing information about needle cleaning to clients. One of the features of the AIDS epidemic is that it has forced us to confront a number of issues that are not only medical, but also social, political, and economic in nature. Intravenous drug use is such an issue, and, therefore, a dilemma nurses must face. Using needles is dangerous. Every time addicts put a needle in a vein, they face death from overdose or from cardiac arrest. Not sharing needles and cleaning equipment will *not* protect against these risks but will protect against HIV and perhaps prevent its transmission to sexual partners and unborn children. Given the current difficulties in providing either drug abuse treatment or sterile needles to drug users, the provision of information about easy, practical ways to prevent HIV transmission by cleaning needles and syringes seems appropriate.

There is a community of drug users but it is often disorganized, chaotic, and politically powerless. News and information spread very rapidly among this network. Frequently, what spread are rumor and misinformation. Nevertheless, this network is our best vehicle for getting the information about HIV and its prevention out into the community of intravenous drug abusers. By sharing what we know with addicts when they are hospitalized, we are also educating the community.

Prevention Education—Sexual Transmission

Unfortunately, it seems that people who use drugs are not as aware or concerned about the risk of acquiring HIV infection sexually as they are about transmission through drug use (Williams et al., 1987). Most heterosexuals with HIV infection are intravenous drug abusers and most children with HIV infection have a parent who has injected drugs. In addition, the nondrug-using sexual partners are also at risk of acquiring infection. For some women who use drugs, prostitution is a source of money to acquire drugs. In this case, sexual behavior is not a question of sexual orientation, but of survival. We should not concentrate on counseling about drug use to the exclusion of sexual counseling for these patients. The principles of safer sex counseling are discussed in Chapter 14 and issues specific to women are covered in Chapter 8.

The Intravenous Drug Abuser as a Person With HIV Infection

Intravenous drug abusers who have HIV carry a double burden. They already suffer from the primary medical and mental health problem of drug addiction. HIV infection is only the most recent in a series of overwhelming health and social problems faced by addicts.

Most drug users have few personal and social resources with which to respond to the physical and social stress of illness. When physically dependent on heroin or in the midst of a cocaine "run," life centers around acquiring and using drugs. There is often little available in the way of family or social support. Users may have antagonized and alienated potentially helpful family members. The most important friends are drug-using comrades on the street.

Taking care of these clients can be frustrating and emotionally draining for the nurse. No one person can begin to address all the needs; a team approach with frequent consultation and communication is essential. But the rewards can be tremendous. People so desperately in need of support often respond with sincere gratitude at being accepted and comforted. Although many intravenous drug abusers have long histories of intractable emotional isolation, others crave genuine concern and respond warmly to kindness and empathy. The intravenous drug abuser with HIV infection is frightened, anxious, and defensive. The nurse may also be uncomfortable and apprehensive. But when respect, communication, and trust are established, providing care becomes a satisfying challenge.

References

Adams, E.H., Gfroerer, J.C., Rouse, B.A., & Kozel, N.J. (1986). Trends in prevalence and consequences of cocaine use. *Advances in Alcohol and Substance Abuse, 6,* 49-71.

Anonymous. (1985). Naltrexone for opioid addiction. *The Medical Letter, 27*(680), 11-12.

Finnegan, L.P. (1979). Drug dependence in pregnancy: Clinical management of mother and child. National Institute on Drug Abuse Services Research Monograph Series, Publication Number ADM 79-678, Rockville, MD.

Gavin, F., & Ellinwood, E.H. (1988). Cocaine and other stimulants. *New England Journal of Medicine, 318*(18), 1173-1182.

Gavin, F. & Kleber, H. (1986) Pharmacological treatments of cocaine abuse. *Psychiatric Clinics of North America, 9,* 573-83.

Gold, M.S., Redmon, E., & Kleber, H.D. (1979). Noradrenergic hyperactivity in opiate withdrawal supported by clonidine reversal of opiate withdrawal. *American Journal of Psychiatry, 136*(1), 100-101.

Jaffe, J.H. (1970a). Drug addiction and drug abuse. In L.S. Goodman & A. Gilman (Eds.), *The pharmacological basis of therapeutics* (pp. 276-313). New York: Macmillan.

Jaffe, J.H. (1970b). Narcotic analgesics. In L.S. Goodman & A. Gilman (Eds.), *The pharmacological basis of therapeutics* (pp. 237-275). New York: Macmillan.

Kreek, M.J. (1983). Health consequences associated with the use of methadone. In J.R. Cooper et al. (Eds.), *Research on the Treatment of Narcotic Addiction.* National Institute of Drug Abuse Treatment Research Monograph Series, Publication Number ADM 83-1281, Rockville, MD.

Rounsaville, B.J., Weissman, M.M., Crits-Christoph, K., Wilber, C., Kleber, H. (1982). Diagnosis and symptoms of depression in opiate addicts. *Archives of General Psychiatry, 39,* 151-156.

Rounsaville, B.J., Weissman, M.M., Kleber, H., & Wilber, C. (1982). Heterogeneity of psychiatric diagnosis in treated opiate addicts. *Archives of General Psychiatry, 39,* 161-166.

Schoenbaum, E.E., Selwyn, P.A., Klein, R.S., Rogers, M.F., Freeman, K., Friedland, G.H., et al. (1986, June). Prevalence of and risk factors associated with HTLV-III antibodies among intravenous drug abusers in methadone programs in New York City. Poster presented at the III International Conference on AIDS, Paris, France.

Selwyn, P.A., Feiner, C., Cox, C.P., Lipshultz, C., & Cohen, R.L. (1987). Knowledge about AIDS and high-risk behavior among intravenous drug users in New York City. *AIDS, 1*(4), 247-254.

VanDyke, C., & Buck, R. (1983). Cocaine. *Scientific American, 246,* 128-141.

Williams, A.B., D'Aquila, R.T., & Williams, A.E. (1987). HIV infection in intravenous drug abusers. *IMAGE, 19*(4), 179-183.

Chapter 7

Breaking Down Barriers: HIV Infection and Communities of Color

Kattie Portis

Kathie is a young, single mother who is suffering with HIV infection along with her three-year-old son. When her child began to have difficulty breathing, Kathie, feeling ill herself, used all her energy to get her son to a hospital for treatment. Kathie and her child were placed in a room and left there for more than two hours. As the word spread that her child had AIDS, Kathie saw hospital staff come to the door and peek in at them, but no one offered assistance, not even to take the child's pulse or blood pressure, until the doctor entered the room. Kathie was deeply hurt. She went home feeling sick, vulnerable, worried. She knew that she as well as her child needed medical care, but she couldn't face the possibility of another rejection when she was feeling so weak. After feeling ill all night, she came to Women Incorporated for moral support before seeking health care services for herself. Her health is further compromised by a lack of child-care support. Kathie has had her child's name on every day care center list in her area, but no center will accept him. Kathie misses many of her own medical appointments because she has no one to look after her son. Since he feels well most of the time, he is usually an active little boy. On the days when she is not feeling well, the child is more than she can handle. Kathie worries about how she can take care of herself, how she can care for her child, and who else cares about them both. Kathie is one of the people who needs our help, who needs the barriers broken, who needs our care.

My Experience With Breaking Down Barriers

Working in communities of color has been an incredible learning experience. I find myself in a continuous struggle to access services for members of communities that historically have never received ample resources to meet their needs. I have had to break down barriers every step of the way.

When I first realized that I was in a major struggle, I sat in my room and cried. From that moment, I could feel my strength become real in my soul, I became stubborn to the point of anger, for I knew that I had one long fight ahead of me.

The target population that I chose to work with was women. I have been working with substance-abusing women and their children for seventeen years, teaching them to live substance-free, take control of their lives, and keep their families together. When I first began working with women, I was excited. I thought everyone knew that when you help women, you automatically help their children. I was not prepared for the first barrier I encountered in the community. I was told that women did not need specialized treatment. The human services people could not understand why substance-abusing women needed services that included their family members. The existing organizations boasted that the community had services available to women, but the women failed to use these resources. I saw that the existing services were designed for men, run by men, and dominated by men. The issue of children was not addressed. The existing services assumed that women who violated society's norms were undeserving of their children. My own community was denying some of the basic problems and needs of women within their community.

When I discovered this major denial from my own people, I felt alone and afraid. I was also angry that these women were not being given a chance. I had to convince the community that these women were worth saving and had a right to have their children with them while they got their lives together. I realize now that making a decision to work exclusively with women in the early 1970s was a threatening statement to society. Someone who had known me for a long time and who knew that I was not gay gave me the label "a black, radical lesbian," because he was so threatened by my advocacy for women.

We had a major research and demonstration project to prove that women responded if the treatment was designed for women and included their children. The community has accepted that a family-oriented approach works better for serving women. After all these years, I am still not sure if society at large believes that these women deserve a second chance. These are examples of social barriers. Breaking down economic barriers to provide services in communities of color is an ongoing struggle.

I take great pleasure in watching the women take control of their lives. Watching them grow is like watching a tulip, which sleeps in the cold, dark earth all winter, but when spring comes, bursts through the earth bringing forth such beautiful colors. I have the same feeling of joy at the renewal of life when I see people grow and become productive members of the community. Seeing these lives change has given me strength to continue to break down the barriers for communities of color.

Barriers for Communities of Color

People in communities of color face the barriers of discrimination and poverty every day of their lives. These are the people who make up the statistics of the homeless, the raped, the murdered. Infants born in communities of color have a lower chance of survival in the first year of life. The elderly are targets for theft and other crimes. The young adults make up the list of homicides, due to the rampant drug using and selling in the community of color.

Society at large tends to blame poor people for their poverty. Poor people, in particular those of color, have no rights. It is widely believed that poor people should be happy with the handouts they get from a system that is designed to keep them poor and oppressed.

The lack of resources that pervades communities of color leaves people hopeless and desperate. For example, the educational system has failed to meet the needs of the communities of color. Since education is the major tool for raising oneself out of poverty—the only means of escape—the lack of education feeds the despair. When the public education system fails those whose only option is the public school, society finds itself dealing with a population of people who are illiterate and not prepared to break the barriers. Without the necessary educational tools, the reality of poverty falls far below the poverty level, below the average income of poor people. When you have generation after generation of illiteracy, the cycle of deep poverty continues. Without reading and writing skills, even filling out a job application becomes impossible. Without a home address, no one will employ you. Many members of the communities of color have no options for survival other than using and selling drugs to meet their economic needs.

Everyone who lives in communities of color is affected by poverty, because those who don't have any resources will take from those who do have resources within the same community. The crime list consists of mostly people of color, both victims and perpetrators. The individual who commits the crime in the community of color is an individual who does not have the necessary resources and strength to penetrate the barriers that keep one hostage in oppression. Thus, all are victims of the discrimination that keeps people trapped in the despair of poverty and that corners them into the escape of drugs.

The 1980s have brought a right-wing power, a government system in which the rich are richer and the poor have less than ever before. We are confronted with more racial incidents than before because the atmosphere in the eighties says, it's "OK" to discriminate against individuals because of their educational level, economic status, or skin color. When the media give detailed reports of negative incidents in the communities of color, most people lose sight of the real issues. In my anger and helplessness during this long period of devastating violence among our young people, even I forget that a person who is illiterate and lives in poverty has the same need to survive and the same greed as the new breed of upper-middle-class yuppie drug dealers.

In addition to social, economic, and educational barriers, language is another barrier in our community. There are many different cultures in the community of color. Even within the same race, there are different languages, social customs, and beliefs. Not all black people are the same, not all Hispanics are the same. All of the different cultures of people in the community share only one thing: discrimination. They are united only by the barriers of poverty built by a prejudiced society.

AIDS and Communities of Color

AIDS has had a devastating impact on the people in communities of color. For years, I have worked with people whose lives are completely out of control due to substance abuse. I have learned that substance abuse is only one of the issues of poverty, illiteracy, discrimination, and low self-esteem that threw their lives into a crisis. My greatest joy has been to fight through those issues, seeing people take control of their lives and live drug-free.

Now I find myself helping to prepare them for death. These are the same people who make up the lists of high school dropouts, illiterates, unemployed, homeless, raped, and teenage mothers. It is not surprising that women of color are dying of HIV infection in disproportional numbers.

As I watched the progression of the AIDS virus in the media, I have said to myself, "My God, why doesn't someone do something?" It never occurred to me that the client population I have been working with for all these years would be the hardest hit. Now I find myself teaching them how to clean their needles by using bleach.

In 1987, when I accepted the job as coordinator for the National Women's AIDS Risk Network (WARN), I found myself again confronting many barriers, the largest of which was denial. This virus is so frightening that society at large went into total denial, which angered many members of the communities of color. People of the majority felt safe because the virus was killing two groups that society sees as undesirable: homosexuals and IV drug users. Not only was the mainstream denying its vulnerability, so were people in the communities of color. I knew I had a long fight ahead of me again. People in the communities of color were so overwhelmed at the horror of AIDS, they denied its severity. They were saying, "It can't be that bad; it's just another form of racism. It's just one more thing that society puts on us."

AIDS, like substance abuse, is just one more entry onto a list of life-threatening issues: poverty, homelessness, illiteracy, violence. When you live below the poverty level, which means that you are poorer than the average poor, you live with a high risk of violent incidents. When there are so many crises confronting a community, mobilizing people to fight yet another crisis is difficult. Already overwhelmed with the danger confronting them, people in the community use denial as a way of coping with the emotional overload of so many threats to their survival.

Many people who use drugs believe they will die from violence before they will die from AIDS. People are concerned but they have so many other issues affecting their lives that they hide from the horror of AIDS with denial. Since the high-risk groups for AIDS are viewed as leeches of society, the only hope for my people had to come from their own community. Therefore, when the communities of color are in denial, no one does anything. We have worked long and hard to break this barrier of denial within our communities.

In addition to denial, there is also the barrier of cultural values. In the communities of color, there is a judgmental atmosphere that almost reaches the extreme of homophobia. Just like people in society at large, people in communities of color want to disassociate themselves from AIDS because of the connotations of sexuality. The communities of color are composed of a very mixed cultural population with a wide diversity of values and beliefs. We are Afro-American blacks, Haitian blacks, black West Indians, Latinos, Puerto Ricans, Cape Verdeans, Portuguese, and Asian Americans. The variety of cultures and the pervading taboo of homosexuality hinder AIDS education. Transmission of the virus must be explained carefully, within the context of the cultural values by someone from the same background as the people in the audience. People need to hear about AIDS in their own language from one of their own people, because the discussion of sexual issues is handled so differently in each ethnic group. AIDS education in communities of color is not just one program, but multiple programs to each cultural entity. After months of work, the people have begun to get the message that the virus is not only killing gays and drug addicts, but it is a threat to all members of the community.

Although people of color comprise 18 percent of all people in the United States, we comprise 39 percent of all people with AIDS. Women of color are the majority of all women with AIDS, 52 percent of whom are black women. Sixty-one percent of all children born with AIDS are black. The people in these categories will be coming to the local health centers and hospitals in need of care. Most of the time, they will be without family support, especially if they are addicted or gay, which is often socially unacceptable to the family. Many people who may be at risk for HIV infection refuse to get tested for fear of rejection from their families and communities.

Communities of Color and the Health Care System

One of the most devastating experiences that confronts us constantly is the lack of housing or services to persons with HIV infection. People who are well enough to go home from the hospital, but still need emotional and physical support, often have no place to go. Without family support, without financial resources, they have no home, no one to care for them.

People of color often present to the health care system more acutely ill, since health maintenance is not a part of their survival agenda. By the time they arrive in an emergency room, they are usually in severe crisis, acutely ill, vulnerable, alone, and frightened. They may fail to disclose their seropositive status because they deny their infection to themselves in order to avoid having to change their behavior. People living with HIV infection expect rejection in the health care system, their only means of help. Some people, such as Kathie, have shared with me the discrimination and ostracism they have perceived.

When these people are in your nursing care, you become more than just the person with the thermometer: You are often their only hope for support. In addition to the lack of financial resources, many people lack emotional support to sustain them through the shock of accepting that they are HIV-infected. Because of the stigma of this disease, they are afraid to discuss AIDS with family members. Most often, they have already been rejected by family members because of their lifestyle or high-risk behavior. Since many people in communities of color are uneducated about AIDS, they often have unnecessary fears of catching AIDS from the infected family member. The family withdraws out of fear and out of shame. As in other communities, family members try to hide and keep the secret in order to avoid public disgrace. Therefore, by the time these individuals seek health care service and come under your care, they are without emotional support or necessary resources to help them through the crisis of their illness. The only source of help they have is the health care system, and even here they fear rejection. Your ability to show your sincere acceptance, concern, and respect may make all the difference in the quality of life in their last days.

The AIDS virus has a very rare affect on people. I have seen individuals become empowered by the disease. I am reminded of a woman I have known for at least twenty years. She was abandoned by her mother when she was an infant and has spent the rest of her life looking for someone to love her. After being passed around from foster home to foster home throughout her childhood, by the age of thirteen, she had given up on ever finding loving parents. She went to school one day and never returned home. By the time she was fourteen, she was placed with the Department of Youth Services for prostitution. Her search for love brought her to men who exploited her childhood and vulnerability. After she was released from the Department of Youth Services, she returned to the streets and prostitution, the only life she knew. Eventually she landed in the state correctional institution for women, addicted to drugs. From prison, she entered a drug treatment program and stayed for a few months. After treatment, she went back to the streets and started the cycle all over again. As I watched her constantly repeating the same downward spiral, I asked her, "What do you want out of life?" She replied, "All I want is a family." She was still looking for someone to love her. She proceeded to get pregnant and had two children. Since she never received loving care as a child, she had no idea how to take care of her own children. With her consent, they were placed in foster care and eventually adopted. She had lost her last chance for love.

In 1987, she showed up at my office to tell me she was positive with the HIV virus. A few months later, I received a call from the hospital where she had been admitted. I went to see her, feeling both angry and sad, for life had been so unfair to her. Over the years I wanted so much to stop her pain but I could not. The one thing she wanted was a family, which I could not give her.

As I sat in her room talking with her, I watched all the hospital personnel avoid her. The housekeeper would stand in the hallway and push the mop in only as far as she could. Therefore, the room was not cleaned properly. To my surprise, I found as I talked with my friend that she was preparing for her death. I have never witnessed so much courage, so much power. For the first time in her life, she felt in charge. She was not afraid to die. She had planned how she would leave when the time came. She seemed to be at peace. I asked her to help me understand the peace she was experiencing. She said, "I never felt in control of how I lived before, but now I will be in control of how I die." She wanted to go quickly when the time came. She planned to refuse life support systems and wanted a brief funeral.

After her stay in the hospital, she was released and went to one of the local shelters. This woman was sick with no home or family. She had never had any dignity in her life. I am sad because she will die with no respect as a human being. As her executor, I will make sure that all of her requests are met. I will do this with all respect for her as a person. If you happen to meet her, please respect her, for it costs nothing. I know that the virus does not discriminate. Everything seems to happen to poor people, including AIDS. I hope and pray that my friend keeps the peace inside her and finds true happiness with her family in the next world.

There are many people in the same situation as my friend: without family, without the necessary skills for survival. My friend does not want pity or sympathy, she just wants to go to sleep in the way she chooses. Although she knows that laws protect her from discrimination, what she seeks cannot be legislated. Professional people cannot be forced to have compassion, kindness, or concern. I have met many individuals who had the highest degrees from the best educational institutions in the country, but they had very little compassion or tolerance for people. They failed to be effective in their roles. I know that care givers choose their profession because they like the job, which is fine. However, when you choose to work with people with HIV infection, the work is more than a job; it's a commitment to give all you have to people who need your help. I have met many wonderful, committed, compassionate people determined to fight the AIDS virus. Compassion and tolerance are necessary. Kindness and tenderness are critical. Acceptance and respect are essential.

Chapter 8

Counseling Women With HIV Infection

Ann Williams

Gloria is a tiny black woman with a warm, appealing smile. At age thirty-eight, she has raised three children in a rough inner-city ghetto and now lives alone. Gloria is dying of AIDS. She has been hospitalized numerous times and suffers from severe peripheral neuropathies, fatigue, and weakness. She says one of the most difficult things for her is the vulnerability she now feels. She is afraid to go out because she is an easy target for muggers. After all these years of surviving the street, she's helpless.

Elaine is a young white woman, the daughter of a prominent suburban lawyer. Last year she discovered that she was pregnant; the same week her HIV test came back positive. Elaine very much wanted to have a baby and she decided against an abortion. Her son is healthy and HIV-negative. Now Elaine, whose family has disowned her, worries about who will care for her son if she becomes ill.

Gloria and Elaine are members of a hidden minority. Most Americans with AIDS are young men. But since the beginning of the epidemic, women have also suffered. And although the proportion of cases of AIDS in women has increased only slightly, the absolute number of women with HIV infection is growing rapidly with the epidemic. In some parts of the United States, AIDS is now the number-one cause of death in women between the ages of twenty-five and twenty-nine.

Women with AIDS or HIV infection differ from most men at risk in a number of ways. They are women who, to a large extent, have been disenfranchised by the larger society. Women with AIDS are not organized; they have no one to speak for them in the political forums where the AIDS epidemic is being debated. There are few voices raised to protect their interests when research and treatment protocols are being designed. Most of the health professionals who manage AIDS patients have little experience in caring for these women and, unfortunately, often have little understanding or empathy for them. They are too often seen as "noncompliant," frustrating, and difficult patients who are of interest or concern chiefly as transmitters of AIDS to their unborn children.

Women with AIDS or HIV infection need special attention from nurses who care for women for a variety of reasons. First, women with AIDS are sicker and survive a shorter time after diagnosis than do men (Rothenberg et al., 1987; Verdegem, Sattler, & Boylen, 1988). Second, many women with AIDS are single mothers who care for, and eventually leave behind, small children. Third, these same children may themselves be infected with HIV. The tragedy of a dying woman whose last wish is that she live long enough to be with her child when the child dies is unspeakably painful and becoming all too common in our inner cities. It is most often the nurse who shares the pain of these mothers, who helps them say good-bye to their children. And it is nurses who are best placed to identify women at risk when they interact with the health care system, particularly in emergency rooms, gynecologic and prenatal facilities, and pediatric clinics.

Epidemiology of AIDS in Women

The proportion of reported cases of AIDS in women has remained fairly constant throughout the epidemic. As of June 20, 1988, the 5,155 women with AIDS represented 8 percent of all AIDS cases in the United States (Centers for Disease Control [CDC], 1988). A little over half of these women were intravenous drug abusers. Another large subgroup of women with AIDS are women whose male sex partners have injected drugs. These two groups together make up more than two-thirds of the women with AIDS in the United States (CDC, 1988).

The geographic distribution of women with AIDS is tied to that of intravenous drug users with AIDS; most women with AIDS are living on the East Coast of the United States (Guinan & Hardy, 1987). Although nationally only 8 percent of AIDS cases are in women, in some parts of the urban Northeast they represent almost onethird of the persons with AIDS. The overwhelming majority of women with AIDS are members of minority groups: black Americans or Hispanics (Guinan & Hardy, 1987).

HIV Transmission in Women

Intravenous Drug Abuse

Most women with AIDS are women whose lives have been touched in some way by intravenous drug abuse. AIDS is a blood-borne, sexually transmitted disease. This simple message bears repeating. The basics of HIV transmission are the same for women as they are for men. The virus is transmitted through intimate contact with sexual secretions or blood.

Although half the women with AIDS in the United States at present are women who have used intravenous drugs, we can not actually say for sure that they all acquired their infection through their own drug use. This is because the sexual partners of most women who use intravenous drugs are also drug users; thus, these women are at risk for HIV infection via two routes: contaminated drug injection equipment and heterosexual contact with men at risk for AIDS.

Heterosexual Transmission

Heterosexual transmission clearly plays a major role in the epidemic of AIDS in women. Heterosexual-contact cases represented over one-quarter of the cumulative number of women with AIDS who had been reported to the CDC (CDC, 1988). Most of these women had had sexual contact with a man who had AIDS or was at risk for AIDS. On the East Coast, this man was likely to have been someone who used intravenous drugs.

Currently, in the United States, there are many more women than men with heterosexually acquired AIDS. The relative efficiency of male-to-female versus female-to-male transmission of HIV has been an area of controversy. Some studies of heterosexual couples in which one partner is infected suggest that the risk of acquiring infection may be equal for men and women (Steigbigel et al., 1988); in other studies, the uninfected female partners appear at greater risk (Padian, Glass, Marquis, Wiley, & Winkelstein, 1988). Nevertheless, HIV has been cultured from cervical secretions (Vogt et al., 1987), and there is no doubt that heterosexual transmission of the virus can be bidirectional.

Prostitution

The concern about heterosexual transmission of AIDS from women to men has led to some of the ugliest episodes in the social history of the epidemic. The stigma of AIDS was attached to prostitutes in many cities and there were calls for involuntary testing and confinement or quarantine of prostitutes who continued to work after testing positive. Prostitutes with AIDS or HIV infection have had their names published in newspapers, have been placed under house arrest, have been threatened with death.

Prostitutes are not yet playing a major role in the growth of the AIDS epidemic but they are themselves vulnerable and in need of safer sex education, as are all women with multiple sex partners. Seroprevalence studies of HIV infection in prostitutes have confirmed that for these women too, the major risk is intravenous drug abuse, their own or that of a sexual partner (CDC, 1987).

Sexual Transmission Between Women

One percent of women reported with AIDS identified their sexual orientation as lesbian; another 1 percent considered themselves bisexuals. These women were at risk mainly through intravenous drug use (Drotman & Mays, 1988). There have been a few case reports of HIV transmitted sexually between women when sexual activities included contact with blood (Marmor et al., 1986). Although, as with other sexually transmitted diseases, the risk is low, it is real and is of great concern to lesbian couples in which one partner has HIV infection or is at risk of acquiring it.

Reproductive Concerns

Pregnancy and AIDS

Pediatric AIDS devastates the entire family unit. Its distinct features are discussed in detail in Chapter 13. Most children with AIDS are born to women who are at risk for HIV infection (CDC, 1988). The virus may be transmitted transplacentally or perinatally (CDC, 1985). Unfortunately, the questions of greatest importance to women with AIDS or HIV infection remain largely unanswered. What exactly is the rate of HIV transmission in pregnancy? At what point in the pregnancy is the virus transmitted? Are there clinical features in the mother that might help predict the outcome for her child? We need the answers to these and many other questions in order to help women like Elaine make informed decisions about their childbearing options.

Determining the frequency of true infection in the child is complicated by the presence of maternal antibody to HIV in the infant. The rate of maternal-infant transmission may actually be as low as 20 percent and the development of severe, early-onset pediatric AIDS may be unusual (Andiman, Simpson, Dember, Fraulino, & Miller, 1988). But very little is understood about the role of possible co-factors such as the mother's clinical status or the impact of social and economic variables. Most women with AIDS are economically disadvantaged and both they and their children are likely to have had limited access to health care. As a rule of thumb, counselors working with women who are HIV-positive usually tell them that there is a fifty-fifty chance of the virus being transmitted to an unborn child.

Another area of concern is the impact of pregnancy on the immune system of a woman with HIV infection or AIDS. Pregnancy is associated with a decreased T-helper to T-suppressor cell ratio and there has been speculation that pregnancy might trigger clinical AIDS in a previously asymptomatic woman (CDC, 1985). Prospective studies have not supported this hypothesis to date although the question is far from answered.

Childbearing Options

The U.S. Public Health Service currently recommends that women who are infected with HIV postpone pregnancy until more is known about the risk of perinatal HIV transmission. Women who are not infected but who are the sexual partners of men at risk are also advised to postpone pregnancy (CDC, 1985). This is quite a lot to ask of women. As far as we now know, HIV infection is lifelong; in effect, women are being told to forgo childbearing without much hope that this recommendation will be lifted in the near future.

In the absence of more concrete data, some women will choose, as Elaine did, to bear a child. They may feel that a one-in-five chance of having an infected baby, or even fifty-fifty odds, is worth the risk. Most women with HIV infection have had to survive very hard times on the street. They have taken many risks just to survive; if they use drugs, they risk death every time they shoot heroin or cocaine. These odds with childbearing don't look too bad. It may seem to be a chance worth taking.

They often desperately want their babies. In many cases, they have been isolated and rejected by their families. Their sexual relationships may have been abusive and exploitative. A child holds the promise of love and possibly even the restoration of family ties. The grandmother who washed her hands of a drug-using daughter will often open her heart again to a grandchild. Preliminary results from a prospective study of pregnant women who had a history of intravenous drug abuse suggest that for some women, knowing their HIV-antibody status and being worried about AIDS was not associated with decisions about terminating a pregnancy. A more important issue for these women was whether or not the pregnancy was planned (Selwyn et al., 1988).

For many women who use drugs such as heroin and cocaine, pregnancies are not planned. The drugs themselves disrupt the menstrual cycle, often causing long periods of amenorrhea that lead the women to believe that they are incapable of conception. Even women who do not want more children frequently fail to practice effective contraception (Selwyn et al., 1988; Williams, 1981). Also as a result of irregular menstrual cycles, women may not realize they are pregnant until four or five months after conception. Limited access to health care facilities, long waiting periods for clinic appointments, and the chaotic lifestyle associated with a dependence on heroin or cocaine work together to ensure that large numbers of women at risk for HIV infection enter the prenatal care system late, when terminating the pregnancy is no longer an option even if that is the choice they would like to make.

Contraception and abortion are two areas of women's lives that have changed dramatically in the past twenty years. Women today are empowered to make choices that were not available to their mothers. The goal in counseling these women must be to support them in making choices that reflect their individual situation. We need to share the information we have, which is incomplete and inadequate, and then we need to respect their decisions. Nurses must not assume that women who do not make the same choices as they would make, or as the Public Health Service recommends, are unaware, uneducated, or noncompliant. If we understand some of the dynamics behind the decision to risk, or not to risk, a baby with HIV, then we can better defend women's right to quality health care, whatever their choice.

Breast Feeding

In the United States and other parts of the so-called developed world, HIV-positive women who do bear children are counseled not to breast feed their babies. HIV has been cultured from breast milk (Thiry, Sprecher-Goldberger, Jonckheer, et al., 1985) and case reports have documented transmission of infection to infants through breast feeding (Ziegler, Stewart, Penny, Stuckey, & Good, 1988). The exact risk of acquiring infection via this route is unknown and the question is particularly serious for the Third World where breast feeding is the best defense against infant mortality due to malnutrition and diarrhea.

Risk-Reduction Strategies for Women

Role of Intravenous Drug Abuse

Women who use drugs intravenously run the same risk of acquiring HIV infection as men who use drugs. Half the women with AIDS in the United States have a history of intravenous drug use. If we are to slow the epidemic, women who use drugs must be identified before they are infected and must be given the prevention education discussed in Chapter 6. Unfortunately, women who use drugs are elusive and difficult to identify. In the hospital women at risk will be found particularly in the emergency room, the pediatric and gynecologic clinics, and on the inpatient units with cellulitis, endocarditis, pelvic inflammatory disease, and hepatitis.

Women who don't use drugs themselves may be able to influence their drug-using sexual partners not to share needles and to clean their equipment, thus decreasing their own risk of heterosexually acquired infection. Information about the dangers of shooting galleries and needle sharing and instructions on how to clean drug injection equipment ("paraphernalia" or "works") should be widely available in emergency rooms, ambulatory clinics, and inpatient units. As nurses, we need to be comfortable talking about this information with all of our patients. It can be prefaced with a statement such as, "I know you don't use drugs, but we are hoping that by sharing this information with everyone, it will reach the people in the community who need it."

One of the most difficult prevention problems is presented by women who don't use drugs themselves and who are unaware of their partners' drug use, either past or present. In some subcultures men and women lead very separate social lives and it is considered inappropriate for women to question men about what they do when they are not at home. Women who have been placed at risk this way report feeling very angry when they discovered their partners' behavior and suggest that other women should be alert to signs of intravenous drug use and be willing to confront men early with their fears. This is by no means an uncommon situation and the ultimate solution lies with the male partners who must acknowledge the risk their behavior poses and take responsibility for it.

Choosing Sexual Partners

Women have been told to choose their partners carefully and to avoid having sex with men who may have used drugs or who may be bisexual. For women living in areas where there is a high incidence of drug abuse, this has led to feelings of frustration and helplessness, a sense that no one can be trusted and that all sexual encounters might be deadly.

Women who use drugs themselves are very unlikely to be able to make the choice to avoid partners at risk for HIV. It is unusual for a woman who uses intravenous drugs to have a spouse or male companion who does not use drugs. Most women are introduced to drugs by a man and many remain dependent on men for their supply of drugs. Women in this situation have little power or control.

Condoms

Condoms are recommended for all sexually active persons who are not involved in a strictly monogamous relationship with a partner who is known to be uninfected with HIV. There is good reason to believe that the consistent and proper use of condoms will substantially reduce the risk of heterosexual HIV transmission (Fischl et al., 1987). Chapter 14 talks about condom use and other safer sex techniques in greater detail.

Since the advent of birth control pills and IUDs, condoms have not been a popular method of birth control in the United States. Most women under forty-five have had little experience with condoms. As a society, we do not support women who are direct about their sexuality or assertive about protecting themselves during sexual encounters. Being prepared for sex, carrying condoms, suggests to many people a looseness about sex; it has implications of immorality. It is a hard thing for some women to do.

Women don't use condoms; men do. It's not enough for a woman to buy and carry or bring home the condoms; she must get the man she is involved with to use them. This may raise difficult issues of power and control within the relationship. Women who do *not* ask men to use condoms say that they are afraid the men will accuse them either of having other sexual partners or of not trusting the men. The risk of physical violence for some women may outweigh the risk of acquiring HIV infection.

Even before the HIV epidemic, many prostitutes used condoms at work with their paying sex customers. The same women generally do not use condoms for sexual activities with their spouses or regular partners, yet these men are often intravenous drug users (Cohen et al., 1988). This pattern may be difficult to change because of the association of condoms with nonaffectionate sexual activity. In addition, not all women who exchange sex for money are professionals. Women who need money for drugs for themselves or their significant male partners may engage only occasionally in this sort of sexual behavior. Women in this situation may be desperate and unlikely to insist on condom use if the man refuses.

Women are aware of the high failure rate of condoms when the goal is pregnancy prevention; they, therefore, have little faith in their effectiveness in HIV prevention. When one member of a couple knows for certain that he or she is infected with HIV, the couple often chooses to abstain from sex entirely rather than rely on condoms.

HIV Testing for Women

Testing for antibodies to HIV has become widely available in the past three years. We now know more about what the test means and it is increasingly used for clinical as well as epidemiologic and research purposes. The clinical and ethical implications of this test are explored in Chapters 3 and 9; however, there are some specific issues for women to consider.

The HIV antibody test is most often recommended for women at risk as a decision-making aid in reproductive planning. The suggested ideal is that women at risk be tested before becoming pregnant; failing that, that they be tested early in the pregnancy so that they have the option of terminating the pregnancy if they are infected. As we have seen, these recommendations are useful only for that minority of at-risk women who plan their pregnancies.

There are sound clinical reasons for identifying pregnant women who are HIV-positive; both the mother and the child deserve to have the pregnancy especially closely monitored. Blinded studies of cord blood samples suggest that women are not being appropriately identified on the basis of history and risk assessment alone in prenatal clinics (Landesman, Minkoff, Holman, McCalla, & Odalis, 1987). The trend, therefore, is toward more frequent use of HIV testing as part of prenatal evaluations in geographic areas where the AIDS risk is thought to be high. It is essential that all nonblinded tests be conducted only with informed consent and that sensitive and appropriate counseling be provided.

Psychosocial Issues for Women With AIDS

Self-esteem and Drug Abuse

When we talk about women and AIDS, we must realize that currently most women with AIDS are women who have abused drugs. Drug abuse in women can not be understood without first acknowledging the fact that gender plays a fundamental role in personality development in our society. Gender helps to define individual identity, the structure of a person's life cycle, the nature of his or her life experiences, and the opportunities and resources available.

Women's patterns of drug use have been influenced by the social context in which they live. Society has different expectations about appropriate male/female roles and behavior, with specifically negative feelings and attitudes toward women drug users. There is a significant stigma associated with drug use, particularly intravenous drug use, by a woman. A man who injects heroin or cocaine may be seen as "bad," as a criminal, but he is not "unmanly." A woman who injects drugs, however, is viewed as violating her feminine nature. A woman with a drug abuse problem may be seen as "sicker" than a man because she not only has a drug problem, she has a "male" disease.

The HIV epidemic has reinforced this attitude. In addition, the assumption that only men participate in high-risk activities may be contributing to the poorer prognosis for women with AIDS when it precludes early diagnosis. One study has noted that AIDS was less likely to be considered as a prehospitalization diagnosis in women hospitalized with Pneumocystis Carinii Pneumonia (PCP) (Verdegem et al., 1988) than in men presenting with similar complaints. Practitioners tend to be less sensitive to the possibility of HIV infection in women.

When caring for or counseling women with AIDS who are intravenous drug abusers, it will be helpful to review many of the issues raised in Chapter 6. Some points deserve emphasis. People don't go out on their own and begin injecting heroin or cocaine. Drug users are introduced to drugs by other users. For women this introduction is almost always performed by a man. Many women continue to remain dependent on men for their drug supplies. Relationships may become dominated by the need to secure drugs. If a woman is still using drugs and is in this position, counseling her to insist on condoms or choose another partner is not realistic and adds considerably to her stress.

Addicted women have lower self-esteem and higher levels of anxiety and depression than do addicted men or nonaddicted women from similar socioeconomic backgrounds (Colten, 1979). They are generally not assertive and have little sense of control. Society's attitude toward, and perceptions of, addicted women are generally negative and the women mirror this attitude. They hold very traditional beliefs about sex-role behaviors and see themselves often as failures in maintaining these standards. For instance, they believe in heterosexuality, monogamy, marriage, being a good mother, and are antiabortion (Williams, 1981).

Social Networks

Little has been written about the support systems that exist for women with AIDS. Again we must rely on what we know about drug-addicted women. Women who use drugs have fewer social networks and less support from their spouses than male addicts or nonaddicted women from similar backgrounds (Tucker, 1979). Most are of childbearing age and have children who live with them. Their strongest connection may be with their own mothers who, if available, often help with child rearing. They also have fewer psychological and practical resources and skills for coping with the problems of daily life than do their male counterparts or comparison women (Tucker, 1979). When HIV enters the picture, these resources are severely strained.

Women who discover that they have AIDS or HIV infection feel extremely isolated. They frequently are terrified and have no one to talk to other than the counselor who breaks the news. They do not talk to family or friends for fear of being ostracized. They are reluctant to attend support groups because they do not wish to be identified either as drug abusers or as people with HIV infection (Williams, 1988). Their position is somewhat similar to that of gay men who are not yet "out of the closet," but it is more difficult. Should they choose to come out, there is no supportive community waiting to help. They are forced to depend for support on health care professionals but cultural differences and attitudes of mistrust limit the usefulness of this resource.

Mothering

Women are very concerned about their children. Women who do not take care of themselves will go to great lengths to protect their children. Women who have little self-esteem can feel good about themselves if they feel that they are good mothers. A woman who takes good care of her children in spite of her drug habit is respected in the world of heroin. The HIV epidemic directly attacks women in this very vulnerable area.

Whether it is the mother or the child who first receives the diagnosis of HIV disease, both are threatened. The woman must face her own impending death as well as that of her child. She must also be concerned for her other children; she worries about whether or not they are also infected and who will care for them when she cannot. For mothers with HIV, concern about their children is the most painful and difficult issue they face (Williams, 1988).

When confronted with AIDS, women who have used drugs are overwhelmed by feelings of guilt about their behavior. One way of dealing with guilt and anxiety is denial. Women may deny that they are sick, may deny that they have AIDS or that their child has AIDS. This denial can lead to frequently missed medical appointments and inadequate follow-up care. Health care providers see only a noncompliant patient or a mother who doesn't care. If, when a woman does present for care or becomes so ill as to be hospitalized, she encounters a disbelieving and judgmental attitude, she is much less likely to return. On the other hand, sensitive and caring responses from professionals will encourage her to seek help sooner the next time.

Conclusion

HIV-prevention and-education activities must be directed at all women, heterosexual and lesbian, rich and poor, professionals, working women, and housewives. But AIDS care programs and support services must begin to address the needs of the women who are infected and sick today and who represent the community of women most at risk in the foreseeable future. They are for the most part poor women whose lives have been touched by intravenous drug abuse and who exist outside the established structures of society. We have not successfully reached these women in the past but we must do so now.

References

Andiman, W.A., Simpson, J., Dember, L., Fraulino, L., & Miller, G. (1988, June). Prospective studies of a cohort of 50 infants born to human immunodeficiency virus (HIV) seropositive mothers. Poster presented at the IV International Conference on AIDS, Stockholm, Sweden.

Centers for Disease Control. (1988, June 20). AIDS weekly surveillance report.

Centers for Disease Control. (1987). Human immunodeficiency virus infection in the United States: A review of current knowledge. *Morbidity and Mortality Weekly Report, 36* (suppl. no. S-6), 8.

Centers for Disease Control. (1985). Recommendations for assisting in the prevention of perinatal transmission of human T-lymphotropic virus type III/lymphadenopathy-associated virus and acquired immunodeficiency syndrome. *Morbidity and Mortality Weekly Report, 34*(48), 721-732.

Cohen, J.B., Poole, L.E., Lyons, C.A., Lockette, G.J., Alexander, P., & Woofsy, C.B. (1988, June). Sexual behavior and HIV infection risk among 354 sex industry women in a participant based research and prevention program. Poster presented at the IV International Conference on AIDS, Stockholm, Sweden.

Colten, M.E. (1979). A descriptive and comparative analysis of self-perceptions and attitudes of heroin-addicted women. *Addicted Women: Family Dynamics, Self Perceptions and Support Systems,* Services Research Monograph Series, National Institute on Drug Abuse, DHEW Publication No. [ADM]80-762.

Drotman, D.P., & Mays, M.A. (1988, June). AIDS and lesbians: IV-drug use is the risk. Poster presented at the IV International Conference on AIDS, Stockholm, Sweden.

Fischl, M.A., Dickinson, G.M., Scott, G.B., Klimas, N., Fletcher, M.A., & Parks, W. (1987). Evaluation of heterosexual partners, children and household contacts of adults with AIDS. *Journal of the American Medical Association, 257,* 640-4.

Guinan, M.E., & Hardy, A. (1987). Epidemiology of AIDS in women in the United States. *Journal of the American Medical Association, 257*(15), 2039-2042.

Landesman, S., Minkoff, H., Holman, S., McCalla, S., & Odalis, S. (1987). Serosurvey of human immunodeficiency virus infection in parturients. *Journal of the American Medical Association, 258*(19), 2701-2703.

Marmor, M., Weiss, L.R., Lyden, M., Weiss, S.H., Saxinger, W.C., Spira, T.J., & Feorine, P.M. (1986). Possible female to female transmission of human immunodeficiency virus [Letter]. *Annals of Internal Medicine, 105*(6), 971.

Padian, N., Glass, S., Marquis, L., Wiley, J., & Winkelstein, W. (1988, June). Heterosexual transmission of HIV in California: Results from a heterosexual partner's study. Poster presented at the IV International Conference on AIDS, Stockholm, Sweden.

Rothenberg, R., Woelfel, M., Stoneburner, R., Milberg, J., Parker, R., & Truman, B. (1987). Survival with the acquired immunodeficiency syndrome. *New England Journal of Medicine, 317*(21), 1297-1302.

Selwyn, P.A., Carter, R.J., Hartel, D., Schoenbaum, E.E., Robertson, V.J., Klein, R.S., et al. (1988, June). Elective termination of pregnancy among HIV seropositive and seronegative intravenous drug users. Poster presented at the IV International Conference on AIDS, Stockholm, Sweden.

Steigbigel, N.H., Maude, D.W., Feiner, C.J., Harris, C.A., Saltzman, B.R., Klein, R.S., et al.(1988, June). Heterosexual transmission of HIV infection. Poster presented at the IV International Conference on AIDS, Stockholm, Sweden.

Thiry, L., Sprecher-Goldberger, S., Jonckheer, T., et al. (1985). Isolation of AIDS virus from cell-free breast milk of three healthy virus carriers. [Letter] *Lancet,* ii:891-2

Tucker, M.B. (1979). A descriptive and comparative analysis of the social support structure of heroin-addicted women. *Addicted Women: Family Dynamics, Self Perceptions and Support Systems,* Services Research Monograph Series, National Institute on Drug Abuse, DHEW Publication No. [ADM]80-762.

Verdegem, T.D., Sattler, F.R., Boylen, C.T. (1988, June). Increased fatality from pneumocystis carinii pneumonia in women with AIDS. Poster presented at the IV International Conference on AIDS, Stockholm, Sweden.

Vogt, M.W., Witt, D.J., Craven, D.E., Byington, R., Crawford, D.F., Hutchinson, M.S., Schooley, R.T., & Hirsch, M.S. (1987). Isolation patterns of the human immunodeficiency virus from cervical secretions during the menstrual cycle of women at risk for the acquired immunodeficiency syndrome. *Annals of Internal Medicine,* 106, 380-382.

Williams, A.B. (1981). Concerns of methadone addicted women about sexuality, contraception, pregnancy and motherhood. Unpublished master's thesis, Yale School of Nursing, New Haven, CT.

Williams, A.B. (1988). Knowledge and attitudes about AIDS among women at risk: An educational needs assessment. Unpublished doctoral dissertation, Teacher's College, Columbia University, New York.

Ziegler, J.B., Stewart, G.J., Penny, R., Stuckey, M., & Good, S. (1988, June). Breast feeding and transmission of HIV from mother to infant. Poster presented at the IV International Conference on AIDS, Stockholm, Sweden.

Part III

Comfort With Physical Needs

Chapter 9

Understanding the Disease

Christopher L. LaCharite
Jeffrey Huyett

A number of opportunistic infections and malignancies are associated with HIV infection. This chapter provides an overview of some of the most common of these, including current treatment trends. Many new drugs are being investigated in a variety of centers, and much data are yet unpublished. For more specific details regarding diagnosis and treatment of HIV-related diseases, one should consult the appropriate medical journals. Additionally, a directory of experimental treatment for AIDS/HIV is published quarterly by the American Foundation for AIDS Research.

Human Immunodeficiency Virus (HIV)

HIV belongs to a classification of virus known as retrovirus. HIV infects T-helper cells (T4 lymphocytes), macrophages, B-cells, and certain cells in the brain and CNS. T-helper cells are the most extensively infected cells and their subsequent depletion is responsible for the wide variety of opportunistic infections.
The following lists the steps in which HIV infects the T-helper cells.
  1. Virus attaches to the T-helper cell via its receptor molecule, CD4.
  2. Virus is internalized and uncoated.
  3. An enzyme known as reverse transcriptase is released, which transcribes the viral RNA into DNA.
  4. The proviral DNA is encoded into host DNA.
  5. Cell activation takes place (mechanism uncertain).

6. DNA transcribes genomic RNA and messenger RNA.
7. Protein synthesis and RNA assembly at cell surface.
8. Budding of HIV "virion" (Fauci, 1988).

Clinical Spectrum of HIV Infection

Transition to Illness

The actual number of individuals who transition to illness and the rate of transition to illness are still unknown. The best data to date are from studies that used the stored sera of gay men in San Francisco from hepatitis research from 1978 to 1980. Of those infected between 1978 and 1980, approximately one-third developed CDC-defined AIDS by 1987, and 25 percent were asymptomatic. The remaining 40 percent had symptoms such as lymphadenopathy, oral thrush, zoster, or other constitutional symptoms (Nessal et al., 1987).

HIV can lie dormant in the body for long periods of time. The mechanism for activation of the immune system and subsequent viral replication are unknown. Therefore, the development of illness after infection can take many years. Factors thought to play some role in transition to illness include genetic factors, other infectious processes, pregnancy, stress, improper nutrition, recreational drugs, and alcohol (Black & Levy, 1988). Scientists now believe that most people with HIV infection will develop illness over a period of time if no effective agent is developed for the treatment of HIV infection (Moss et al., 1988).

HIV disease should be conceptualized as a continuum of infection from asymptomatic to seriously ill with life-threatening opportunistic infections and malignancies.

HIV Positive/ARC/AIDS

Acute infection results from exposure to HIV through well-known risk activities. The acute infectious process can either be symptomatic or asymptomatic. If symptomatic, the individual will generally experience a fever, malaise, aseptic meningitis, and rashes (Cooper et al., 1985). Antibody development generally takes about four to twelve weeks, with the vast majority of individuals developing antibody by six months (Mayer, 1988). Rarely, antibody formation may take up to a year or longer. During this period of time between infection and antibody production, HIV antibody tests will be nonreactive.

Attempts at defining stages along the HIV infection continuum have led to significant amounts of confusion on the part of health care providers and the general public. The CDC has attempted to end this confusion by developing a classification system for HIV infection (see Table 9.1). However, this classification does not represent a continuum (i.e., subgroup E is not the worst-case scenario).

Understanding the Disease

Table 9.1 *Classification System for HIV Infection (CDC)*

Group I	Acute infection
Group II	Asymptomatic infection
Group III	Persistent generalized lymphadenopathy
Group IV	Other diseases
Subgroup A	Constitutional diseases
Subgroup B	Neurological diseases
Subgroup C	Secondary infectious diseases
Category C-1	Specified secondary infectious diseases listed in the CDC surveillance definition for AIDS
Category C-2	Other specified secondary infectious diseases
Subgroup D	Secondary cancers
Subgroup E	Other conditions

The diagnosis of AIDS was developed by the CDC as a case definition for epidemiological surveillance (see Appendix B at the end of this book). Although useful as an epidemiological tool, the usefulness clinically is minimal. The diagnosis of AIDS indicates underlying cellular immunity due to HIV infection in a state serious enough to cause certain infections and malignancies. However, AIDS tells you very little about an individual's condition, life span, or quality of life. It represents a myriad of diseases and must be further defined by a specific opportunistic infection or malignancy. ARC has a variety of definitions and interpretations. Generally, ARC is a "stage" in HIV infection where a number of signs and symptoms or diseases may occur. It is indicative of immune suppression but not to the same degree as CDC-defined AIDS. The signs and symptoms associated with ARC include fever, night sweats, oral thrush, weight loss, persistent diarrhea, and persistent generalized lymphadenopathy. Those with asymptomatic HIV infection are frequently referred to as HIV positive. Although most people refer to asymptomatic patients as "HIV positive," we must remember that these individuals have viral infection. Using terms like *positive* and *carriers* may at times minimize the needs of these individuals.

HIV Testing

HIV testing remains one of the most controversial issues in the HIV epidemic. Clearly, there are advantages and disadvantages to testing.

The only commercially available tests for HIV are the antibody tests. The antibody test does not diagnose AIDS nor can it be used as a prognostic indicator regarding transition to illness. The antibody test indicates presence of HIV antibodies. Although antigen testing does exist, it is currently not available for commercial use.

Antibody testing is generally performed in two steps. The first test, the Enzyme-Linked Immunoabsorbent Assay, or ELISA, is a screening test that was developed to screen the nation's blood supply. There is a high rate of false positivity with this test and it should be run with a more specific test, the Western Blot. While the ELISA is quick and easy to perform, the Western Blot is complex and time-consuming. Generally, if the ELISA is positive, a confirmatory Western Blot will be performed. Table 9.2 gives interpretations of the test.

The importance of counseling and education along with HIV testing cannot be emphasized enough. A mental health assessment should be performed and information regarding risk reduction should be provided. Providing an opportunity for questions and answers is very important. Clearly, there are reasons that the test is important for an individual. Decisions regarding health behaviors may be easier to make if an individual knows his antibody status. Although not in great supply, centers for treating all phases of HIV infection are developing. The literature is replete with cases of HIV discrimination, and the importance of confidentiality is a major issue; anonymous testing is preferable. When a patient is being counseled regarding HIV testing, one of the most important questions to ask is, "What are you going to do with the results?" Other questions include: "If you test positive, how do you think you will handle the information?" When the need to test comes from a provider for clinical decision making, the same sort of counseling and education should be provided. Many times, it may be up to the nurse to assess the client and provide information, especially if the client is in the hospital.

Table 9.2

A positive antibody test can mean:

1. HIV antibodies are present and the person is infected with HIV;
2. a false positive.

A negative antibody test can mean:

1. the individual has no antibody and is, therefore, not infected;
2. the individual has no antibody but has been tested in the "window phase" of infection and has HIV infection but has not developed antibodies;
3. the individual has advanced HIV infection and is no longer capable of producing antibodies;
4. the virus is dormant and no antibodies are being produced despite the fact that the individual may still be infectious (very rare).

Asymptomatic HIV Infection

Currently, there are very few treatment options for individuals with asymptomatic HIV infection. Clinical trials of zidovudine (Retrovir, formerly AZT) for asymptomatic individuals are being conducted across the country. Persons with asymptomatic HIV infection are the most underserved in terms of most traditional medical and mental health services.

Below is advice that may be useful for those with asymptomatic infection.

1. Find a health provider who is sensitive to your needs and experienced in dealing with HIV infection. If you obtain drugs through a buyers club (a pool of individuals who purchase nonapproved drugs for personal use from foreign markets), find a physician who will agree to follow you while on medication. Follow up with regular medical checkups.

2. Maintain a healthy lifestyle. Eat well-balanced meals, get enough sleep and rest, exercise regularly, avoid drugs and alcohol, and quit smoking.

3. Manage stress. Support groups, meditation, relaxation response, etc., are very important in staying well. (See Chapter 15.)

4. Feel good about yourself. Try and manage a positive outlook about yourself and others. Take control of your life. (See Chapter 15.)

5. Stay informed. New treatment options are being developed. There are many newsletters and advocacy organizations that can help you stay in touch.

HIV and Its Effects on the Body

HIV affects every organ system of the body. HIV has been known to cause cardiomyopathy, arthritis, and a number of other rarely discussed or previously mentioned diseases. We will concentrate on the following four broad categories:
  1. effects on the immune system;
  2. effects on the central nervous system;
  3. effects on certain blood cells;
  4. malignancies associated with HIV infection.

Effects on the Immune System

One of the most dramatic abnormalities of the HIV-infected person is the depletion of T4 lymphocytes. It is unknown whether the reduction of these cells is due to the cytopathic effects of HIV on the T4 lymphocytes or if HIV may also have an effect on precursors to T4 lymphocytes. Along with a quantitative reduction in T4 cells, there also seems to be a functional impairment of T4 lymphocytes in persons with HIV infection. This is what is thought to cause predisposition to the number of infectious processes (Fauci, 1988).

Glatt, Chirgwin, and Landesman (1988) describe six basic principles in the diagnosis and treatment of HIV-associated diseases.

1. Infections that are viral, fungal, or parasitic are rarely curable and generally require long-term suppressive therapy.

2. Opportunistic infections resulting from HIV infection are primarily due to reactivation of prior infection resulting from depletion of the immune system and are not contagious to other individuals. The only communicable diseases associated with HIV infection are tuberculosis, herpes zoster, and possibly salmonellosis.

3. Look for multiple concurrent or consecutive infections. Treatment failures may result from other unidentified infectious processes.

4. The frequency of asymptomatic infection with certain fungi or parasites in geographic areas will result in a higher rate of symptomatic infections in HIV-infected individuals. Examples include histoplasmosis (Ohio River basin), strongyloidosis (Puerto Rico), and coccidiomycosis (American Southwest). The travel history of patients may be useful in diagnosing certain infectious processes.

5. HIV-related diseases now include certain bacterial infections. This may be due to abnormalities in B-cell function related to HIV infection.

6. Infections in HIV-infected individuals are serious and can be widespread.

The most common opportunistic infections seen with HIV infection, their diagnosis, treatment, and nursing considerations are given in Appendix 9 at the end of this chapter.

HIV Effects on the Central Nervous System

Neurological complications in persons with HIV disease are caused by opportunistic infections, cerebrovascular events, and direct invasion of HIV on nervous tissues (Elder & Sever, 1988). Neurological symptoms have been reported in about 40 percent of persons with AIDS and are the presenting symptoms in 10 percent. Pathology studies reveal that nearly 75 percent of individuals have some degree of brain pathology. (See Table 9.3.)

Patients with neurological manifestations of HIV disease may present with headache, seizure, altered consciousness, dizziness, behavioral changes, or gait disturbance (see Table 9.4). A work-up for neurological involvement includes history and physical, cerebrospinal fluid studies, and radiological studies including CAT scan and MRI.

Direct Effects of HIV on the CNS

Although the pathogenesis and etiology are uncertain, it appears that HIV has a direct effect on the CNS. HIV encephalitis, aseptic meningitis, vacuolar myelopathy, and peripheral nervous system aberrations are most frequently described.

AIDS Dementia Complex

AIDS Dementia Complex, also referred to as HIV encephalopathy, is the most common neurologic disorder in persons with AIDS (Price et al., 1988). It is charac-

Table 9.3 *Diseases Affecting the Central Nervous System in AIDS*

Primary viral (HIV)
    HIV encephalopathy
    Atypical aseptic meningitis
    Vacuolar myelopathy

Secondary viral (encephalitis, myelitis, retinitis, vasculitis)
    Cytomegalovirus
    Herpes simplex virus types I and II
    Papovavirus (PML)

Nonviral infections (encephalitis, meningitis, abscess)
    Toxoplasma gondii
    Cryptococcus neoformans
    Candida albicans
    Histoplasma capsulatum
    Aspergillus fumigatus
    Coccidioide immitis
    Acremonium alavamensis
    Rhizopus species
    Mycobacterium avium-intercellulare
    Mycobacterium tuberculosis hominis
    Mycobacterium kansasii
    Listeria monocytogenes
    Nocardia asteroides

Neoplasma
    Primary CNS lymphoma
    Metastatic systemic lymphoma
    Metastatic Kaposi's sarcoma

Cerebrovascular
    Infarction
    Hemorrhage
    Vasculitis

Complications of systemic therapy of AIDS

terized early in the disease by its effects on cognition, behavior, and motor function (Gabuzda & Hirsch, 1987). Many individuals complain of memory loss and appear withdrawn and apathetic. Depression may easily be mistaken for HIV dementia due to incidence of apathy, blunted affect, and social withdrawal (Flaskerund, 1987). The dementia may progress to severe intellectual dysfunction, generalized profound weakness, hypokinesia, incontinence, mutism, and death. Some patients may experience hallucinations, paranoia, and hostility.

Table 9.4 *Symptoms of Central Nervous System Illness in AIDS*

Headache	Pain
Altered consciousness or cognition	Seizures
	Aphasia
Weakness	Dizziness
Sensory loss	Visual disturbance
Parasthesias	Disorder gait

Computerized axial tomography generally reveals cortical atrophy and enlarged ventricles. There is no current treatment for HIV encephalitis. Investigational protocols are underway to determine the effects of zidovudine on AIDS dementia.

Aseptic Meningitis

Aseptic meningitis presents with headache, fever, and meningeal signs. This illness is generally self-limiting and recurrent rather than progressive (Elder & Sever, 1988).

Vacuolar Myelopathy

Vacuolar myelopathy is an HIV-related spinal cord degeneration. It results from a loss of myelin and spongy degeneration of the cord substance and frequently coexists with AIDS dementia complex. Vacuolar myelopathy resembles the degeneration present in vitamin B12 deficiency but no metabolic effects have been demonstrated. The most common symptoms are leg weakness and incontinence. Paraparesis, spasticity, and ataxia can also be found (Gabuzda & Hirsch, 1987).

Peripheral Nervous System Effects

Peripheral nervous system effects of HIV are well-documented. The most common form of neuropathy is chronic sensory polyneuropathy. It is characterized by painful dysesthesias, numbness, weakness, and autonomic dysfunction. Chronic inflammatory demyelinating polyneuropathy accounts for the second-most common type of peripheral nervous system disorder. Signs and symptoms include weakness, mild sensory deficits, areflexia, and electrophysiologic evidence of a predominantly demyelinating neuropathy (Gabuzda & Hirsch, 1987). Diagnostic work-up for PNS problems may include CT with contrast, lumbar puncture electromyography, nerve conduction studies, muscle biopsy, and nerve biopsy. The use of plasmapheresis and steroids has been effective (Elder & Sever, 1988).

HIV Effects on Lymphocytes and Platelets

It is suggested that neutropenia and thrombocytopenia in HIV disease is due to an autoimmune destruction of neutrophils and platelets (Murphy et al., 1987). Many drug therapies for opportunistic infection can worsen neutropenia. Although no treatment for neutropenia exists, patients with severe thrombocytopenia have been treated successfully with prednisone, intravenous gammaglobulin, and spleenectomy (Pollak, Janinis, & Green, 1988; Walsh et al., 1985). Vincristine has been successful in the treatment of thrombocytopenia, especially when the patient has coexisting Kaposi's sarcoma (Mintzer et al., 1985).

HIV-Associated Malignancy

Approximately 40 percent of persons with AIDS have malignant diseases. About 90 percent of these diseases are Kaposi's sarcoma and 10 percent are lymphoma (Steiss & Longo, 1988).

Kaposi's Sarcoma

Kaposi's sarcoma has a variable natural course in a person with AIDS. Generally diagnosed by the presence of purple-brownish spots on the skin, patients with KS may remain otherwise asymptomatic. Others may experience rapidly progressing disease that invades the lungs, heart, eyes, GI tract, and other parts of the body, requiring aggressive treatment. Although the causes of death in persons with KS are most often due to other opportunistic infection, the malignancy can cause significant emotional and physical discomfort. The most common and successful treatment is with chemotherapy (Steiss & Longo, 1988).

Interferon. Interferon alpha has been used extensively in investigational protocols in the treatment of KS. Reports have indicated that there is a 30-40 percent response rate. This drug is known for its antiproliferative, immunomodulatory, and antiviral activities (other than HIV). The weekly dosage is generally 30-50 million units administered subcutaneously or intramuscularly. Common side effects include high fever, rigors, nausea, vomiting, myalgia, headache, fatigue, and weight loss (Kaplan et al., 1987). Individuals with a competent immune system at the onset of therapy generally have the best treatment response (Steiss & Longo, 1988).

Chemotherapy. The decision to treat KS with chemotherapy is best approached through a risk/benefit analysis. The use of chemotherapy is associated with high rates of side effects and potential further immunosuppression. For patients whose disease is limited to the skin, the therapy may be worse than the disease. For those with internal and/or life-threatening KS, single or combination agents may be suggested. One should keep in mind, however, that treating the KS will not affect the course of their immunodeficiency and clients are still vulnerable to opportunistic infections.

Vincristine and vinblastine are used frequently because of their low incidence of toxicity, and they are most helpful in the early treatment of the disease. Vinblastine sulfate is administered weekly at a dose of .05 mg to .1 mg/kg per week. Vincristine sulfate is administered intravenously at a dose of 2 mg weekly or every two weeks and may be used for patients who are neutropenic. Some may alternate vincristine and vinblastine (Kaplan et al., 1987).

Drug combination, such as alternating treatments of actinomycin D, vincristine, and DTIC with adriamycin, bleomycin, and vinblastine, has been successful in small studies in patients with life-threatening KS (Steiss & Longo, 1988). Other drugs such as etoposide, and doxyrubicin with or without vincristine or vinblastine, are sometimes used (Kaplan et al., 1987).

Radiation. The role of radiation is generally palliative, especially in those with large, bulky, disfiguring lesions, or those causing obstruction of lymph ducts. Lesions generally respond very well to radiation; however, they may reappear. Some patients have achieved response by undergoing combination chemotherapy and radiation therapy.

Non-Hodgkin's Lymphoma (NHL)

Non-Hodgkin's lymphoma is frequently present in the person with AIDS. The most frequently occurring sites are extranodal, involving the central nervous system, bone marrow, and skin (Ziegler, 1984). Historically, NHL has been very responsive to chemotherapy in the nonimmunocompromised individual; however, in the person with AIDS there is no effective treatment. Some patients have responded to traditional treatment initially; however, there is a high relapse and mortality rate associated with treatment (Kaplan et al., 1987).

Zidovudine (AZT)

Zidovudine (trade name: Retrovir) is currently the only noninvestigational antiviral treatment for HIV infection. In the original studies, zidovudine increased life span, decreased the frequency of opportunistic infections, improved functional status, and promoted weight gain for a short period of time (Fischl et al., 1987). Long-term effects are unknown but it is clear that there is a limited amount of time that the drug seems to be effective.

The Side Effects of Zidovudine

One of the major side effects of zidovudine is neutropenia, which may further compromise the individual's immune system. Anemia accounts for another major side effect of zidovudine therapy. In the original studies, approximately one-third of patients on zidovudine developed anemia requiring blood transfusion. The cause of the anemia is probably bone marrow depression. An increase in the red-cell mean corpuscular volume, an indication of macrocytosis, has been observed in most patients receiving Retrovir. Other side effects of zidovudine include headache, myalgias, nausea, and insomnia (Richman, et al., 1987).

Dosage. The usual dosage of zidovudine is 200 mg every four hours around the clock. However, variations in the dose and frequency are common. Patients on zidovudine must realize the importance of taking it in the method prescribed and must be willing to interrupt their sleep to maintain an effective level.

The appearance of neutropenia and/or anemia may require decreasing the dose or discontinuing the medication temporarily or permanently. Individuals with poor immune status at the onset of treatment are more likely to experience side effects requiring termination of treatment.

Summary

HIV is a retrovirus that causes immune suppression, central nervous system dysfunction, thrombocytopenia and neutropenia, and certain malignancies. The treatment of HIV-related disorders is frequently ineffective and associated with a high rate of side effects. It is important for the nurse to be knowledgeable about HIV disease to function in a collaborative role. Chapter 10 provides information about doing a nursing assessment, which provides a more nursing-oriented structure to assess the client with HIV infection.

References

Black, P., & Levy, E. (1988). The HIV seropositive state and progression to AIDS: An overview of factors promoting progression. *New England Journal of Public Policy, 4*(1), 97-107.

Conant, M.A. (1988). Prophylactic and suppressive treatment with acyclovir and the management of herpes in patients with acquired immunodeficiency syndrome. *Journal of the American Academy of Dermatology, 18*(1, pt 2), 186-188.

Cooper, D.A., Gold, J., MacLean, P., Donovon, B., Barnes, T.G., Michelmore, H.M., Brooke, P., & Penny, R. (1985). Acute AIDS retrovirus infection: Definition of a clinical illness associated with seroconversion. *Lancet, 1,* 537-540.

Dismukes, W.D. (1988, April). Cryptococcal meningitis in patients with AIDS. *The Journal of Infectious Disease, 157*(4), 624-628.

Elder, G.A., & Sever, J.L. (1988, March-April). Neurologic disorders associated with AIDS retroviral infection. *Reviews of Infectious Diseases, 10*(2), 286-302.

Fauci, A.S. (1988, February 5). The human immunodeficiency virus: Infectivity and mechanisms of pathogenesis. *Science, 239*(4840), 617-622.

Fischl, M.A., Richman, D.D., Grieco, M.H., Gottlieb, M.S., Volberding, P.A., Laskin, O.L., Leedom, J.M., Groopman, J.E., Mildvan, D., Schooley, R.T., Jackson, G.G., Durack, D.T., & King, D. (1987, July 23). The efficacy of azidothymidine (AZT) in the treatment of patients with AIDS and AIDS-related complex. *New England Journal of Medicine, 317*(4), 185-191.

Flaskerund, J.H. (1987, December). AIDS: Neuropsychiatric complications. *Journal of Psychosocial Nursing, 25*(12), 17-20.

Gabuzda, D.H., & Hirsch, M.S. (1987, September). Neurologic manifestations of infection with human immunodeficiency virus: Clinical features and pathogenesis. *Annals of Internal Medicine, 107,* 383-391.

Glatt, A.E., Chirgwin, K., & Landesman, S.H. (1988). Treatment of infections associated with human immunodeficiency virus: Current concepts. *New England Journal of Medicine, 318*(22), 1439-1448.

Hopewell, P.C. (1988, June). Pneumocystis carinii pneumonia: Diagnosis. *The Journal of Infectious Diseases, 157*(6), 1115-1119.

Jacobson, M.A., & Mills, J. (1988). Serious cytomegalovirus disease in the acquired immunodeficiency syndrome (AIDS). *Annals of Internal Medicine, 108*(4), 585-594.

Kaplan, L.D., Wofsy, C.B., & Volberding, P.A. (1987, March 13). Treatment of patients with acquired immunodeficiency syndrome and associated manifestations. *Journal of the American Medical Association, 257*(10), 1367-1374.

Kovacs, J.A., & Masur, H. (1987, July). Pneumocystis carinii pneumonia: Therapy and prophylaxis. *The Journal of Infectious Diseases, 158*(1), 254-259.

Luft, B.J., & Remington, J.S. (1988, January). Toxoplasmic encephalitis. *The Journal of Infectious Diseases, 157*(1), 1-5.

Mayer, K. (1988, Winter/Spring). The clinical spectrum of HIV infections: Implications for public policy. *New England Journal of Public Policy, 4*(1), 37-55.

Mintzer, D.M., Real, F., Jovino, L., & Krown, S.E. (1985, February). Treatment of Kaposi's sarcoma and thrombocytopenia with vincristine in patients with the acquired immunodeficiency syndrome. *Annals of Internal Medicine, 102*(2), 200-202.

Montgomery, A.B., Debs, R.J., Luce, J.M., Corkery, K.J., Turner, J., Brunette, E.N., Lin, E.T., & Hopewell, P.C. (1987, August 29). Aerosolized pentamadine as sole therapy for pneumocystis carinii pneumonia in patients with acquired immunodeficiency syndrome. *Lancet,* 480-482.

Moss, A.R., Bacchetti, P., Osmond, D., Krampf, W., Chaisson, R.E., Stites, D., Wilber, J., Allain, J.P., & Carlson, J. (1988, March 12). Seropositivity for HIV and the development of AIDS or AIDS related condition: Three year follow up of the San Francisco General Hospital cohort. *British Medical Journal (Clinical Research), 296*(6624), 745-750.

Murphy, M.F., Metcalfe, P., Waters, A.H., Carne, C.A., Weller, I.V., Linch, D.C., Smith, A. (1987, July). Incidence and mechanism of neutropenia and thrombocytopenia in patients with human immunodeficiency virus infection. *British Journal of Haematology, 66*(3), 337-340.

Nessal, H., Rutherford, G., O'Malley, P.M., Doll, L.S., Darrow, W.W., & Jaffe, H.W. (1987, June 1-5). The natural history of HIV in a cohort of homosexual and bisexual men: A 7-year prospective study. Abstract of the Third International Conference on AIDS, Washington, DC.

Pollak, A.N., Janinis, J., & Green, D. (1988, March). Successful intravenous immune globulin therapy for human immunodeficiency virus-associated thrombocytopenia. *Archives of Internal Medicine, 148*(3), 695-697.

Price, R., Brew, B., Sidtis, J., Rosenblum, M., Scheck, A.C., & Cleary, P. (1988, February 5). The brain in AIDS: Central nervous system HIV-1 infection and AIDS dementia complex. *Science, 239,* 586-591.

Richman, D.D., Fischl, M.A., Grieco, M.H., Gottlieb, M.S., Volberding, P.A., Laskin, O.L., Leedom, J.M., Groopman, J.E., Mildvan, D., Hirsch, M.S., Jackson, G.G., Durack, D.T., & Nusinoff-Lehrman, S. (1987, July 23). The toxicity of azidothymidine (AZT) in the treatment of patients with AIDS and AIDS-related complex. *The New England Journal of Medicine, 317*(4), 192-197.

Steiss, R.G., & Longo, D.L. (1988, April). Clinical, biologic, and therapeutic aspects of malignancies associated with the acquired immunodeficiency syndrome: Parts 1 and 2. *Annals of Allergy, 60*(4), 310-323.

Walsh, C., Krigel, R., Lennette, E., & Karpatkin, S. (1985, October). Thrombocytopenia in homosexual patients. *Annals of Internal Medicine, 103*(4), 542-545.

Young, L.S. (1988, May). Mycobacterium avium complex infection. *Journal of Infectious Diseases, 157*(5), 863-867.

Ziegler, J.L., Beckstead, J.A., Volberding, F.A., Abrams, D.I., Levine, A.M., Lukes, R.J., Gill, P.S., Burkes, R.D., Meyer, P.R., & Metroka, C.E. (1984, August 30). Non-Hodgkin's lymphoma in 90 homosexual men: Relation to generalized lymphadenopathy and the acquired immunodeficiency syndrome. *New England Journal of Medicine, 311*(9), 565, 570.

Appendix 9.1

Opportunistic Infections Associated With HIV Infection

CNS Toxoplasmosis

Presentation	Focal neurological findings Seizures Fever	
Site	Brain	
Diagnosis	Presumptive:	CAT scan/MRI showing ring-enhanced lesions
	Definitive:	Brain biopsy
Treatment	Pyrimethamine/sulfadiazine/leucovorin	
Dose and Route:	Pyrimethamine:	20-50 mg po every day
	Sulfadiazine:	1 gm po qid
	Leucovorin:	5-10 mg po qid
Side Effects	(Generally to sulfadiazine) rash, fever, neutropenia	

Special Considerations:

Treatment is generally initiated on the basis of a presumptive diagnosis.

If allergic reaction to sulfa occurs, Clindamycin 900 mg po qid may be substituted for sulfadiazine.

SOURCE: Kaplan, Wofsy, & Volberding, 1987; Luft & Remington, 1988.

Candida (Thrush)

Presentation and Site
    Oral—white spots in mouth
    Esophagus—dysphagia, substernal burning and pain

Diagnosis Visual inspection
    Esophagoscopy
    Culture

Treatment
Mycostatin
    Route: Oral
    Dose: 5 cc swish and swallow qid
    Side Effects: None

Chlortrimazole troches
    Route: PO
    Dose: 1 qid
    Side Effect: Impaired liver function

Ketaconazole
    Route: PO
    Dose: 200-400 mg qd
    Side Effects: hepatotoxicity, nausea and vomiting, stomach pain, itching, fever, and neutropenia

Special Considerations:

Many individuals will remain on mycostatin or chlortrimazole troches for prophylaxis. Ketaconazole may be given in combination with either mycostatin or chlortrimazole and is usually reserved for refractory thrush.

Cryptococcal Meningitis

Presentation   Fever, headache are most common
               Nausea
               Vomiting
               Malaise

Site   CNS

Diagnosis   LP with CSF culture

Treatment
Amphoteracin B with or without flucytosine
        Route: IV
        Dose: .5-.8 mg/kg/day until 1-1.5 grams of amphoteracin have been infused over six weeks. Requires maintenance of 100 mg/week in divided doses indefinitely.
        Side Effects: Fever
                        Chills
                        Neutropenia
                        Renal dysfunction

    Premedication with Benadryl and Tylenol and the addition of 25-50 mg of hydrocortisone may minimize side effects.

Fluconazole (investigational)
        Route: PO
        Dose: 50-200 mg qd can be used initially and for maintenance
        Side Effects: Well-tolerated in initial studies

Source: Dismukes, 1988; Kaplan et al., 1987.

Cryptospordium

Presentation	Severe watery diarrhea often resulting in weight loss and dehydration
Diagnosis	Culture
Treatment	No effective treatment has been developed. Traditional opiate-derived antidiarrheal medications should be given and hydration be maintained.

Cytomegalovirus Infection

Presentation   Retinitis—decreased visual acuity and blurred vision
  Colon—abdominal pain and diarrhea
  Lungs—dyspnea, cough
  Esophagus—dysphagia, burning, pain

Site   Retina
  Colon
  Lungs
  Esophagus

Diagnosis   Visual examination
  Culture
  Antigen testing

Treatment
Gancyclovir (DHPG) (investigational)
  Route: IV
  Dose: Loading—5 mg/kg IV bid for two weeks
    Maintenance—5-7.5 mg/kg 5-7 days a week
  Side Effect: Neutropenia—most frequent

Special Considerations:

Gancyclovir treatment for CMV pneumonitis has been disappointing. Oral maintenance may be an option in the future.

SOURCE: Jacobson & Mills, 1988.

Herpes Simplex Virus

Presentation   Single or multiple vesicles with clear fluid, may be painful

Site   Genitals, mouth, eyes, can be disseminated

Diagnosis   Visual examination
Culture

Treatment
Acyclovir

    Route: Ointment, PO, IV
    Dose*:   Ointment—Apply liberally six times a day
             PO—200-400 mg five times a day for 10 days
             IV—5 mg/kg TID
    Side Effects: Ointment—burning, stinging, discomfort
             PO—nausea and vomiting, headache (long-term therapy)
             IV—phlebitis, elevated creatinine, rash, and hives

Special Considerations:

During IV acyclovir therapy, adequate hydration must be ensured to prevent renal damage due to collection of acyclovir crystals in the renal tubules.

*May require long-term maintenance therapy.

SOURCE: Conant, 1988; Kaplan et al., 1987.

Mycobacterium Avium Complex (MAC)

Presentation Fever, weight loss, diarrhea, night sweats

Site Disseminated

Diagnosis Culture

Treatment Amikacin, clofazimine, ethambutol, and rifampin in combination

Amikacin
- Route: IV
- Dose: 7.5 mg/kg q 12h
- Side Effects: Neurotoxicity, ototoxicity, and nephrotoxicity

Clofazimine
- Route: PO
- Dose: 50-100 mg po qd
- Side Effects: GI bleeding and colitis

Ethambutol
- Route: PO
- Dose: 600 mg po qd
- Side Effects: Decreased visual acuity

Rifampin
- Route: PO
- Dose: 3 mg/kg qd
- Side Effects: Liver dysfunction; GI disturbances; blood dyscrasias; reddish-brown coloration of sputum, feces, urine, sweat, and tears; and multiple lesser-occurring side effects

Special Considerations:

An increase in survival and a decrease in symptoms have never been shown with above treatment in controlled studies. Generally, an induction phase of about a month is required. If a clinical response is appreciated, maintenance therapy is necessary (Young, 1988).

Pneumocystis Carinii Pneumonia

Presentation Fever
Dry cough
Exertional dyspnea
Hypoxemia
Diffuse pulmonary infiltrates

Site Lungs

Diagnosis Chest X ray
Microbiology
Bronchoscopy
Ultrasonic nebulization for sputum induction
Gallium scan

Treatment
Sulfamethoxazole/trimethoprim (Bactrim)
Route:	IV/PO
Dose:	Trimethoprim 20 mg/kg/day
	Sulfamethoxazole 100 mg/kg/day
Side Effects:	Neutropenia, rash, fever

Pentamadine
Route:	Slow IV (over 1 hour)
Dose:	4 mg/kg/day
Side Effects:	Hypoglycemia, hypotension (especially with rapid infusion), neutropenia, renal and hepatic toxicity
Route:	Inhaled
Dose:	Not established
	Therapeutic = 600 mg/day
	Prophylaxis = 50-120 mg/q 1-2 weeks
Side Effects:	Few reports of systemic side effects

Dapsone/trimethoprim (investigational)
Dose and Route:	Dapsone 100 mg po qd
	Trimethoprim 320 mg po tid
Side Effects:	Rash, fever, methamoglobinemia, hemolysis

SOURCE: Hopewell, 1988; Kovacks & Masur, 1988; Montgomery, et al., 1987.

Chapter 10

Assessing the Client's Needs

David J. Hannabury

The nurse's responsibility is to maximize the client's level of functioning, optimize the quality of the client's life, and, when appropriate, help the client achieve a peaceful and dignified death (Henderson, 1961). HIV infection poses perhaps the greatest challenge to these goals, not only by the extensiveness and pervasiveness of a disease that invades all systems and hinders all functions, but also by the lack of a cure. When medicine has little to offer, nursing becomes the major provider of health care. The first step in giving nursing care is assessment of the client's needs.

Nursing strives to identify the *human response* to illness: how this disease impacts all aspects of the client's life. Medicine seeks to identify the cause of the illness in order to treat and cure. Since nursing and medicine have different goals for providing care, they use the data collected from the assessment differently.

For example, when physicians detect a client's respiratory dysfunction in the course of examination, they attempt to uncover the cause of the respiratory problem and cure it. The nurse, upon detecting the same problem, explores the ways in which respiratory dysfunction affects activity tolerance, self-concept, roles and relationships, sexuality, sleep, and nutrition. The nurse takes a more holistic view of the client. The dysfunction is seen in terms of the effect it has upon the client. The nurse's goal is then to help the client increase the level of function in all the affected areas as well as to adapt to, and possibly improve, the level of respiratory function. In order to achieve this unique nursing focus, a cohesive and comprehensive plan of care must begin with a thorough assessment of the client from a nursing perspective.

Functional health patterns provide us with a framework for structuring our assessments and forming nursing diagnoses (Gordon, 1982). So many of the responses to HIV infection can be hidden; nausea, pain, isolation, spiritual depression, and sexual loss. A systematic, standardized assessment provides a tool for uncovering the most critical needs of these clients, without which the areas of greatest pain might go undetected and untreated. Nursing diagnoses help to articulate these problems and differentiate between problems that are within the province of nursing to treat, and problems that require collaboration between nursing and medicine or other disciplines (Gordon, 1987). Nursing diagnoses enable the nurse to provide better care by standardizing communications among nurses (Herberth & Gosnell, 1987; Burke et al., 1986; Rossi & Haines, 1979; Mundinger, 1978; Gordon, 1982).

A nursing assessment based upon the functional health patterns requires some time to complete. This is especially true when assessing the person with AIDS; indeed, most aspects of care for the person with AIDS are more time-intensive than the care we provide to our other patients (*American Journal of Nursing*, 1987). The time investment of an assessment pays off by crystalizing our priorities and focusing our care so that we can maximize our time and effectiveness with our clients.

Nevertheless, we all must live and work within certain time constraints. If sufficient time isn't available to complete your assessment during a single interview, data collection can be spread out over two or even three contacts with the client. When time is at a premium, it may also be helpful to conduct a "screening assessment" (Gordon, 1982), in which just one or two key questions are asked from each functional pattern area. This method is not a substitute for a thorough nursing assessment; it is simply a stopgap measure that can be used until you have set aside sufficient time and established sufficient rapport with the client to perform a proper assessment. The most important objective is to collect the data, then plan your care based upon what you have learned. Only then can you be sure that you are identifying and meeting your client's needs to the best of your ability.

This assessment tool is based on the functional health patterns of Gordon (1982) with revisions by others (Brigham & Women's Hospital, 1985; Carpenito, 1983; Jones, 1984; Hannabury, 1987; Herberth & Gosnell, 1987). The tool adapts easily to different clinical situations, whether home or inpatient. The more you use it, the more you will adapt it to your own assessment needs. Although the questions on this tool are similar to questions asked any client population, they are critical questions used routinely by nurses experienced in AIDS care. People with HIV infection have the same nursing diagnoses and need the same nursing interventions as people with other health problems. It is not the nursing care that differs with HIV infection. The difference is that client needs may vary more from person to person, since HIV infection manifests itself and impacts in such a variety of ways. This disease often is unpredictable and complex; it changes rapidly. Therefore, you will find a wide range in the combination of problems experienced by these clients. Initial and ongoing assessments enable us to discover each person's problems as they arise.

Keep in mind that a problem identified in one pattern area will often lead you to a problem in another area: Activity intolerance may stem from an ineffective breathing pattern, or pain may contribute to sleep pattern disturbance. Be thorough, and assess your client in all functional areas, but also let your assessment be guided by the data your client provides. Remember that this tool is meant to be used only as a framework for assessment. Never hesitate to omit questions that seem inappropriate or unnecessary or to ask questions beyond those provided here, when cues you receive from the client indicate that further exploration is needed.

Introduce the assessment by explaining why you are asking these questions. You can explain that nurses are concerned about how illness and hospitalization disrupt all aspects of your life. Nurses need to get an idea of what kinds of nursing services are most helpful for the client. Include the family whenever possible, and interview the family when the client is unable to answer questions coherently.

The first six health patterns focus primarily on physical concerns. They give you an opportunity to explore concrete and essentially nonthreatening issues with the client. This part of the assessment allows times for you and the client to become more comfortable with the assessment and each other. The questions pertaining to self-concept, relationships, sexuality, coping, and beliefs contain more sensitive content. Often these questions work best after you have established a *trusting* rapport with the client. Some clinicians use these questions in the process of counseling clients, since they set the stage for intimate and therapeutic interaction.

Functional Health Patterns

1. Health perception/health management pattern

These questions explore how clients perceive the immediate health problem and their health in general. Health promotion/health maintenance behaviors are assessed, including the client's use of therapeutic regimens.

Suggested questions:

How do you feel regarding your condition/illness?

How has your health been over the last year?

Have you had previous hospitalizations? Have they been positive or negative experiences? Have contacts with health care providers been positive or negative?

What actions did you take when you first perceived signs or symptoms? What results did they have? What do you think may have caused signs or symptoms?

What was your general health like before the onset of signs/symptoms?

Are you on medication at home? What medication? What for? What are the side effects?

Do you use any home care services (VNA, etc.)? Any family members, friends helping with care at home?

Where do you receive outpatient care? When was your last visit? Do you generally find it easy to follow the suggestions of doctors, nurses?

Do you have any allergies?

Do you use alcohol? How much? How often? For how long?

Do you use recreational drugs? What kind? How much? How often? For how long? (If IV drug user) Do you share needles? Do you clean works before shooting drugs?

Do you use tobacco? How much? How often? For how long?

Do you have any specific health maintenance practices (breast self-exam, testicular self-exam, etc.)?

Do you use complementary therapies, such as acupuncture, massage, relaxation therapies? Do you plan to continue them in the hospital?

Are you a client of AIDS service organizations?

What can *we* do for you? What do you expect from us?

2. Nutritional/Metabolic Pattern

Nutritional problems are very common in persons with HIV infection, as outlined in detail in Chapter 11. Initial problems may be related to anorexia, nausea, vomiting, or the inability to prepare food due to fatigue. Opportunistic infections and cellular changes in gastric absorption from the HIV further compromise nutrition. Many clients experience serious dehydration secondary to fever, diarrhea, nausea, and vomiting. Nutrition directly impacts skin integrity. Since so many persons with HIV infection experience decreased mobility, poor nutrition further increases their risk of skin breakdown. Thrombocytopenia, rashes secondary to drug reactions, lesions from Kaposi's sarcoma, and dry skin secondary to dehydration are all common problems that warrant assessment.

Suggested questions:

Do you follow a special diet? Any dietary restrictions? Any food allergies? Most favorite/least favorite foods?

Who shops for, prepares food? Do you have enough food?

Do you have any problems chewing? Swallowing? Nausea/vomiting? Last dental exam?

Have there been any recent changes in your appetite or weight? How much over what period of time?

Do you currently have any cuts, lesions, rashes, dry skin? (Confirm with physical exam.) Do cuts, lesions seem to take unusually long time to heal? Do you bruise easily? Do you bleed easily or for unusually long time before clotting?

Do you want your family to bring in food?

Do you usually get meals provided by a community service organization?

3. Elimination Pattern

People with HIV infection routinely experience diarrhea. However, some clients suffer with constipation due to dehydration, decreased activity, and hypomotility of the bowel (see Chapter 11).

Suggested questions:

How frequently do you move your bowels? What is the consistency of your stools? Do you currently or frequently experience diarrhea/constipation? Do you use anything (medication, enemas, diet, etc.) to control it? When was you last bowel movement? Do you ever have blood in stools? Pain upon moving bowels? Incontinence of stools?

How frequently do you urinate (day/night)? Any pain, burning upon urination? Urgency to urinate? Straining to urinate? Are you able to empty bladder of urine? Incontinence of urine? Unusual appearance, unusual or strong odor to urine? Blood in urine?

Have you noted recent changes in the amount or characteristics of your perspiration? Any night sweats?

4. Activity/Exercise Pattern

Mobility becomes compromised by shortness of breath due to both pneumocystis carinii and bacterial pneumonia, cytomegalovirus (CMV) pneumonitis, and pulmonary lesions of Kaposi's sarcoma. Peripheral neuropathy and arthritis also limit movement in HIV-infected people. The fatigue of HIV infection further impairs clients' ability to care for themselves. You may use a functional level code to record ability to perform ADLs, as follows:

0 = independent
1 = requires assistive equipment or device
2 = requires assistance or supervision
3 = requires assistive equipment or device *and* assistance or supervision
4 = fully dependent

Suggested questions:

Do you have sufficient energy for your desired or required activities? Have you noted recent changes in energy level, amount of activity tolerated?

Do you have a regular exercise regimen? Please describe.

What are your leisure, recreational activities?

Nurse's/client's perception of ability for (before and after onset of symptoms):

bathing	feeding	ambulation
skin care	dressing	housekeeping
mouth care	toileting	cooking
hair	mobility in bed	transportation

(Supplement data in this pattern area with physical exam including range of motion, extremity strength, coordination, dexterity, etc.)

When you are doing something and you have to stop and rest, what is it that makes you stop (pain, shortness of breath, fatigue)?

5. Sleep/Rest Pattern

Anxiety and pain may disrupt the sleep/rest pattern of people with HIV infection. However, even if these patterns are intact, clients may still feel fatigued due to the general impact of HIV infection. Many people with HIV infection routinely use relaxation tapes, guided imagery, or other forms of complementary therapy at bedtime for sleep induction (see Chapter 15).

Suggested questions:

How many hours do you sleep each night? Has there been any recent change in sleep patterns? Duration of sleep? Onset of sleep? Interruptions of sleep? Ability to awaken?

Do you take anything or do anything special to help yourself sleep?

Do you dream frequently? Do your dreams disturb your sleep? Do you have frequent nightmares?

Do you have night sweats? Do they require sheet changes?

Do you take naps or rest periods during the day?

6. Cognitive/Perceptual Pattern

Most people with HIV infection experience neurological involvement. Memory loss and disorientation commonly progress to dementia. Visual disturbances occur from retinitis secondary to cytomegaloviral infection. In addition to assessing impairments, explore learning needs for both the client and family.

Suggested questions:

Client's level of consciousness/orientation?

Client's primary language and degree of literacy?

What is your understanding/description of your health problem?

What information do you feel you need before you go home? Which method do you prefer for learning (reading, demonstration, discussion, etc.)?

Have you noticed recent changes in your memory? Has anyone pointed out to you changes in your memory?

Do you have any pain? Location? Description? Severity (on scale of 1-10)? Does anything seem to bring it on? Does anything seem to alleviate it? Are there any other symptoms associated with it (nausea, visual disturbances, etc.)?

Do you have any deficits in/use any aids for:

vision?	taste?
hearing?	touch?
smell?	memory?

Do you ever see or hear things that are not really there?

7. Self-Perception/Self-Concept Pattern

One of the major responses to the diagnoses of AIDS is changes in self-esteem and self-concept. Kaposi's sarcoma, weight loss, and diarrhea seriously threaten body image and self-worth. Chapters 16 and 17 describe the self-concept issues of people with HIV infection.

Suggested questions:

How do you feel about yourself? Have those feelings changed since the onset of your symptoms/illness?

Have there been any changes in your body or the way you think of your body since the onset of your symptoms/illness? Any changes in your capabilities? Have these changes been a problem?

Do you find that you frequently feel angry? Frustrated? Depressed? Anxious? Frightened? More so than before onset of symptoms/illness? What do you find helpful when you have these feelings?

Do you ever feel a loss of control? A loss of hope? What helps when you have these feelings?

What makes you feel good about yourself?

8. Role/Relationship Pattern

The diagnosis of HIV infection almost always impacts roles and relationships. AIDS threatens people with the loss of lovers, parents, children, friends. Families may be nontraditional, fractioned, or hostile. Chapters 5, 13, and 17 explore some of these dynamics in detail.

Suggested questions:

Who is/ whom do you consider your family?
Do you have a lover or are you married?
From whom do you get the most support?
Are you responsible for anyone else's care?
How do family/friends feel about your illness?
Are you concerned about the effect your illness is having on your family?
How do you handle problems when they arise in your family/ with friends? Is it difficult to handle these problems?
Do you belong to any social groups?
Do you frequently feel lonely?
What kind of work do/did you do? Are/were you happy with your job?
Is your income sufficient for your needs? Do you have any financial concerns?
Do you have any concerns about housing? Do you have health insurance?
Do you have one person to whom you look for support more than others? If you

become unable to make decisions for yourself, is there someone whom you wish to make decisions for you regarding your care?

Whom do you wish to be involved in your discharge planning?

9. Sexuality/Reproductive Pattern

Although safer sex is a concern, the biggest sexual issue for HIV-infected people is the disruption of their sexuality by this disease. For some people, loss of sexuality becomes one of the most painful aspects of AIDS, yet it is so easily overlooked by care givers. Chapter 14 provides detailed guidelines on sexual assessment, ways to approach the subject, and content for safer sex teaching.

Suggested questions:

Are you sexually active? With men, women, or both?

Are you currently satisfied with your sexual activity, sexuality? Has your sexual activity, sexuality changed since onset of symptoms/illness? Has this been a problem?

Do you use contraception? Date of last menstrual period? Dysmenorrhea? Date of last GYN exam?

Has your HIV status affected your plans for childbearing?

10. Coping/Stress Tolerance Pattern

People with AIDS display the full gamut of coping mechanisms, from denial to spiritual healing. Chapters 15, 16, and 17 equip you with methods for responding to clients' coping reactions as well as various coping strategies to offer.

Suggested questions:

You have just been diagnosed with HIV infection. How do you cope with this diagnosis?

Are there other recent changes or crises in your life?

Do you find your way of coping effective?

When problems arose in the past, how did you handle them? Is there someone with whom you find it helpful to talk? Is that person available to you now?

Do you find drugs, alcohol, medication helpful in coping with problems?

Are you in a support group? If not, are you interested in one?

11. Value/Belief Pattern

The incurability of AIDS pushes people to examine existential questions about the meaning of their lives, as well as pulls them toward more nontraditional therapies as a source of hope. Chapters 15 and 16 identify some of the pathways of faith that people travel. For some people, this area may be the major source of comfort.

Suggested questions:

Do you have any religious or spiritual practices? Is illness/symptoms/presence in hospital, etc., interfering with your engaging in these practices?

Do you find speaking with clergy helpful? Would you like to speak with clergy while in hospital?

Do you have plans for the future?

Physical Assessment

Table 10.1 offers suggestions for points to be covered in the physical examination of the person with, or at risk for, HIV infection. Nurses with advanced skills in physical assessment may wish to expand upon this list.

Table 10.1 *Physical Examination Guidelines for the Person With or at Risk for HIV Infection*

Blood pressure
Apical pulse
    Rhythm
Peripheral pulses
Breath sounds
Cough
    Productive/nonproductive
Temperature
Weight
Edema
Oral mucosa
    Lesions
    Bleeding
    Dryness
Other lesions
    Location, description
Easy bruising, bleeding
Skin turgor
Memory loss
Word-finding difficulty
Decreased acuity of thought

The literature is alerting us almost weekly to newly discovered ways in which HIV infection may manifest itself: cardiac abnormalities (*Medical Week*, 1988); dysphagia (*Cope*, 1987); psychoneurological symptoms (*Nursing 88*, 1988); the seemingly minor dry cough that may precede an episode of pneumocystis carinii pneumonia. A physical assessment determines whether signs of HIV infection are currently present and establishes baseline data for future comparison. Assess your client thoroughly and frequently so that changes are noted and interventions are started as early as possible.

Compiling the Data

Once you have collected the data, you can identify the problems and create a list of nursing diagnoses. Table 10.2 lists common nursing diagnoses associated with HIV infection. Discuss the nursing diagnoses with the client either at the conclusion of the interview or after you have had time to formalize the list. You might say, "This is how I am seeing your needs, and here are some ideas of what we can do for you." Then get the client's input on your recommendations for care. Clients often appreciate hearing your perspective of their problems, which teaches them about your role as a nurse and helps them to solicit your skills more appropriately.

Table 10.2 *Nursing Diagnosis to Consider for People With HIV Infection*

Impaired nutritional status—less than required

Alteration in climination—diarrhea

Self-concept disturbance

Decreased activity tolerance

Self-care deficit (specify)

Memory deficit

Knowledge deficit

Social isolation

Spiritual distress

Impaired home management

Ineffective coping, individual and family

Sensory deficit

Altered skin integrity

Your assessment provides the foundation for all other care that you give. A systematic, comprehensive assessment enables you to provide an holistic approach to care with confidence. Once you have formulated your diagnosis, care of the person with

HIV infection will be similar to care of any client. The assessment and diagnosis provide a secure base with which to be comfortable giving care.

References

American Journal of Nursing (1987). AIDS patients need more (nursing) time. *87,* 1540-1541.

Brigham & Women's Hospital, Boston (1985). Nursing assessment form.

Burke, L.J., Gabriel, L.M., Fischer, L.E., & Zemke, S.L. (1986). Nursing diagnoses, indicators, and interventions in an out-patient cardiac rehabilitation program. *Heart and Lung, 15 ,* 70-76.

Carpenito, L.J. (1983). *Nursing diagnosis: Application to clinical practice.* Philadelphia: Lippincott.

COPE Oncology Magazine (1987). Pain swallowing a clue to HIV? 2(3), 13.

Gordon, M. (1982). *Nursing diagnoses: Process and application.* New York: McGraw-Hill.

Gordon, M. (1987). *Manual of nursing diagnosis:* New York: McGraw-Hill.

Hannabury, D.J. (1987). [A univariate exploratory-descriptive study of nursing diagnoses in acute and ambulatory male patients with AIDS.] Unpublished master's thesis, Boston College, Boston, MA.

Henderson, V. (1961). *The nature of nursing: A definition and its implications for practice, research, and education.* New York: Macmillan.

Herberth, L., & Gosnell, D.J. (1987). Nursing diagnosis for oncology nursing practice. *Cancer Nursing, 10*(1), 41-51.

Jones, D.A. (1984). *Health assessment across the life span.* New York: McGraw-Hill.

Medical Week (1988, May 16). Cardiac disease may indicate AIDS. *10.*

Mundinger, M.O. (1978). Nursing diagnoses for cancer patients. *Cancer Nursing, 1,* 221-226.

Nursing 88 (1988, March). Know the early signs of HIV dementia complex. *18,* 18.

Rossi, L.P., & Haines, V.M. (1979). Nursing diagnoses related to acute myocardial infarction. *Cardio-Vascular Nursing, 15,* 11-15.

Appendix 10.1

Example: Nursing Care Plan for Person With AIDS

Problem or Need	Intervention	Expected Outcome
1. Anxiety, anger, depression, and/or fear due to • nonspecific diagnosis, prognosis, and/or treatments; • self-image changes and/or disfigurement; • concepts of death and dying.	1. Provide an atmosphere of individual acceptance. 2. Provide opportunities for patient to express feelings. 3. Involve Shanti,* chaplaincy, and/or psychiatric liaison as appropriate for patient, significant others, and family. 4. Encourage honest, consistent communication by all members of caretaking team. 5. Assess need for psychopharmacologic intervention.	1. Expression of feelings. 2. Feelings of adequate support. 3. Integration of significant others, family, and friends into care and support. 4. Awareness and use of community resources.
2. Alterations in mental status due to • disease process; • opportunistic infections; • medications.	1. Clarify baseline mental status. 2. Monitor for changes in neurologic status at least every four hours. 3. Assess possible drug-related causes. 4. Provide safe environment (see Problem 13).	1. Etiology is identified where possible. 2. Further deterioration is minimized.

*The Shanti Project of San Francisco is a volunteer community project that offers emotional support, practical support, and residential support to persons with AIDS.

Problem or Need	Intervention	Expected Outcome
3. Fatigue and malaise due to • disease process; • change in nutritional status; • medications.	1. a) Provide restful and quiet environment. b) Assess need for pharmaceutical intervention. c) Monitor tolerance for visits and telephone calls; suggest limits as appropriate. d) Avoid awakening patient except as necessary. e) Encourage frequent naps. 2. a) Titrate doses of symptom-relieving medications to achieve optimal benefits. b) Assist with activities of daily living. 3. See interventions for Problem 5.	1. Patient feels rested and gets adequate sleep. 2. Side effects of medication are minimized. 3. Admission weight is maintained or increased.
4. Respiratory distress including shortness of breath, dyspnea on exertion, tachypnea, cough, cyanosis due to • infiltrates; • effusions; • cavitations; • pneumothorax; • anemia; • hypoxemia.	1. Assess respiratory status every four hours or more frequently as indicated. 2. Monitor vital signs, chest sounds, color, and nail beds for relevant changes. 3. Assess need for respiratory therapy and evaluate efficacy of therapy administered.	1. Optimal respiratory status is achieved and maintained.

Problem or Need	Intervention	Expected Outcome
5. Anorexia, nausea/vomiting, diarrhea, dehydration due to • disease process; • gastrointestinal infection and/or masses; • medications.	1. Monitor weights, intake and output, and calorie counts as appropriate. 2. Monitor for signs of dehydration. 3. Encourage nutritional supplements as tolerated. 4. Encourage significant others to provide appealing and nutritious foods. 5. Consult dietician as appropriate.	1. Optimal nutrition is received. 2. Optimal electrolyte balance and hydration are achieved and maintained.
6. Inadequate resistance to infection due to • disease process; • neutropenia.	1. Initiate precautions against neutropenia per hospital protocol. 2. Wash hands before entering room. 3. Monitor vital signs, especially temperature, as appropriate. 4. Monitor white blood cell counts and differentials for changes. 5. Monitor skin integrity every shift, including intravenous line sites, rectum, mouth. 6. Instruct patient and significant others regarding infection control.	1. Nosocomial infection is prevented.
7. Fevers due to • disease process; • infection; • drug reaction.	1. Monitor temperature every four hours, or more frequently as needed.	1. Fevers are optimally controlled.

Problem or Need	Intervention	Expected Outcome
7. Fevers (continued)	2. Administer antipyretics as ordered and evaluate efficacy. 3. Evaluate need for cooling measures (i.e., cooling blankets, alcohol rubs, ice packs) and institute as needed. 4. Encourage fluid intake.	1. Fevers are optimally controlled.

8. Bleeding due to
• disease process;
• medication.
	1. Monitor vital signs and note tachycardia, hypotension, pallor, anxiety, restlessness at least every four hours.
	2. Monitor body surfaces for ecchymosis, petechiae, hematomas every shift.
	3. Check urine, stool, vomit for heme.
	4. Use safety precautions if platelet count is low (i.e., under 20,000 per cu mm):
	  a) No tooth brushing; use alternative oral hygiene.
	  b) Use electric razor.
	  c) Use side rail and fall precautions.
	5. Instruct patient and significant others about safety precautions.
		1. Bleeding is minimized.

Problem or Need	Intervention	Expected Outcome
9. Alteration in skin integrity due to • disease process; • immobility; • poor nutritional status; • incontinence.	1. Assess skin surfaces at least once per shift, documenting any breakdown and daily changes in breakdown. 2. Assist patient with position change as necessary. 3. Encourage mobility within functional limits. 4. Assist with or provide bath and massage with soap, lotions, or oils. 5. Use appropriate beds or appliances for pressure relief. 6. Implement pressure-sore care as indicated. 7. See interventions for Problem 5.	1. Skin integrity is maintained.
10. Pain due to • disease process; • other (specify).	1. Assess character and intensity of pain. 2. Administer analgesics as ordered and assess efficacy and side effects. 3. Consider benefits of routine versus as-needed use of analgesics.	1. Patient is maximally pain-free.

Problem or Need	Intervention	Expected Outcome
11. Need for intravenous therapy due to • dehydration; • medication administration; • electrolyte imbalances; • total parenteral nutrition.	1. Examine site every shift for infiltration and inflammation. 2. Change site, bag, tubing, and dressing per hospital policy. 3. Teach patient and significant others signs and symptoms of inflammation and infiltration.	1. Intravenous line is maintained without inflammation, infiltration, or infection.
12. Local and systemic reactions to medications: • nausea/vomiting, diarrhea; • fever; • hypotension or hypertension; • orthostasis; • hypoglycemia or hyperglycemia; • rash; • neutropenia.	1. Monitor appropriate laboratory test values (i.e., complete blood count, serum glucose, liver function tests, renal panel, and so on). 2. Assess need for premedication preparation with antihistamines or antiemetics and evaluate efficacy of those administered. 3. Assess need for antidiarrheals and assess efficacy of those administered. 4. Monitor skin and mucous membranes for location and nature of rash. 5. Assess hydration status and fluid balance to restrict or encourage fluid as needed.	1. Reactions are minimized.

Problem or Need	Intervention	Expected Outcome

13. Injury due to falls.	1. Identify risk factors:
	   a) weakness;
	   b) sedation;
	   c) mental confusion;
	   d) diarrhea.
	2. For weak patients:
	   a) encourage use of call lights;
	   b) assist with ambulation;
	   c) leave belongings within reach.
	3. Evaluate patient for effects of sedation; check drug interactions.
	4. For patients with mental confusion:
	   a) restrain as appropriate;
	   b) reorient frequently and remind to call for assistance.
	5. For patients with diarrhea, provide bedside commode and/or place bedpan within reach.
	6. For patients with orthostasis:
	   a) monitor for side effects of medications;
	   b) encourage use of call light;
	   c) assist with standing and walking.	

Assessing the Client's Needs **127**

Problem or Need	Intervention	Expected Outcome
14. Substance abuse.	1. Evaluate patient for substance use. 2. Provide information about AIDS Substance Abuse Program (ASAP). 3. Refer directly to Alcohol Evaluation and Treatment Center (AETC) if indicated. 4. Consult with AETC when ASAP is not available.	1. Information regarding interrelationship between substance abuse and AIDS is accessible. 2. Patient demonstrates knowledge of treatment options and referrals.

15. Need for education of patient, significant others, family regarding
• disease process;
• infection control;
• transmissibility of virus;
• safer sex practices;
• medication and side effects;
• other (specify).
	1. Teach patient and significant others about
	  a) disease process;
	  b) infection control;
	  c) safer sex practices;
	  d) medication and side effects;
	  e) other (specify).
	2. Assess and document efficacy of teaching in nursing progress notes.
		1. Patient and significant others are knowledgeable, to the extent of their ability, regarding pertinent information.

16. Need for clarification of resuscitation status.	1. Coordinate process of decision making and ensure appropriate documentation. 2. Involve significant others, Shanti, chaplain, and medical and nursing ethicists as appropriate.	1. Patient makes informed consent with regard to resuscitation status.

Problem or Need	Intervention	Expected Outcome
16. Need for clarification of resuscitation status.	3. Assess patient's understanding of currently ordered resuscitation status to ensure informed consent. 4. Support patient decision.	1. Patient makes informed consent with regard to resuscitation status.
17. Need for identification of legal issues: • wills; • power of attorney.	1. Assess knowledge of legal options. 2. Coordinate with Shanti to provide legal aid.	1. Patient is maximally comfortable. 2. Focus is on palliative care.
18. Terminal care.	1. Use appropriate pharmacological interventions for pain control, sedation, feelings of air hunger. 2. Bathe, provide oral hygiene, turn, and reposition for comfort. 3. Attend to psychosocial needs of significant others.	1. Patient is given opportunity to complete legal documents as appropriate.

SOURCE: Reprinted with permission from San Fransisco General Hospital's Special Care Unit for Persons with AIDS.

Chapter 11

Nutrition: Controlling the "Slims"

Tara Coghlin
Margaret Benak

For the person with HIV infection, nutrition plays a vital role in the fight for wellness. Eating well improves the immune system, maintains a normal lifestyle, promotes socialization, provides enjoyment, reinforces a "healthy" self-image, and gives clients control over an aspect of treatment. The wasting and inability to eat common with AIDS can result in depression, anxiety, withdrawal, and body-image disturbance. Malnutrition directly undermines the immune system. As a group of rapidly reproducing cells, the immune system needs sufficient daily intake of protein, fat, carbohydrates, vitamins, and minerals or it becomes depleted and *further* compromised. One of the best defenses against a weakened immune system, threatening infection, and compromising medications is a well-balanced diet.

How AIDS Undermines Nutrition

Weight Loss

People with HIV infection commonly lose an alarming 20 percent or more of their usual weight, probably due to increased energy requirements, basal metabolism, and/or stress. Weight loss increases infections, end-organ damage, and intolerance to therapy. Any weight loss of greater than 10 percent of clients' *usual* weight places them at nutritional risk. Such a weight loss could set off a vicious cycle of immune deficiency, repeated infections, and progressive deterioration.

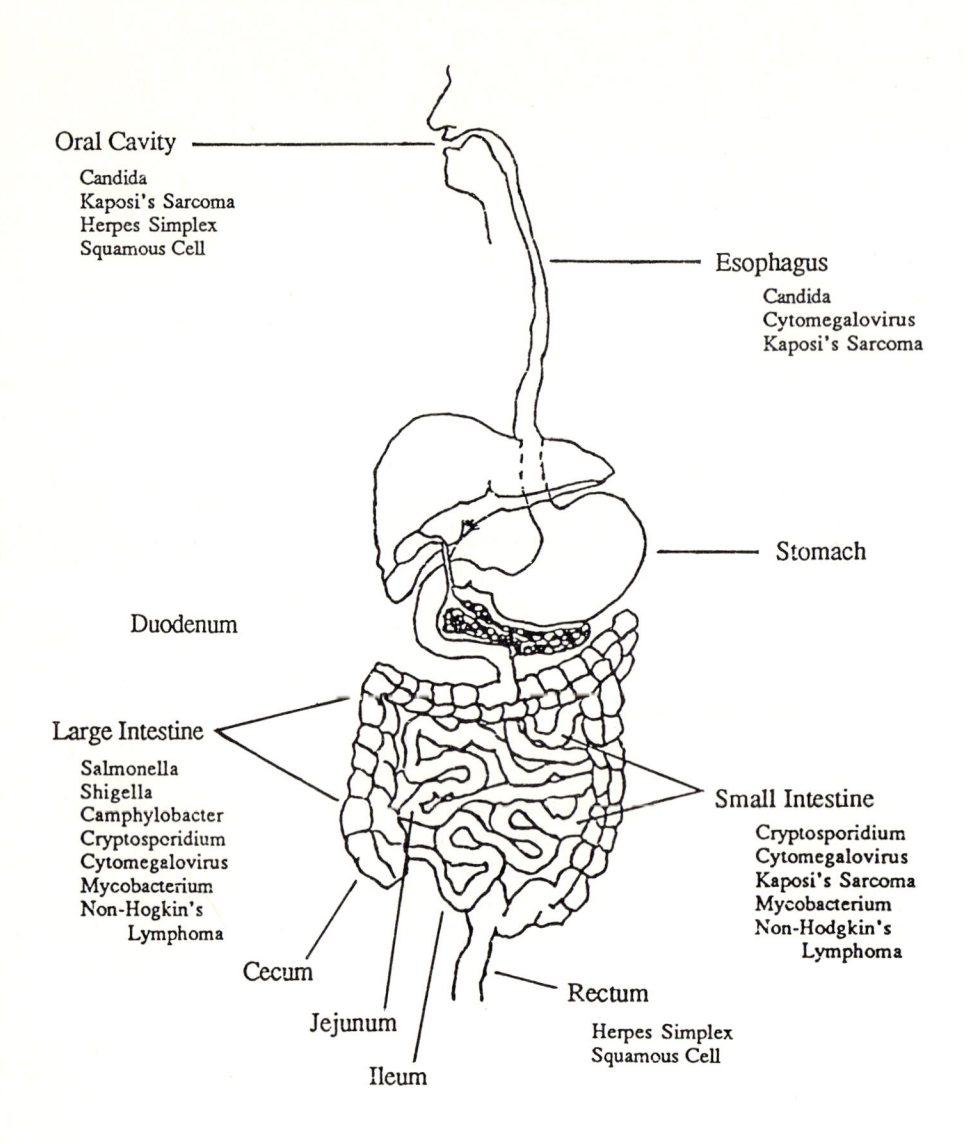

Oral Cavity
  Candida
  Kaposi's Sarcoma
  Herpes Simplex
  Squamous Cell

Esophagus
  Candida
  Cytomegalovirus
  Kaposi's Sarcoma

Stomach

Duodenum

Large Intestine
  Salmonella
  Shigella
  Camphylobacter
  Cryptosporidium
  Cytomegalovirus
  Mycobacterium
  Non-Hogkin's
    Lymphoma

Small Intestine
  Cryptosporidium
  Cytomegalovirus
  Kaposi's Sarcoma
  Mycobacterium
  Non-Hodgkin's
    Lymphoma

Cecum
Jejunum
Ileum

Rectum
  Herpes Simplex
  Squamous Cell

Figure 11.1 Commonly Affected Areas Related to Infections and Diseases

Gastrointestinal Disorders

Figure 11.1 illustrates the commonly affected areas of the gastrointestinal tract. Upper gastrointestinal disorders common with AIDS include anorexia, nausea, vomiting, fevers, oral lesions, mucositis, dysphagia, odynophagia, and persistent generalized lymphadenopathy (PGL). All of these compromise nutrition. Lower GI disorders, mainly diarrhea and malabsorption, commonly result from infectious diseases (i.e., cytomegalovirus, cryptosporidium, and mycobacterium) as well as the medications used to treat them. Dietary intolerances develop as a result of enzyme insufficiencies, mucosal abnormalities, tissue breakdown, atrophy, inflammation, bacterial overgrowth, osmotic changes, hypoproteinemia, or gut hypomotility. These problems result from HIV infection directly, infectious organisms, and *malnutrition itself*. Thus, many of the above disorders are sometimes reversible with adequate nutritional intake. For example, malnutrition causes lactase enzyme deficiency, which furthers protein energy malnutrition. Maintaining adequate daily nutritional intake helps to prevent the GI tract from being further compromised.

Assessing the Client at Nutritional Risk

Given the above devastating effects of HIV infection on the body's nutritional competency, the very diagnosis of HIV infection warrants immediate attention to a well-balanced diet. The goal of maintaining body weight and fortifying the immune system with necessary nutrients at once becomes a lifetime goal for these clients. Equip clients with information on how to eat well and stress the importance of doing so in spite of fatigue, depression, or finance. Their health depends on it.

Clients at risk are those who experience any symptoms that compromise intake or absorption of food, as listed in the section above, or a weight loss of 10 percent or more of their usual weight. Table 11.1 contains the assessment criteria for determining the extent of nutritional risk. Since they vary in their sensitivity, specificity, practicality, and usage, these measures combined help to tell us the extent of metabolic impairment due to malnutrition.

The nurse's role includes:

1. Teaching basic nutrition to all HIV-infected persons, emphasizing the importance of eating well to maintain immune function.

2. Identifying any nutritional problems experienced by the client such as stomatitis or diarrhea.

3. Equipping the client with strategies for overcoming common problems, as listed in Appendix 11.1.

4. Identifying the client at risk by history of weight loss and other measurements listed on Table 11.1.

5. Identifying clients who need aggressive nutritional therapy, such as enteral, nasoenteric, or parenteral feedings, according to the assessment chart outlined in Figure 11.2.

6. Consulting a registered dietitian (RD) for nutritional planning in any or all of the above.

Appendix 11.1 outlines specific problems often confronting persons with HIV infection and strategies to overcome each. This appendix can be used as a reference list for the nurse as well as helpful handouts for clients.

Table 11.1 *Measures of Nutritional Risk*

Measures		Mild	Moderate	Severe
Anthropometric				
weight change (from usual)		≤5%	≤10%	≤20%
tricep skinfold thickness		90-81	80-70	<70
midarm muscle circumference		90-51	50-30	<30
Biochemical*				
visceral proteins*	Tp	6.5-6.4	6.4-6.0	<6.0
	Alb	3.5-3.2	3.2-2.2	2.0
	TIBC	214-182	182-152	152
hematologic*	Transferrin	200-180	180-160	<160
	Total lymphocytes	1500-1200	1200-800	<800
Clinical*				
determining adequacy of dietary intake*			less than needs	
physical appearance			cachectic	
Miscellaneous				
taste acuity			depressed	
dark adaptation			prolonged	
hand grip strength			decreased	

*Assessment taking into account needs with stress factors to be provided for, protein needs at a 150:1 ratio (Kcals:grams nitrogen) with basal energy requirements increased 13% per degree Celsius above normal, and vitamins and minerals meeting the Recommended Daily Allowance (RDA) for the individual.

Source: Adapted from Zeman, F.J. (1983). *Clinical Nutrition and Dietetics.* Lexington, MA: Collamore Press.

Unproven Nutritional Regimes

In the absence of a cure or definitive treatment, people with HIV infection frequently use complementary therapy for their disease, including a variety of dietary therapies. These therapies can offer hope in the face of terminal illness and, in many cases, provide good nutrition (see Chapter 15). However, some dietary therapies can lead to weight loss, gastrointestinal distress, vitamin/mineral deficiencies, and electrolyte imbalances (see Table 11.2). Provide clients with accurate information on specific treatments, continue to monitor their nutritional status, and support their decision to deal with their disease in their own way.

Nutrition: Controlling the "Slims" 133

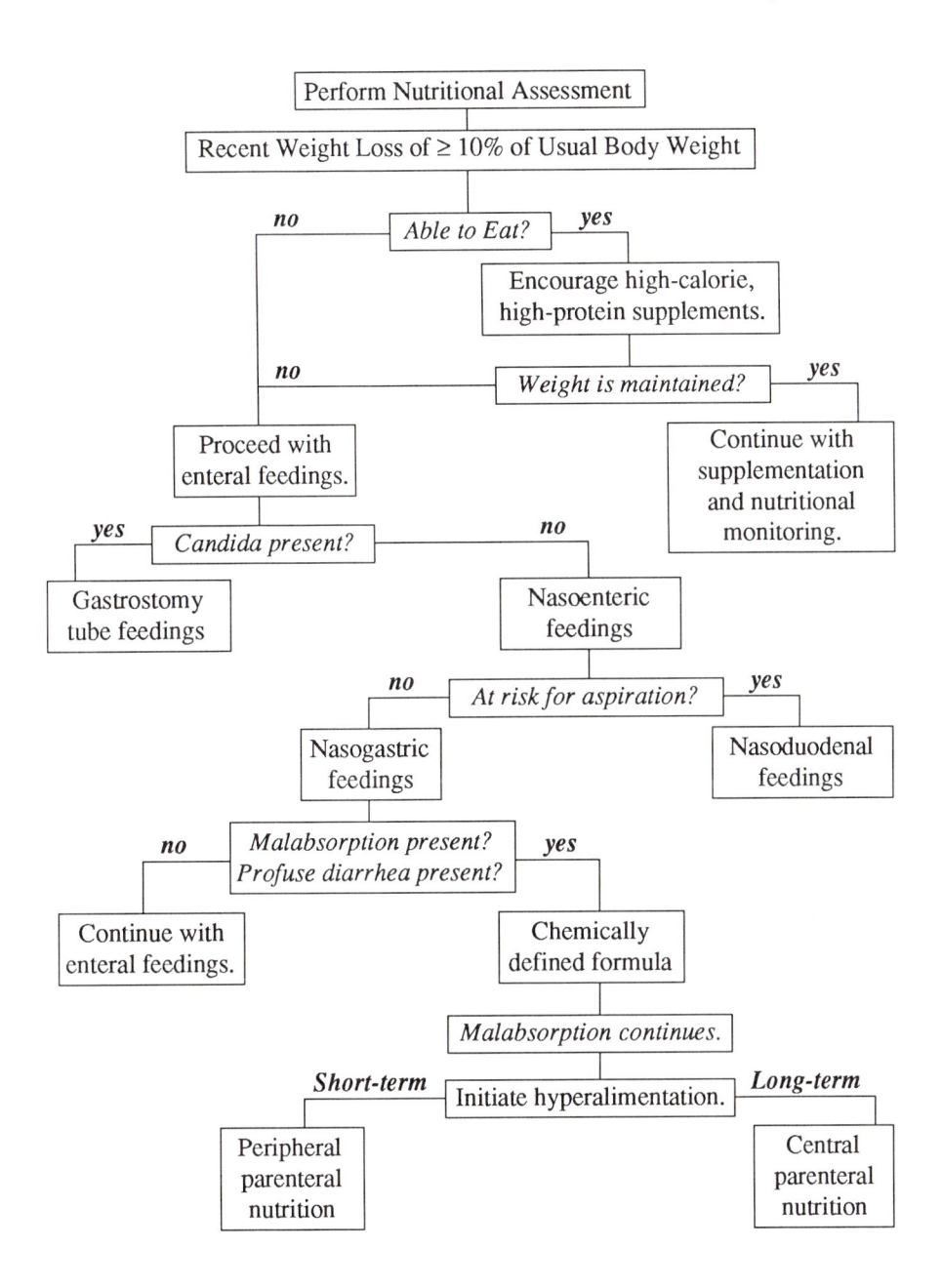

```
                    Perform Nutritional Assessment
            Recent Weight Loss of ≥ 10% of Usual Body Weight

                 no                       yes
                         Able to Eat?
                                          │
                              Encourage high-calorie,
                              high-protein supplements.

                 no                                        yes
                         Weight is maintained?

    Proceed with                                    Continue with
    enteral feedings.                               supplementation
                                                    and nutritional
     yes                              no            monitoring.
           Candida present?

    Gastrostomy              Nasoenteric
    tube feedings            feedings

                  no                        yes
                       At risk for aspiration?

            Nasogastric                    Nasoduodenal
            feedings                       feedings

       no      Malabsorption present?     yes
               Profuse diarrhea present?

    Continue with                   Chemically
    enteral feedings.               defined formula

                         Malabsorption continues.

         Short-term    Initiate hyperalimentation.   Long-term

    Peripheral                                   Central
    parenteral                                   parenteral
    nutrition                                    nutrition
```

Figure 11.2 Decision Making for Initiating Enteral Nutrition/Hyperalimentation

Table 11.2 Unproven Nutritional Therapies for AIDS/ARC

Type of Therapy	Regime	Claim	Safety	Efficacy
A. Immunological				
1. Vitamin/Mineral Therapy	Megadosing	Restores cell-mediated immunity by increasing T-cell number and activity	Toxicities, vitamin/mineral imbalance	Undemonstrated
2. Coenzyme Q	Oral supplement	Aids in regulating the immune system	Undetermined	Undemonstrated
B. Inhibitors of Cancer Growth				
1. Mistletoe Extract	Injections	Inhibits tumor growth	Toxicities can occur.	Undemonstrated
C. Antiviral				
1. Homemade AL721	Recipe made from soy or egg lecithin, taken orally	Inhibits HIV replication in vitro	AL721 approved by FDA for clinical trials. (Lecithin in large doses can cause nausea, vomiting, diarrhea.)	Undemonstrated; not known if active substance in AL721 can attack AIDS virus in human body after being digested
2. Butylated-hydroxytoluene (BHT)	Oral supplement	Attacks coating of AIDS virus	Large doses can cause nausea, vomiting, diarrhea.	Undemonstrated
D. Antiinfective				
1. Anti-Yeast Diet	Eliminates sugar and foods containing sugar; also restricts cheese, alcoholic beverages, coffee, tea	Prevents opportunistic yeast (candida) infections	Restricts food choices, which can lead to calorie deficit and weight loss.	Undemonstrated
E. Homeostatic				
1. Macrobiotic Diet	Diet composed of: 50% by volume whole-grain cereals, 20-30% vegetables, 10-15% cooked beans or seaweed	Restores balance and harmony between yin and yang forces to ameliorate disease	Fluid restricts, possible protein-calorie malnutrition; inadequate intake of riboflavin, niacin, calcium in adults; inadequate intake of above as well as vitamins B6, B12, and D in children.	None for cancer; undemonstrated for AIDS patients

SOURCE: Adapted from Dwyer, J., Bye, R., Holt, P., Lauze, S. (1988). Unproven nutritional therapies: What is the evidence? *Nutrition Today*, 23(2), 31.

Meal Plans

Appendixes 11.2 and 11.3 provide an example diet and supplement products for maximizing nutrition, a high-calorie/high-protein diet, often termed "power packing" by AIDS community groups. Encourage clients to eat as much as possible of these nutritious foods. Supplemental feedings, listed at the end of the chapter, are another way of adding calories and critical nutrients. A well-balanced diet is one major defense against the siege of HIV infection.

Appendix 11.1

Difficulties Meeting Nutrition Requirements: Some Solutions

It is important for you to eat well. Protein and calorie needs are greater during illness, treatment, and recovery than they normally are. When you eat less, your body uses its own nutrient stores, putting you at nutritional risk. Also, it has been found that those who eat diets high in protein and calories are better able to withstand side effects or higher doses of certain therapies. Maintaining your body weight is a good way to be fairly certain you are getting enough calories each day.

At times you may lose your appetite or experience other discomforts that affect how much you eat. There may be many reasons for your decreased intake, including anxiety, fatigue, personal and emotional problems, or complications associated with AIDS.

The purpose of this section is to offer suggestions to help maximize your nutritional intake.

Get full too fast?

Try these tips to provide a larger number of calories in small servings:

- Add butter or margarine (45 cals per tsp) to soups, hot cereal, mashed potatoes, rice, and bread.
- Add an extra serving of mayonnaise (100 cals per tbsp) to salads, eggs, and sandwiches.
- Try peanut butter (90 cals per tbsp) on apples, bananas, pears, celery, or on sandwiches with cream cheese, jelly, mayonnaise, or honey.
- Add honey (65 cals per tbsp) to tea, coffee, cereal (hot or cold), fruit, and bread with peanut butter.
- Try sour cream (30 cals per tbsp) on vegetables, potatoes, beans, carrots, squash, and as a dressing for fruit or a dip for vegetables.
- Try marshmallows (25 cals ea) in hot chocolate and with peanut butter, chocolate, and Jell-O.
- Try whipped cream (60 cals per tbsp) with pie, fruit, cake, pudding, and hot chocolate.
- Add powdered coffee creamer (30 cals per tbsp) to gravies, soups, milk shakes, and hot cereal.

Too tired to eat?

- Take advantage of the up times when you're feeling well by preparing meals

in large batches so you can freeze them for the down days. Eat even if it isn't meal time, and choose foods of increased nutritional value.
- Try eating smaller portions of easily digested foods and slowly work back to normal.
- Make dishes that don't require a lot of clean-up—use foil containers, paper, and plastic.
- Use canned creamed soups for nutritious, tasty sauces. Combine with chicken or fish and serve on toast.

Not hungry?

- Rely on food that you really love during your "not hungry" periods.
- Concentrate on making your meals more enjoyable; let someone else do the cooking. Accept gifts of food and offers to help prepare meals.
- Try ice cream mixed with ginger ale or your favorite carbonated beverage as a drink. Try eggnog, milk shakes, frappes, or frozen yogurt. (See daily meal plans in Appendix 11.2 for ideas.)

Mouth Soreness/Difficulty Chewing and Swallowing?

The lining of the mouth and throat are among the most sensitive areas of the body. Soreness and difficulty chewing and swallowing due to oral candidiasis is not uncommon with HIV infection. Remember, however, that part of the healing process in this area of the body depends upon your eating well and drinking fluids. If your mouth is dry, ask your physician whether medicines you are taking are causing the dryness. If your gums, tongue, and throat become dry or sore, be sure to follow a mouth-cleaning regimen prescribed by your doctor.

Some Do's and Don'ts for Proper Mouth Care

Do:

- eat foods lukewarm.
- try cold foods.
- try tilting your head back or moving it forward to make swallowing easier.
- use a straw or drink your food from a cup instead of using a spoon.
- rinse your mouth whenever you feel you need to remove debris, stimulate your gums, lubricate your mouth, or put a fresh taste in your mouth. Try rinsing every two hours while you are awake, especially before and after eating. Use a solution of 1/2 tsp salt and 1 tsp of baking soda to one quart of lukewarm water, or the cleaning regimen prescribed by your doctor.
- have your doctor prescribe artificial saliva for severe dryness; also, try sugarless candy, mints, or sour balls to stimulate saliva.

- soften or moisten foods by dipping them in liquid or taking a swallow of beverage with food.
- choose soft foods such as mashed potatoes, yogurt, scrambled or poached eggs, custards, egg salad, ricotta cheese, milk shakes, puddings, creamy soups and cereals, cheese and rice casseroles, macaroni and cheese, and meat loaf.
- eat soft fruits such as bananas, canned pears or peaches, and applesauce.
- try blending hard-to-chew meats with gravies or creamed soup.
- eat ice cream or yogurt, or make Popsicles with milk or milk substitutes.

Don't:

- use spices.
- smoke; it can irritate your mouth and throat.
- lick your lips; this increases dryness and chapping.
- drink citrus, acidic, or alcoholic beverages (they can be irritating).
- eat hard, dry, or fried foods; raw vegetables; bran; or foods with seeds or tough skins.
- eat citrus foods; too much may sting and burn.

Getting Enough Protein

You can improve your protein intake without increasing the amount of food you eat.

- Use skim milk powder to add protein to foods. Drink fortified milk or use it in your recipes (1 c powdered skim milk to 1 qt regular milk). Add skim milk powder to hot cereals, soups, scrambled eggs, gravies, ground meats (for meatballs, meat patties, meat loaf), and casserole dishes.
- Use whole or fortified milk or half-and-half instead of water when making soups, cereals, pudding, and instant cocoa.
- Add ground meat to soups and casseroles.
- Add grated cheese or cheese chunks to sauces, vegetables, soups, and casseroles.
- Add cheese spread or peanut butter to bread, sauces, waffles, and crackers.
- Add tuna, shrimp, crabmeat, diced ham, or sliced boiled eggs to sauces, rice, noodles, buttered toast, and hot biscuits.
- Choose dessert recipes that contain eggs, such as sponge cake, custard, and rice puddings.
- Try meat substitutes, such as tofu, dried peas and beans, and soy milk.

Taste Changes

Some PWAs/PWARCs experience a bitter or metallic taste in their mouths due to medications. Often, foods may have lost their taste or taste differently. Sweet foods can be less sweet, bitter foods taste stronger than before, and red meats are no longer enjoyable. This is caused by changes in your taste buds and because you are producing less saliva.

- Eat small, frequent meals and snacks. Try new foods; they may appeal to you now.
- Check with your physician about a zinc supplement. Zinc is needed by the body for proper taste sensation.
- Set a colorful table and make meals appetizing to the eye.
- Drink liquids such as tea or tonic and eat foods that leave their own taste in your mouth, such as fresh fruits and hard candies.
- Clean your mouth thoroughly, including brushing your gums and tongue. (See Do's and Don'ts for Proper Mouth Care on pages 137-138.)
- Experiment with herbs and spices: Basil, oregano, rosemary, tarragon, or mint added to meat and meat substitutes can be delicious. Add bacon bits, sliced almonds, ham strips, and pieces of onion to enhance flavor.
- Add wine or beer to soups and stews for a better taste.
- Eat foods with sauces and gravies to improve their flavor. Tart foods such as pickles, orange juice, lemonade, vinegar, and lemon juice may enhance flavor, especially for those who have no mouth or throat problems.
- Try other protein sources such as chicken, turkey, and fish if red meat does not taste the same. Also try eggs and dairy products such as cheese and yogurt. Tofu, or soybean curd, is another good protein source.

Nausea

- Talk with your physician about antinausea medication.
- Sip liquids through a straw. Take liquids thirty to sixty minutes before eating to avoid filling up at meal time.
- Don't eat foods you really like if you know specific times when you're going to be nauseated. Later you may be turned off by these favorite foods.
- Try staying out of the kitchen while meals are being prepared if your sense of smell is altered.
- Try to eat small meals frequently throughout the day (every two to three hours is suggested).
- Eat salty foods and avoid overly sweet ones.
- Eat plain, dry foods such as toast and crackers, especially when getting up in the morning.
- Try clear, cool beverages, flavored gelatin, Popsicles, and ice cubes made from flavored juice.
- Try carbonated beverages (club soda or cola helps settle your stomach; let the beverage sit for thirty minutes to lose some of its carbonation).

- Try cold-meat plates, sandwiches, fruit plates, cottage cheese, and other cold foods that don't have a strong aroma.

Heartburn

- Don't lie down for two hours after eating, if possible; otherwise, elevate the head of the bed four inches.
- Take liquid antacids one to three hours after meals, at bedtime, and upon waking in the middle of the night. (If you take antacids, keep them chilled; they will taste better.)
- Use mildly seasoned foods, and avoid fried, greasy, or heavily spiced ones.

Diarrhea

Pathogens associated with AIDS/ARC such as cryptosporidium, mycobacterium avian intercellulare (MAI), or cytomegalovirus can cause diarrhea. To help alleviate this:

- Make sure you drink plenty of fluids such as juices and broths.
- Use less fiber (roughage). Fiber is the fibrous material in your food that doesn't digest and is passed on in a bowel movement. If your intestines are irritated, the normal amount of fiber may be too much for them.
- Eat foods high in potassium since it is an important mineral that is lost when you have diarrhea. Some high-potassium foods include bananas, apricots, peach nectar, avocado, broccoli, potatoes (no skin), and nectarines (no skin). If you are unable to eat these foods, talk to your physician about a potassium supplement.
- Use only cooked fruits and vegetables, omitting those with seeds and tough skins and such high-fiber foods as broccoli, corn, beans, onions, and nuts. Also, some foods tend to be more binding and you may want to include these in your diet: bananas, fruit nectars, whipped potatoes, applesauce, and avocados.

Constipation

Some drugs, such as pain medications, may cause the bowel to slow down, resulting in constipation. Also, a diet low in fiber can contribute to constipation. Three ways to prevent or relieve constipation are: 1) gradually increase fiber, 2) increase fluids (6-8 c per day) and 3) exercise regularly.

The skins of many fruits and vegetables contain fiber, minerals, and vitamins. They will keep your stools soft as fiber soaks up the water. Try to eat one serving of a high-fiber food at each meal (see list below). In addition, unprocessed bran can be added to foods or liquids to increase dietary fiber. Hot beverages such as regular or decaffeinated coffee, Postum, and tea can sometimes help promote a bowel movement. Also, prunes and prune juice can help keep you regular since they contain a natural laxative.

High-Fiber Foods

Cereals & Starches	Vegetables	Fruits & Nuts
bran cereal/muffins	artichokes	apples
bran fiber	broccoli	avocados
brown rice	Brussels sprouts	black cherries
corn	cabbage	blueberries
cornmeal	carrots	dates
dried beans	cauliflower	figs
lentils	green beans	guava
oat bran	kale	grapes
potato with skin	lettuce	nuts
shredded wheat	mustard greens	peaches
wheat germ	okra	peanut butter
whole-grain bread	onions	pears
whole-grain cereal	parsnips	raisins
	peas	raspberries
	pumpkin	rhubarb
	turnip	strawberries

Dehydration

There may be times when you don't feel like eating at all because of frequent nausea, vomiting, or diarrhea. At this time, you are at risk of becoming fluid-depleted and it is very important for you to take measures to prevent dehydration. Signs of dehydration can include dark-colored urine, decreased appetite, weakness, weight loss, confusion, and poor skin appearance. Drinking fluids throughout the day equal to the amount that is lost is important. A healthy person at rest and not perspiring needs 1800 cc-2500 cc (8-10 c per day) daily to replace losses. For water loss through vomiting, diarrhea, and excessive sweating, additional fluids must be added. Fluids such as fruit juices, Gatorade, tonic, and bouillon, which supply calories as well as some vitamins and minerals, are strongly encouraged. Keep liquids by your bedside and sip them frequently throughout the day.

Lactose Intolerance

Lactose, or milk sugar, is found in all milk products. Individuals with lactose intolerance do not have enough lactase enzyme in their intestines to digest milk products. Foods containing lactose may cause problems such as abdominal cramping, bloating, or diarrhea for these persons. Lactose intolerance varies greatly from client to client, and may be temporary. Milk products may be tolerated at a later date. Make sure you add them back gradually.

Foods that contain lactose should be monitored closely when you have an intolerance. They include all milk and milk products, ice cream, puddings, desserts containing milk or milk products, scrambled eggs, omelets or other eggs prepared with milk, cream, half-and-half, whipping cream, creamed soups, chowders, and all commercially prepared soups that contain milk or milk products. Artificial fruit drinks may contain lactose, and canned or frozen juices sometimes are processed with lactose. Potatoes, rice, and pasta prepared with milk may also contain lactose. Be aware that not everyone has an intolerance to all these foods. Many people experience problems only with milk.

A product in the supermarket called Lactaid Milk contains digested lactose. You may find this product easy to tolerate. In addition, lactase enzyme pills or drops are available in most drugstores. They break down lactose for easy digestion. These should be taken with meals that contain milk products. Read the label carefully before using.

Abdominal Cramping

- Avoid foods that produce gas or cramps such as carbonated drinks, beer, beans, cabbage, broccoli, cauliflower, highly spiced foods, too many sweets, chewing gum, cooked dried beans, and onions.
- Avoid fatty foods.
- Eat smaller amounts of food more often.
- Don't skip meals.
- Try to chew with your mouth closed. Talking while you are chewing may cause you to swallow excess air.
- Limit large volumes of cold beverages and ice in beverages.
- Try warm food instead of hot food since hot food can increase the natural movement of the intestinal tract.

Appendix 11.2

Daily Meal Plans

Day 1

	Calories	Protein (gm)
Breakfast		
1 cooked egg and 1 oz cheese on English muffin	319	19
1 c fruit nectar	144	0
Mid-morning		
1 slice of bread with 2 tbsp peanut butter and 1 tsp honey	277	10
1 c chocolate eggnog	400	12
Lunch		
1 c cream of tomato soup	114	7
tuna melt	514	32
1 c enriched milk	224	16
1/2 c vanilla ice cream with sliced fruit	203	4
Mid-afternoon		
1/2 c dried fruit and nuts	284	8
1 c fruit-and-yogurt milk shake (3/4 c fruited yogurt and 1/4 c whole milk)	371	17
Dinner		
1 turkey and avocado sandwich with 1 tbsp mayonnaise	423	34
1 c canned peaches	96	0
2 peanut butter cookies	150	3
1 c Carnation Instant Breakfast milk shake	370	17
Evening		
1 c chocolate milk	180	8
1 slice banana bread with 1 tbsp cream cheese	300	3
TOTAL	4369	190

Day 2

	Calories	Protein (gm)
Breakfast		
1/2 c oatmeal with 2 tbsp maple syrup	230	10
1/2 c enriched milk	115	8
1 c canned peaches	200	0
4 oz (1/2 c) cranberry juice	85	0
Mid-morning		
1 c strawberry Carnation Instant Breakfast milk shake	380	17
Lunch		
3 oz sliced ham with 1 oz Swiss cheese on rye bread	515	31
1/2 c fruit cocktail	96	0
1/2 c butterscotch pudding	140	2
Mid-afternoon		
1 c fruited yogurt	245	8
1 bran muffin with 1 tbsp margarine or butter	300	5
Dinner		
1 c macaroni and cheese	423	34
1 1/2 c seedless grapes	96	0
1 c raspberry sorbet	150	3
Evening		
3 fig bars	150	1
1 c chocolate milk	190	8
TOTAL	3315	127

Day 3

	Calories	Protein (gm)
Breakfast		
1 c apricot nectar	152	0
1 2-egg omelet with 1 oz cheese	336	24
1 bagel with margarine and jelly	239	4
Mid-morning		
1 c cold cereal (granola) with banana and sugar	492	4
1 c enriched milk	224	16
Lunch		
1 cheeseburger on bun	310	15
1 c French fries with catsup	270	4
1 c chocolate milk	208	8
1/2 c fruit cocktail	96	0
Mid-afternoon		
1 c chocolate peanut butter milk shake	456	19
1/2 box animal crackers	120	2
Dinner		
4 oz broiled fish with lemon butter	282	28
1/2 c mashed potatoes with butter, sour cream	150	2
1/2 c mixed vegetables with butter	100	1
1 slice carrot cake (1/12)	403	5
1 c enriched milk	224	16
Evening		
1 c peach milk shake (3/4 c enriched milk with 1/2 c peaches)	262	12
2 oatmeal cookies	130	2
TOTAL	4454	162

Day 4

	Calories	Protein (gm)
Breakfast		
1/2 c grape juice	84	0
3 apple cinnamon pancakes with butter and maple syrup	500	8
1/2 c fruited yogurt	113	10
Mid-morning		
1 c Carnation Instant Breakfast milk shake	371	17
2 graham crackers	110	2
2 tbsp peanut butter	172	4
Lunch		
1 c cream of chicken soup	191	4
1 open-faced ham and melted cheese sandwich	380	23
1/2 c vanilla ice cream with 1/2 c sliced fruit	165	2
1/2 c enriched milk with malted milk powder	142	8
Mid-afternoon		
1 c pineapple tapioca pudding	176	5
Dinner		
1 slice quiche or cheese pie	240	34
1 c cooked carrots with butter and mint jelly	50	0
1 slice apple pie with 1-oz slice cheddar cheese	485	11
Evening		
1/2 c cottage cheese	100	14
1/4 c canned pineapple chunks	76	0
TOTAL	3355	142

Day 5

	Calories	Protein (gm)
Breakfast		
1/2 c sliced apple	60	0
1 c hot cereal with cream and molasses	213	2
1 c hot cocoa made with enriched milk	252	14
Mid-morning		
1 c banana eggnog	282	17
1 blueberry muffin with butter	300	4
Lunch		
2 toasted English muffin halves topped with spaghetti sauce and cheese (1-oz slice each)	470	25
1 c enriched milk	224	16
1 c chocolate pudding with whipped cream	440	9
Mid-afternoon		
1 c sliced strawberries	60	0
1/4 c cream and brown sugar (1 tbsp)	83	0
Dinner		
1/2 c cranberry juice	84	0
3 oz meat loaf with gravy	305	21
1 baked potato with sour cream and butter	179	2
1 c tossed salad with salad dressing (1 tbsp)	100	0
1 c rice pudding	350	10
Evening		
1 c root beer float (ice cream)	279	2
1 slice pound cake	200	2
TOTAL	3881	124

Appendix 11.3

Supplements

If you are unable to consume enough calories from regular foods, you might want to include a commercially available supplement. These supplements not only provide calories and protein but also vitamins and minerals. They are available in your local pharmacy or grocery store.

Product	Manufacturer	Description	Flavors	Cals/ (8 oz)	Prot/ (8 oz)
Ensure	Ross	liquid nutrition; ready-to-use; lactose-free	chocolate vanilla	264	9.5
Ensure Plus	Ross	high-calorie nutrition; ready-to-use; lactose-free	chocolate coffee eggnog strawberry vanilla	360	13.2
Sustacal	Mead-Johnson	liquid nutrition; ready-to-use; lactose-free	chocolate eggnog vanilla	240	14.7
Sustacal HC	Mead-Johnson	high-calorie nutrition; ready-to-use; lactose-free	chocolate eggnog vanilla	360	14.7
Carnation Instant Breakfast (made with whole milk)	Carnation	high-calorie; high-protein; contains lactose	chocolate eggnog strawberry vanilla	288	16.1
Meritene Liquid	Sandoz	liquid nutrition; ready-to-use; contains lactose	chocolate eggnog vanilla vanilla supreme	230	13.8
Nutrament	Carnation	liquid nutrition; ready-to-use; contains lactose	chocolate strawberry vanilla	240	12.0
Polycose Liquid	Ross	liquid carbohydrate supplement; lactose-free	———	480	———
Polycose Powder	Ross	powder carbohydrate supplement; lactose-free	———	480	———

Chapter 12

Getting Them Home: Discharge Planning

Berit Pratt

Discharge planning for clients with HIV infection starts with you, the nurse, in the hospital. Your knowledge of the clients and their needs serves as the springboard for a successful plan that will get clients home with the services they need. With a diagnosis of AIDS, a person's depressed immune system renders him susceptible to numerous opportunistic infections and malignancies. The varieties of disabling diagnoses, as well as frequent changes in condition, require increased case management and warrant a thorough plan for discharge. Well-planned discharges for clients with AIDS can also decrease the frequency and length of hospital readmission. People with HIV infection often prefer to be cared for in the home setting where they can benefit from familiar surroundings, a supportive network of care givers, and increased privacy and control over their lives.

The Need for Home Care

In the early part of the AIDS epidemic, it was common to see people with HIV disease spend the entire course of their illness in a hospital setting. This can be attributed to many factors, among them the fact that little was known about AIDS and few treatments for opportunistic infections were available. Clients would often spend the terminal stages of their illness in the ICU and die in the hospital. The majority of people were, in fact, more acutely ill than now, having been diagnosed later in the course of their illness. Now, with the advent of life-prolonging drugs such as AZT, we see people living longer in more chronic phases of HIV illness. The cost of caring for people with AIDS was initially high, with original estimates from diagnosis to death running as high as $147,000. Home care for persons with AIDS was simply not considered as a viable option. Home care agencies and hospices did not have the staff needed, nor were staff trained in the needs of people with HIV infection. The first city in the United States to develop extensive home care services for persons with AIDS was San Francisco, one of the hardest-hit cities in numbers of AIDS cases in the beginning of the epidemic. The San Francisco Department of Public Health developed a comprehensive approach to caring for people with AIDS that was based in the community. The program was comprised of a network of services including hospitals, home care agencies, and volunteers. Through a combination of state and city funding, a team approach utilizing a broad base of community support allowed persons with AIDS to spend a majority of their time in the home setting with services provided. The estimates of cost from diagnosis to death were startlingly different from previous estimates. In San Francisco, the average cost was $27,571. Some of the differences in cost can be attributed to the fact that home care is significantly less expensive than hospital care (Bloom & Carlinger, 1988; Scitovsky et al., 1986).

Not all people with HIV infection are appropriate for home care. Depending on their level of physical disability and dementia, a long-term care facility may be a better option. Often, because people with AIDS become sick and weaken quickly, it is difficult for them and their significant others to accept the option of long-term care. However, in some instances, it is much better to send a person to a facility that provides supervision around the clock. For example, people who live alone with scant support systems who need twenty-four-hour care, are very difficult to service successfully with home care. Careful evaluation of a client's needs will help you to determine whether a residential hospice, nursing home, or long-term care hospital is justified.

The Discharge Process

Discharge planning for people with AIDS from the hospital back into the community involves a six-step process beginning while the client is still hospitalized:
1. Identify the key players.
2. Evaluate the home situation.
3. Evaluate patient's level of home care needs.
4. Evaluate reimbursement sources.
5. Develop a home care package.
6. Implement the home care package.

This process is further detailed in the following sections:

1. Identify the Key Players.

The first step in discharge planning is to identify the key players. Who are the significant people in the patient's life who will be involved with care once the patient returns home? Does the patient have a lover, a roommate, or spouse already sharing the home? When is this person home, during the day or evening? What about family members and friends? Who have been pitching in or would be willing to help as the client becomes sicker and more dependent on others? Does the person have a volunteer from a local AIDS service organization or other volunteer base such as a church group? There is a significant possibility of burnout among key players due to several factors: the cumulative loss of others to AIDS, being sick with HIV themselves, or simply feeling overwhelmed and helpless while watching a loved one become ill. Therefore, key players prior to the patient's hospitalization may discontinue in the role after discharge, resulting in a loss of physical support (see Chapters 5 and 17).

Once you have identified the key players on a personal level, determine the key service providers who will be involved with the client's home care. Agencies such as Visiting Nurse Associations, hospices, IV infusion providers, social work services, and AIDS service providers together can help the client stay at home with adequate care.

Because of the increased amount of daily coordination involved in caring for people with AIDS, it is important to identify one primary home case manager. The case manager is the person responsible for the daily assessment and coordination of home care services. This person would monitor the adequacy of services, including the quality, consistency, and need for services. The case manager could be a family member (lover, parent, or friend) or a professional from one of the service agencies involved, such as a home care or inpatient primary nurse, or the discharge planning coordinator of a hospital. Since agencies differ in the roles created for discharge planning and community coordination, the job title of the case manager could be the same person for both inpatient and home care setting, but this is sometimes impossible to do due to agency policies. As nurses in the hospital environment, you are often in a good position to recommend the best person to act as the case manager. Identifying one person ultimately responsible for communicating and coordinating all care helps to eliminate confusion, surplus, or insufficient services.

If the client will be needing a number of services at home, arrange a discharge planning meeting prior to discharge. Included at this meeting should be all the key players, both personal and professional: lover, friends, family, the client's physician, primary nurse, representatives from relevant AIDS community organizations, and hospital discharge planning staff as identified by your hospital (social worker or discharge planning nurse). The meeting offers all key players a chance to meet one another and to clarify goals in developing a home care plan.

2. Evaluate the Home Situation.

The second step in the discharge planning process is to evaluate the home situation. To what kind of home environment will this person be returning in the community? An evaluation of the physical environment is necessary to determine whether discharge home is a reasonable option. Questions to ask are: Does the client live alone or with others? Does the client have an adequate, stable housing situation? Does the client have laundry facilities in close proximity? Are the housemates receptive and supportive of this person returning home in a state of ill health? An increasing number of patients with AIDS are from the IV drug-using community and may have been hospitalized from the street or from homeless shelters. They will not have housing to return to upon discharge so that other alternatives must be sought.

Alternative housing will also be needed for clients who can no longer access their home, such as the weakened person who lives in a fourth-floor walk-up apartment. For economically disadvantaged people, finding alternative housing is one of the biggest problems of discharge planning. A social worker may function as a liaison to community housing. Contact both private organizations and government departments for housing in your area. Since resources in most communities are limited, it takes determined perseverance to track down whatever might be available to the client.

3. Evaluate Patient's Level of Home Care Needs.

Hospital discharge is a stressful time for clients. During hospitalization, clients experience the crisis of acute illness. They may have been away from home for some time and will be returning in a weakened state. Many AIDS diagnoses will impact on the patients' ability to be independent at home (see Chapter 9). Some of these diagnoses are:

AIDS Dementia: Client will not be able to be left alone; may wander, forget to cook or eat.

Neurological Manifestation of HIV (such as toxoplasmosis meningitis, brain abscesses, or spinal cord lesions): Client may be physically or psychologically disabled by these conditions, warranting more supervision at home.

Fatigue: In a younger person accustomed to high levels of strength and physical fitness, fatigue can take clients and care givers by surprise. These needs require advance arrangements for homemaking, etc.

Diarrhea: In-house or nearby laundry facilities are essential.

Pneumocystis Pneumonia or Pulmonary KS: Respiratory symptoms will add to weakness and shortness of breath, decreasing mobility.

Once you have evaluated your clients' home care needs based on their physical and emotional conditions, do an assessment of specific services needed. The more services you can set up ahead of time, the more smoothly the discharge will go. Here is a list of the service categories to be considered.

Specific service assessment:
Home health aide—personal care
Homemaker—shopping, cooking, cleaning

Skilled nursing—case management, physical assessment, medications
High-tech nursing—IV therapy, aerosolized pentamadine
Hospice services—case management, terminal care
Rehab services—PT, OT, speech therapy
Social work/counseling—financing care, housing, etc.
Private duty nursing
Community-based AIDS organizations—shopping, cooking, cleaning, transportation, running errands

Ideally, you want these services to be in place on the day of the client's discharge. The discharge planning meeting will help to expedite this evaluation process.

4. Evaluate Reimbursement Sources.

"Will my insurance pay for home care?" This is a commonly asked question that you will need to answer as part of the discharge planning process. Many third-party reimbursement sources are unaware of the complex home care needs of a client with HIV infection. Insurance companies often have restrictive policies that ration unrealistically small portions of services, insufficient for home care of a person with HIV infection. Even insurance companies will change when given a sound, cost-containment rationale. Since it is still significantly less expensive to care for a person at home than in the hospital, it is worth approaching providers and negotiating for services initially not covered. Reimbursers are restrictive, partly as a matter of policy and partly out of ignorance of the wide variety of needs of clients with HIV infection. A little AIDS education for insurers can often help produce better coverage at home.

5. Develop the Home Care Package.

After you have collected the information from the first four steps, the next step is to develop the home care package. Through utilizing a primary home care case manager, key players, and home care agencies, a realistic home care package for the individual patient can be devised. The availability of the key players must be taken into account. Check with those who will carry the most responsibility and make certain they have agreed to their role. Many home care packages have been unsuccessful because the commitment of lovers, friends, and family members was not confirmed prior to discharge.

Allow sufficient time during the hospitalization for the client, lover, or family to learn their responsibilities for home care. They often need several days to learn how to mix intravenous medications or manipulate IV equipment. Clients/families need to practice on the same equipment they will be using at home. Most companies who supply home IV equipment will come into the hospital and teach people before discharge. (See Table 12.1.)

Table 12.1 *Sending the Client Home With an IV Infusion*

1. Obtain exact information regarding medication dosage, frequency, and line maintenance, such as how often the line needs to be flushed.
2. Determine who will administer the medication (nurse, client, family member, or other).
3. If the client is self-administering, determine if someone else needs to be present while the infusion is running, in case of emergency. This will depend on the predictability of the client's reaction to the drug.
4. A pharmaceutical company will be needed to supply the drug and the necessary equipment. Generally, the hospital's continuing care department will be able to secure this service.
5. Determine who will do the teaching and to whom. If the client is self-administering, have another person included in the teaching to serve as a back-up if the client becomes too ill to self-administer the medication.
6. Make the referral to the pharmaceutical company as much in advance as possible, since it may take several days to secure their services for inpatient teaching and home equipment.
7. If possible, allow the client/family to participate in the presentation and administration of the medication while in the hospital.
8. Evaluate the readiness of all care givers concerned as well as the completeness of the plan before implementing.

In addition to the availability of family/friends, also check the availability of home care. Many times, home health aides or homemakers are unattainable. Also, it can take several days to coordinate these services, so advanced planning becomes essential. Try to discharge clients on a Monday rather than a Friday. Securing adequate home care services over a weekend can be impossible.

6. Implement the Home Care Package.

Implementation of the home care package will be primarily out of your hands once the client leaves the hospital. However, since you have a large body of knowledge about the client that will be helpful to home care service providers, contact the primary home care case manager the day the client goes home. Your telephone call to the home care or hospice nurse can provide an update on the client's latest condition as well as answer questions on the course of the hospital stay.

Confidentiality must also be taken into consideration with the diagnosis of AIDS. Discrimination in housing, employment, and even health care is widespread for persons with HIV infection. Be aware of clients' wishes concerning confidentiality about their diagnosis. For example, clients may have informed some family or household members but not others that they have HIV infection. Omitting this information on an intake form at a home care agency or during phone contact with the agency will ensure that information about a client's diagnosis remains confidential (see Chapter 3).

Summary

Once you've taken steps to evaluate, plan, develop, and implement a discharge package for your clients, you will be able to get them home knowing that needed services are in place. Discharge planning for people with HIV infection often involves a number of key players. You as the hospital nurse can play an instrumental role in pulling the key players together for a successful discharge.

References

Bloom, D.E., & Carlinger, G. (1988). The economic impact of AIDS in the United States. *Science, 239,* 604-609

Scitovsky, A.A., Cline, M., & Lee, P.R. (1986). Medical care costs of patients with AIDS in San Francisco. *Journal of the American Medical Association, 256*(22), 3103-3106.

Chapter 13

Identifying Special Needs: Children With HIV Infection

Nancy Karthas

A seventeen-year-old mother brings her eighteen-month-old child into the infectious disease clinic for the first time. Her husband died of AIDS the previous week. She has been tested and is HIV-positive, though currently she is asymptomatic. As we walk down the hall, she begins to tell her story. Both she and her husband were intravenous drug users. They got married when she found out she was pregnant. Not knowing about AIDS, they were excited at the prospect of having a child. Much of her pregnancy centered around drugs. In her last trimester, she and her husband entered a detoxification program. Reportedly, she has been "clean" ever since. Several months ago, her husband became ill and was found to be HIV-positive. Her testing brought the same result. It was not until her husband's death that the issue of the potential for her daughter to have been infected came to light.

Although her daughter appeared healthy, she did have some physical findings that pointed to the probability of HIV infection: diffuse adenopathy, parotitis, frequent diarrhea, and a striking hepatomegaly. Two weeks later, her daughter's positive HIV status was confirmed by both ELISA and Western Blot. In a follow-up meeting, looking pale, thin, and vulnerable, this mother shared her feelings that even in death there was no relief: Not having yet grieved the loss of her husband or the issue of her own mortality, she now faces the loss of her child. The loss of her husband was not an end, rather only the beginning of the demise of her family.

The HIV-Infected Family

When a child is diagnosed with AIDS, a family is diagnosed with HIV infection. Although a small percentage of children acquire the infection through blood transfusions or sexual abuse, the majority of children receive the virus from their mother perinatally (Barrett, 1988; Boland, 1987; Rogers, 1987). The child is often the index case for diagnosing the disease within a family. Since the care of the child depends on the family's ability to give care, nursing care of the child with HIV infection means giving extensive support to the needs of the parents or care givers. As nurses, we strive to maintain an intact, functioning family system to provide care for the child's lifetime. In order to facilitate family coping, we need to understand families' emotional responses to HIV infection.

The initial reaction of parents is often shock, anger, and blame. The child's diagnosis may be the first realization that not only does the child have a terminal illness, but so does the mother, and possibly the father and siblings. The child's diagnosis may also confront the family for the first time with the high-risk behavior involved, often bisexual activity or intravenous drug use. Parents simultaneously face the threat of loss of a child, loss of their own lives, loss of trust in a relationship, feelings of having failed a child, anxiety at the resources they need to cope with catastrophic illness, and anger at the family member who introduced the virus to the others. In a small number of cases, a parent may have acquired the infection from a blood transfusion prior to the universal screening begun in April 1985. Regardless of the mode of entry, parents most often experience anger and rage at the blood bank, spouse, society, whomever they perceive as responsible for the tragedy. It's hard to imagine the unique kind of torture parents face, realizing that they have unknowingly infected their child with a deadly virus, which will now cause the most precious person in their lives to suffer and die. In order for the family to function, they must move beyond trying to lay blame or guilt, and begin the process of learning to live with HIV infection.

Families with AIDS experience fear: fear of losing their most precious possessions, their lives and the life of their child. One parent lives in fear that she will walk into her child's room one day and find her dead. To cope with this fear, she avoids entering the child's room at night or during nap time. Rather, she waits for the child to wake on her own, get up, and come to her. This fear prevents the mother from sleeping herself, wondering if this is the day her daughter won't wake up. She survives each day from waking period to waking period.

Fear of rejection sometimes stops families from sharing the diagnosis with other family members and friends. Instead of turning to their social network for support, these families bury themselves in isolation, which often leads to depression. Even after the death of the child, families keep their secret, cutting off support for the grief of their child and anticipated grief of their own possible fate.

The diagnosis confronts parents with their own mortality as well as that of their child. Parents frequently experience symptoms that make it difficult or impossible to continue to take care of their child. Parents may need to make arrangements for who will care for their child as well as funeral arrangements for themselves and their child.

When, for whatever reason, parents reach a point of being unable to care for their child, a grandparent or aunt or uncle may assume responsibility. When this happens, parents may feel inadequate and guilty for "failing" their child, thereby increasing their feelings of worthlessness. As much as they need the help and support of the extended family, such assistance confronts them with their own progressing illness and subsequent dependence. The loss of their most important role, caring for their sick child, may be the ultimate insult to an already low self-esteem. This loss may render them dysfunctional: They may refuse to make plans for their lives or that of their child. They may withdraw from all support, isolating themselves in their despair.

The demands on the family with HIV infection may so drain them of their emotional and physical resources that uninfected siblings unintentionally get pushed aside, lost in the crisis. Frequent medical appointments and recurrent, often lengthy hospitalizations of possibly more than one family member block the parents' attempts to spend time with, and address the needs of, the other children in the family. This may lead to school problems, changes in behavior, and sleep disturbances in the uninfected sibling. Therefore, siblings need to be included in the nursing plan of care, helping them feel a part of the care rather than isolated from it.

With all the intense emotions emerging with HIV diagnosis, families need to experience the feelings and work through the pain with the hope that they will reach a point of acceptance where they can function. We need to listen, accept whatever feelings are voiced, validate both the tragedy and the parents' and child's right to feel anger, depression, grief, fear. Some families will get past the emotions sufficiently to remain functional: able to make decisions regarding their child, even if they can no longer be the primary care givers. These families need reinforcement for whatever level of involvement they can maintain with the child. Other families may become dysfunctional, unable to care for the infected child at all. In this case, the health care team may need to refer to social service agencies for meeting the child's needs, as described in the end of this chapter.

The Clinical Picture

At the time this book goes to press, fewer than 2,000 cases of pediatric AIDS have been reported in the United States (CDC, June 20, 1988). An estimated 5,000 more children may be infected but are not yet symptomatic or diagnosed with AIDS (see Tables 13.1 and 13.2). An estimated 35-50 percent of offspring of HIV-positive women will probably develop the infection, which is spread both transplacentally and as the child moves through the birth canal during delivery (Hoff et al., 1988; Rogers, 1987; Willoughby et al., 1988). A child can retain maternal antibodies for

Table 13.1 *Laboratory Findings in Infants and Children*

Hypergammaglobulinemia/ Hypogammaglobulinemia	Anemia
Depressed T-helper cells	Leukopenia
Reversed lymphocyte subset ratio	Thrombocytopenia
Depressed lymphocyte responses to mitogens	Elevated level of circulating immune complexes
Decreased specific antibody responses	Elevated serum transaminase levels

SOURCE: Oleske, J. (1987). Natural history of HIV infection II. In B.K. Silverman & A. Waddell (Eds.), *Report of the Surgeon General's Workshop on Children with HIV Infection and Their Families*. (DHHS Publication No. HRS-D-MC 87-1). Rockville, MD: U.S. Dept. of Health and Human Services.

Table 13.2 *Differences Between Pediatric and Adult AIDS*

1. Kaposi's sarcoma and B cell lymphoma are rare in children.
2. Hepatitis B infection is less frequent than in adults.
3. Hypergammaglobulinemia is more pronounced in children.
4. Peripheral lymphopenia is uncommon in children.
5. Lymphoid interstitial pneumonitis (LIP) is much more common in children.
6. Some children will have normal ratio of helper to suppressor T cells (although quantitatively T helper cells are diminished).
7. Serious bacterial sepsis is a major problem in children.
8. Dysmorphic features may be found in some children.
9. Acute mononucleosis-like presentation is rare in children.
10. Progressive neurologic disease secondary to primary HIV CNS infection is more pronounced in children.

SOURCE: Oleske, J. (1987). Natural history of HIV infection II. In B.K. Silverman & A. Waddell (Eds.), *Report of the Surgeon General's Workshop on Children with HIV Infection and Their Families*. (DHHS Publication No. HRS-D-MC 87-1). Rockville, MD: U.S. Dept. of Health and Human Services.

HIV infection as long as fifteen months. Thus, unless an infant develops an AIDS-defining illness, identifying HIV infection prior to fifteen months of age is difficult. This uncertainty puts tremendous stress on the family, who may wonder if every minor illness is a result of HIV infection or simply part of the common childhood experience.

For children over fifteen months, positive test results for antibodies to HIV are considered to be reliable indicators of infection (see Chapter 9). A positive HIV culture also provides a definitive diagnosis. However, a negative culture or a negative test for antigens does not necessarily rule out the presence of HIV infection. Antibodies may not appear until after fifteen months. A culture may be falsely negative if the blood sample contained insufficient virus to culture. Therefore, testing for seropositivity and culturing for HIV are useful in identifying HIV infection primarily when the results are positive. Signs and symptoms of infection can occur at any time, usually within the first two years of life. The mechanism that triggers the virus to become active within a given host is unknown.

Children with HIV infection commonly present with failure to thrive, which may be the first indication of illness. Unlike adults who may lose 10 percent of baseline weight, children tend to fall off the growth curve. Rather than losing weight, children fail to *gain* weight or grow according to normal standards. Children with HIV infection may also have serious recurrent bacterial infections, chronic diarrhea, recurrent thrush, lymphadenopathy, hepatomegaly, and splenomegaly. They may also exhibit signs of cardiomyopathy, neurologic deterioration, chronic anemia, hypergammaglobulinemia, and renal disease (Barrett, 1988; Scott, 1987). Kaposi's sarcoma, frequently found in adults, is rare in children (Oleske, 1987). Pediatric AIDS is a terminal illness. The diagnosis of lymphoid interstitial pneumonitis (LIP), seen primarily in children, indicates a 25 percent mortality rate. Pneumocystis carinii pneumonia (PCP) indicates an 85 percent mortality rate (Scott, 1987).

The Nursing Role

Symptom Management

The nursing goal for physical care includes minimizing the symptoms and helping each child reach maximum potential, whatever that may be. We need to encourage parents to seek medical help for their child at the first sign of illness, since hospitalizations may sometimes be avoided by early diagnosis and treatment. When the child is hospitalized, we need to treat the current illness, protect from nosocomial infections, and return the child home as soon as possible. The specific goals for care center on the symptoms that the child presents and need to be continually reassessed according to changes in the clinical condition. Some common symptoms are outlined below.

1. Alterations in Nutrition

Nutritional management becomes a challenge for many reasons. Persistent oral thrush and esophageal candidiasis may make eating or drinking extremely painful (Boland & Klug, 1986). Decreased intestinal absorption, decreased appetite, and a wasting syndrome require aggressive nutritional management including high-caloric meals, supplementary enteral feedings at night, and, eventually, total parenteral nutrition through a central venous line. Chapter 11 outlines such problems as well as strategies for managing them. Despite all interventions, many children continue to fail to thrive.

2. Alterations in Breathing Patterns

Alterations in breathing patterns stem from chronic illnesses such as upper respiratory infections, frequent viral or bacterial pneumonias, and sinusitis. Children who recover from acute episodes of PCP and LIP may experience residual respiratory impairment, requiring ongoing chest physical therapy and oxygen dependency. Despite aggressive antibiotic therapy, a child with pneumonia may need ventilator support during the acute phase of illness. Weaning a child from a respirator is a slow and difficult process, requiring frequent monitoring and continuous adjustments as the child's oxygenation needs change.

3. Alterations in Cardiac Output

Up to 90 percent of all children with HIV infection may exhibit changes in cardiac function, usually by a decreased left ventricular function and a high afterload (Lipshultz et al., 1988). Such decreased ability of the heart to pump sometimes results in signs and symptoms of heart failure such as shortness of breath, fatigue, and pedal edema. However, a child may have compromised cardiac function without manifesting any clinical symptoms (Lipshultz et al., 1988). Severe complications may be prevented by early screening, detection, and treatment. Echocardiograms and electrocardiograms are needed every six months for the asymptomatic child, and every three months for the symptomatic child. Children experiencing cardiac problems are treated with digoxin and diuretics in much the same way as any type of heart failure.

4. Alterations in Cognitive Perception

Since the HIV invades neurons, children also experience such neurological disorders as cortical atrophy, chronic encephalopathy, and acquired microcephaly. Such organic damage can result in serious loss of developmental milestones (Belman, 1988; Kastner & Friedman, 1988; Oleske, 1987).

Zidovudine (Retrovir, formerly AZT) is the only antiretroviral drug shown effective in adults with HIV infection. In the first pediatric research studies, zidovudine seems to improve mainly neurological functions, not only regaining lost developmental tasks but even acquiring new ones. Although promising, zidovudine is a possible treatment, not a cure (Pizzo et al., 1988).

Supporting the Family

The child's well-being, regardless of physical condition, depends on the family's ability to love and care for the child. Thus, another nursing goal entails facilitating the family's supportive role in the care of the child. Interventions to meet this goal include the following:

1. Assess the emotions, capabilities, and resources of the family. Help the family work through the emotions described above. Determine the family members who most strongly support the child and are capable of giving care. Often, these people will be extended-family members such as grandparents. When extended-family support is missing and the parents may not be able to care for the child indefinitely, determine the agency and community resources that may enable the family to continue as a unit for as long as possible.

2. Engage the family in all decision making. Parents need to feel a part of a team. This includes not only treatment decisions regarding their child, but also placement and home care issues. We may be the people who first confront parents with the need to appoint guardians or make wills in order to protect their child's future. Parents also need encouragement to care for themselves. Refer parents to appropriate adult health care, emphasizing the importance of their own health in order to care for their child. Parents often push their own health needs aside to focus on the crisis of losing a child.

3. Teach the family to care for the child. Parents need to know symptom management, when to call the physician, how to give medication and other treatments. They need to understand their child's physical illness and how to manage appropriate infection control procedures in the home. A complete outline of essential teaching content as well as examples of teaching tools are included in Chapter 18.

4. Advocate for the rights of the client and family. Families in crisis are vulnerable, more likely to follow any suggestions and less likely to express their needs. For example, only those intimately involved in the child's care need to know about the diagnosis. Often the nurse is in the key position to ensure confidentiality, protecting the child against potential discrimination.

The HIV-Infected Child in the Community

One of the major issues of community living is who needs to know the child's diagnosis. Since many parents work outside the home, they often need day care services for their children. Some parents fear that telling the day care providers about the child's HIV status would result in a loss of the service, forcing the parent to leave work and lose their only source of livelihood. Current recommendations state that children with HIV infection under the age of three or those not in control of their body fluids should not be in a group setting (Commonwealth of Massachusetts, 1986b). Therefore, since the cost of one-to-one child care is prohibitive for many families, the parent following these recommendations is left without a job, without a source of income in the face of huge medical expenses. These recommendations may change, since continuing research supports that only blood and bloody secretions are infectious. Barrier precautions with nonbloody urine, feces, tears, and sputum have been declared unnecessary for avoiding HIV transmission (CDC, June 24, 1988).

A similar situation occurs with school-age children who are well enough to attend school. Since some families have endured threats to their homes and picketing or boycotting of schools that allowed their HIV-infected children to attend, many other families legitimately fear similar rejection. Children in control of their body fluids may safely attend school without any threat of contagion to other children or teachers. One state department of health recommends that the principal, school nurse, and child's teacher know the child's diagnosis (Commonwealth of Massachusetts, 1986a). This enables the school nurse to provide ongoing assessments of the child's health in school and protect the child from any outbreak of communicable disease in the school, such as chicken pox or measles.

When an HIV-infected child is left without parental or family support for whatever reason, the child is placed in custody of the state Department of Social Services. The need for foster care again raises the issue of information concerning diagnosis, and withdrawal of services once that information is disclosed. Since the HIV-infected children are often refused by foster care homes, these children often spend long, unnecessary hospital stays, up to months at a time. In response to the need for competent, comfortable care givers, a combined effort of both the City of Boston and the Commonwealth of Massachusetts resulted in the opening of the first residential program for HIV-infected children in the United States, caring for children from birth to five years of age. This five-bed home serves children who are well enough to be in the community but who have no home or care giver. The residents of this program receive care from specially trained staff knowledgeable about pediatric AIDS: modes of transmission, infection control, and signs and symptoms of the illness (Karthas & Dodwell, 1988; Karthas et al., 1988). Similar programs are now being developed in other areas of the country.

Our role as nurses includes informing the family about recommendations for community living and helping them secure the resources needed (Boland & Klug, 1986). Since often these services or community support remain nonexistent, our role as patient advocates calls on us to be vocal and active in policies in our schools and government agencies. As we increase our comfort and knowledge with caring, we can help create more supportive environments in both our places of work and our communities to meet the needs of families with HIV infection.

References

Barrett, D. (1988, January). The clinician's guide to pediatric AIDS. *Contemporary Pediatrics, 5,* 24-47.

Belman, A., Diamond, G., Dickson, D., Horoupin, D., Llena, J., Lantos, G., & Reinstein, A. (1988, January). Pediatric acquired immunodeficiency syndrome: Neurologic syndromes. *American Journal of Diseases of Children, 142,* 29-35.

Boland, M. (1987). Management of children with HIV infection. In B.K. Silverman & A. Waddell (Eds.), *Report of the surgeon general's workshop on children with HIV infection and their families.* (DHHS Publication No. HRS-D-MC87-1). Rockville, MD: U.S. Dept. of Health and Human Services.

Boland, M., & Klug, P.M. (1986, November/December). AIDS: The implications for home care. *Journal of Maternal Child Nursing, 11,* 404-411.

Centers for Disease Control (1988, June 20). *AIDS Weekly Surveillance Report.* Atlanta, GA.

Centers for Disease Control (1988, June 24). Update: Universal precautions for prevention of transmission of human immunodeficiency virus, hepatitis B virus, and other bloodborne pathogens in health-care settings. *Morbidity & Mortality Weekly Report, 37*(24), 377-392.

Commonwealth of Massachusetts (1986a). AIDS/acquired immune deficiency syndrome and school attendance policy. In *AIDS: Governor's task force on AIDS: Policies and recommendations.* Pp. 1-1 to 1-3. (Available from the Commonwealth of Massachusetts Executive Office of Human Services, Department of Public Health, 150 Tremont Street, Boston, MA.)

Commonwealth of Massachusetts (1986b). Recommendations for caretakers of children with clinical AIDS or evidence of infection with HIV infection. In *AIDS: Governor's task force on AIDS: Policies and recommendations.* Pp. 2-1 to 2-6. (Available from the Commonwealth of Massachusetts Executive Office of Human Services, Department of Public Health, 150 Tremont Street, Boston, MA.)

Hoff, R., Berardi, V., Weiblen, B., Mahoney-Trout, L., Mitchell, M., & Grady, G. (1988, March 3). Seroprevalence of human immunodeficiency virus among childbearing women. *New England Journal of Medicine, 318,* 525-529.

Karthas, N., & Dodwell, A. (1988). The children's AIDS program: Nursing challenges. In R. Schinazi & A. Nahmias (Eds.), *AIDS in children, adolescents & heterosexual adults: An interdisciplinary approach to prevention,* pp. 288-289. New York: Elsevier Science Publishing Co.

Karthas, N., Dodwell, A., Foschia, J., Lamb, G., & Liebling, L. (1988). The Children's AIDS program—A model for the development and implementation of a comprehensive residential program for children with HIV infection. In R. Schinazi & A. Nahmias (Eds.), *AIDS in children, adolescents & heterosexual adults: An interdisciplinary approach to prevention,* pp. 313-314. New York: Elsevier Science Publishing Co.

Kastner, T., & Friedman, B.A. (1988). Pediatric acquired immune deficiency syndrome and the prevention of mental retardation. *Journal of Developmental and Behavioral Pediatrics, 9*(1), 47-48.

Lipshultz, S., Chanock, S., Sanders, S., Colan, S., Perez-Atayde, A., & McIntosh, K. (1988). Cardiac manifestation of pediatric human immunodeficiency virus (HIV) infection. *IV International Conference on AIDS. Book 1. Final Program, Abstracts,* 400. (Abstract No. 7091.) Stockholm, Sweden: Stockholm International Fairs.

Oleske, J. (1987). Natural history of HIV infection II. In B.K. Silverman & A. Waddell (Eds.), *Report of the surgeon general's workshop on children with*

HIV infection and their families. (DHHS Publication No. HRS-D-MC87-1). Rockville, MD: U.S. Dept. of Health and Human Services.

Pizzo, P.A., Eddy, J., Falloon, J., Balis, F., Maha, M., Lehrman, S., Yarchoan, R., Broder, S., & Poplack, D.G. (1988). Continuous intravenous administration of AZT to children with symptomatic HIV infection. *IV International Conference on AIDS. Book 1. Final Program, Abstracts,* 256. (Abstract No. 3146.) Stockholm, Sweden: Stockholm International Fairs.

Rogers, M. (1987). Transmission of human immunodeficiency virus in the United States. In B.K. Silverman & A. Waddell (Eds.), *Report of the surgeon general's workshop on children with HIV infection and their families.* (DHHS Publication No. HRS-D-MC87-1). Rockville, MD: U.S. Dept. of Health and Human Services.

Scott, G. (1987). Natural history of HIV infection I. In B.K. Silverman & A. Waddell (Eds.), *Report of the surgeon general's workshop on children with HIV infection and their families.* (DHHS Publication No. HRS-D-MC87-1). Rockville, MD: U.S. Dept. of Health and Human Services.

Willoughby, A., Mendez, H., Hittelman, J., Holman, S., Goeder, J., Novello, A., & Landesman, S. (1988). Epidemiology of the perinatal transmission of human immunodeficiency virus (HIV). *IV International Conference on AIDS. Book 2. Program and Abstracts,* 293. (Abstract No. 6588.) Stockholm, Sweden: Stockholm International Fairs.

Chapter 14

Teaching Safer Sex

Jeanne Watson Driscoll

- A woman of conservative sexual and religious background is married to a man with previous homosexual experiences, who recently engaged in some episodic homosexual encounters. Now recommitted to each other, they decline any method of birth control due to their religious beliefs. What are their teaching needs?

- A man with a previous history of intravenous drug use has been free from addiction for two years. He is now engaged to be married. What are his teaching needs?

- A young woman in her first year of college is just beginning to become sexually active. She is certain that none of the men she knows could have ever engaged in intravenous drug use or homosexual activity. What are her teaching needs?

The above situations describe people who probably do *not* want to hear about their risk for human immunodeficiency virus. Awareness of their risk threatens their religious practices, childbearing plans, or trust in relationships. Allowing these people to slip through the health care system without equipping them with accurate knowledge for decision making about safer sex constitutes negligence in nursing practice. Yet, assessing, teaching, and counseling clients about sexual issues feels uncomfortable for many of us. This chapter aims to increase confidence in sexual assessment and teaching by outlining the information needed as well as addressing the feelings involved when discussing sexual concerns.

Gaining Comfort in Teaching and Counseling

As nurses, our effectiveness in sexual counseling depends on our awareness of our attitudes and how they influence our nursing practice (Hogan, 1985; Mandel, 1982). Ask yourself these questions:
- Do I feel that sex is a private matter, outside the nursing domain?
- Was I brought up to believe that sexual discussions are taboo?
- Do I have strong views about sexual standards of behavior and lack of respect for others whose views are different?
- Do I tend to deny my own sexual vulnerability to HIV exposure and, therefore, minimize my clients' vulnerability?

We do not need to change our viewpoints in order to be effective in our nursing care, just be *aware* of them. The more comfortably we claim our own value systems, the easier it becomes to accept and reinforce others in whatever choices they make. When we are aware of our own attitudes, we can more readily separate them from our practice, acknowledging each individual's right to choose behavior for oneself.

We can increase comfort with discussing sexual issues if we think of sex in the same line as other physiological and relational functions. We easily question clients on such personal issues as bowel and bladder function, yet questions about sexual behaviors often seem like an intrusion. However, sex serves many needs, all of which are vulnerable to illness and disease. As a method of intimate communication, sexual behavior can be critical to role and relational needs, an important mode for emotional expression. People also view their sexuality as a measurement of their desirability or ability to be loved (Strawn, 1987). By giving the client the option to discuss sexual concerns, we create opportunities to build the client's self-esteem, interpersonal communications, and the social support network.

We can begin to overcome self-consciousness about sexual issues by seeking professional situations that allow us to discuss and explore clients' sexual needs. Often, we lack an example or a role model for how to present sexual issues in a professional, objective, and clinical way. By attending professional workshops, courses, even videotapes that deal with various aspects of sexuality, we gain skill and experience in a safe, colleagueal environment, equipping us to discuss more comfortably sexual concerns with our clients. The more comfortable we feel in initiating a conversation about sexual behavior, the more comfortable our clients will feel in using us as a resource.

Conducting a Sexual Assessment

Why

We do a sexual assessment for the same reason we assess other physiological and relational patterns: to discover and help solve problems that may be unrelated to the medical diagnosis. The AIDS epidemic has made sexual assessment even more of a critical nursing function. By identifying people who might be putting themselves at risk and by providing information and counseling, we can help prevent further infection and save lives.

A sexual assessment not only helps us to identify clients' needs, but also allows clients to bring their concerns to us. Just as clients hesitate to talk about death, they are also afraid to ask about sexual concerns unless the health care professional indicates permission to do so. Many people are more comfortable discussing their personal concerns or seeking information from an objective professional than from sexual partners or other personal contacts. By initiating the topic of sexual concerns, we offer ourselves as a resource.

How To Do a Sexual Assessment

1. Create a comfortable environment; ensure privacy. Close doors, draw curtains, or keep voice tones softly audible. If family members are present, discuss with the client whether or not to ask them to leave, thus allowing the client both privacy and control of the environment.

2. Incorporate the sexual assessment into the overall nursing assessment. Begin with a statement such as: "As nurses, we want to understand how the illness/hospitalization has affected your life and, if possible, suggest strategies to promote healthy sexuality, when needed."

3. Approach in a nonjudgmental, open interviewing style. Encourage the client to disclose sexual orientation (homosexual, heterosexual, or bisexual). Due to the social prejudice against gay men and lesbians, many clients are reluctant to divulge this information unless they sense permission and acceptance from the nurse. By allowing clients to identify themselves, we affirm that identity and self-concept.

4. Collaborate with the client regarding health needs, education, and counseling. Allow the client to control the interview. Explain to clients their right to refuse to answer any questions and emphasize their right to confidentiality and privacy. This conveys respect for the client and helps to build trust. Discuss with clients what you plan to disclose in the chart.

5. Progress from general to specific questions that introduce sexual topics smoothly as well as give the client more control over topics to be discussed. The critical questions move easily from reproductive areas to issues of sexual functioning and behavior, as outlined in Tables 14.1 and 14.2 on pages 170-171.

6. Use language that is comfortable for you, but check that the client understands your meaning. Many people are unaware of the physiological terminology for sexual practices, but are afraid or embarrassed to admit their lack of knowledge. Table 14.3 on page 171 provides common terms used to describe sexual functioning (Elmassian & Wilson, 1982; Hogan, 1985; Krozy, 1978).

Compiling the Information

Having gathered a data base, you can identify any problems in collaboration with the client. Clients may decline to discuss sexual issues, leaving you with little or no

Table 14.1 *Sexual Assessment: Female*

- Do you remember when you got your first period?
- Do you have any problem with your periods? Do you experience heavy bleeding, pain, irregularity?
- When did you have your last period? (This information will allow the nurse to provide sanitary products, if necessary, during the hospitalization.)
- Have you ever been pregnant? If yes, how often? Any live children, abortions, miscarriages, stillbirths?
- When was your last Pap smear or GYN examination? Do you have regular GYN checkups?
- Do you perform breast self-exams? Any lumps, discomfort in the breasts? Any discharges?
- Currently, are you sexually active?
- Do you practice contraceptive methods/birth control? If yes, what type? Are you satisfied with this method? If no, is there a reason why you don't?
- Have you had any problems with vaginal infection, discharge, burning, or itching? If yes, encourage discussion regarding problem.
- Have you ever had any sexually transmitted diseases, e.g., syphilis, gonorrhea, chlamydia, trichomonas?
- Are you satisfied with your sexual abilities? If yes, proceed with next question. If no, is there anything you would like to share with me?
- Have you had more than one partner/lover in the last ten years?
- Are you aware of the AIDS epidemic?
- Can you share with me your understanding of how the AIDS virus is transmitted?
- Have you heard of safer sex techniques and/or risk reduction behaviors? If yes, please share with me your understanding of these. If no, it will be important to educate prior to discharge.
- Has this illness affected your sexual functioning?
- Do you have any questions/concerns regarding sexual behaviors and sexuality?
- Do you have any additional questions/concerns?

Table 14.2 *Sexual Assessment: Male*

- Have you ever had any urinary tract infections?
- Any problems with urination (difficulty starting to urinate, pain, dribbling)?
- Have you noticed any lumps or changes in your testicles? Do you perform testicular examinations on yourself or does your partner?

Table 14.2 *Sexual Assessment: Male* (continued)

- Have you ever been diagnosed with any sexually transmitted diseases? If yes, when and what treatment?
- Currently, are you sexually active?
- Have you had more than one partner/lover in the last ten years?
- Currently, do you use contraceptive methods during intercourse, i.e., condoms?
- Are you aware of the AIDS epidemic?
- Can you share with me your understanding of how the AIDS virus is transmitted?
- Have you heard of safer sex techniques and/or risk reduction behaviors? If yes, please share with me your understanding of these. If no, it will be important to educate prior to discharge.
- Are you satisfied with your sexual functioning? If yes, proceed with next question. If no, is there anything you would like to share with me?
- Has this illness affected your sexual functioning? If yes, is there anything you would like to share?
- Do you have any additional questions/concerns?

Table 14.3 *Sexual Expressions (Slang)*

breasts	boobs, bosom, bust, jugs, knockers, sacks, tits
climax	come, orgasm
clitoris	clit
cunnilingus	eat, give head, go down
erection	bone, hard-on, stiff
fellatio	blow job, cocksucking, give head, go down, suck
intercourse	ball, bang, coitus, fuck, get laid, make love, score, screw, sleep with
masturbation	beat the meat, hand fuck, hand job, jerk off
menstruation	curse, friend, on the rag, period
penis	cock, dick, john, joint, organ, peter, prick, rod, thing
pubic hair	beaver, bush
semen	cum, juice
testes	balls, nuts
vagina	beaver, box, cunt, hole, pussy, snatch, twat

SOURCE: Adapted from Hogan, R., 1985.

information. People may need time to develop a sense of trust in us, waiting for a later opportunity to tap us for sexual information. Others have no need for our services or seek help elsewhere. Our role is to offer our services and allow our clients options. By introducing the topic, we communicate to our clients respect for their choices and our willingness to be a resource.

Any problems identified from the assessment form nursing diagnoses, from which goals and plans flow for the nursing care plan (Elmassian & Wilson, 1982; Gordon, 1982). Examples of potential nursing diagnoses include:

- knowledge deficit regarding safer sex techniques/risk reduction behaviors
- sexual concerns regarding safer sex techniques, decreased ability to eroticize
- concerns regarding intimacy and sexuality based on alterations in body image due to specific disease state
- grief reaction secondary to changes in sexual functioning
- celibacy secondary to ineffective coping with the fear of AIDS
- sexual dysfunction secondary to ___ (specify)

Teaching Safer Sex

All clients need to be made aware of how to avoid the transmission of HIV regardless of their risk potential. By disseminating accurate information about HIV transmission, we enhance the protection of everyone as well as decrease the myths and fantasies surrounding AIDS that so cruelly contribute to discrimination. By providing consistent, correct information, we empower clients to make positive choices regarding their sexual practices after discharge.

Table 14.4 outlines the content for teaching safer sexual practices, while Table 14.5 provides specific guidelines for condom use. These guidelines can be summarized as: *Do not allow one person's semen, blood, vaginal secretions, or lactating mother's milk into another person's body* (Shaw & Paleo, 1986). Many public health departments and local AIDS community organizations provide excellent audiovisual materials as well as pamphlets for teaching aides, as shown in Figure 14.1 on page 175. Be sure to provide time for clients to *discuss* issues with you.

Determining what is safe and what is not calls for an understanding of probability, the foundation of scientific investigation. As nurses, we need to assess our clients' needs in regard to self-determination versus concrete black and white guidelines. The highly educated person will probably comprehend that "possibly safer sex practices" means there might be a low risk of transmission: Few, if any, cases of HIV transmission have been documented by these modes. However, some clients will need simple, basic do's and don'ts. We need to evaluate our clients' needs and individualize the content according to their ability to comprehend the information, their need to make choices, and their willingness to comply. With the more reluctant client, we might want to stress reduction of only high-risk practices, thus setting realistic goals for behavior change.

Table 14.4 *Safer Sex Guidelines*

1. Risk-free behaviors:
   - Massage (without genital stimulation): As you discuss this behavior, you may also want to discuss with the client how massage can be a method of relaxation as well as shared intimacy. It may be helpful to discuss how both client and partner can use oils and lotions as well as create the environment to promote sensuality and eroticism.
   - Mutual masturbation/pleasuring techniques: These behaviors are relatively safe as long as the skin is healthy and free of lesions/open areas. Many people have not learned to masturbate, or may view these behaviors as "dirty" or "sinful," depending on their cultural/religious upbringing. If this is the case, they may need to be referred to a counselor or sex therapist.
   - Social kissing and hugging.
   - Frottage (body-to-body rubbing): This behavior utilizes the erotic sensations of touch and can be combined with massage.
   - The use of sex toys (dildos) that are not shared with partners
   - Casual contact: hand holding, arm holding, shaking hands, etc.
   - Voyeurism and fantasy

2. Low-risk behaviors:
   - Intimate kissing (also known as deep kissing and/or French kissing): Penetration of tongue into partner's mouth. It is important that the mouth not have any open sores or lesions or any evidence of bleeding gums.
   - Fellatio (oral sex) without ingestion of seminal fluid or semen. Risk is further reduced with use of condom.
   - Cunnilingus (oral stimulation of the female genitals): Protective covering of the female genitalia will further reduce risk (dental dams, Saran wrap).
   - Vaginal intercourse with the use of a properly applied condom
   - Rectal intercourse with the use of a properly applied condom
   - Use of shared sex toys that are cleaned in between uses and covered with a condom for penetration
   - External water sports: urination on one's partner

3. High-risk behaviors:
   - Ingestion of semen or vaginal/cervical secretions
   - Vaginal and/or anal intercourse without the use of a condom
   - Sharing sex toys
   - Analingus (oral-anal contact, also known as "rimming")
   - Piercing or drawing blood during sexual behaviors
   - Fisting: Penetration of the anus with one's fist

SOURCE: Adapted from Bay Area Physicians for Human Rights, 1985; Bjorklund, 1987.

Table 14.5 *Guidelines for Condom Use*

Important Information About Condoms

1. Condoms can be very effective in preventing the spread of HIV if used correctly.
2. Condoms can break—breakage can be eliminated with proper use.
3. Condoms decrease sensation—orgasm can be delayed.
4. Use only water-based lubricants. Lubricants with nonoxynol-9 can kill HIV if condoms should break.
5. Condoms should be used only once.
6. Lambskin condoms should be avoided because they may leak virus.
7. Initially, condom use can be anxiety provoking. Many men have found that masturbating while wearing them has made them more comfortable before trying them out with a partner.
8. Condom use can be more erotic if worked into foreplay.
9. Condoms have slight variations in sizes and shapes. Users should be encouraged to experiment with different brands.
10. Reservoir-tip condoms are preferred because there is space to ejaculate.

Instructions for Use

1. Slightly unroll condom.
2. Fill the reservoir tip with lubricant with or without nonoxynol-9. If no lubricant is being used, pinch the reservoir tip to prevent air from occupying the reservoir—air in the tip may promote breakage.
3. Unroll condom as far as it will go.
4. Withdraw immediately after intercourse, holding onto the base of the condom.

Christopher L. LaCharite, unpublished work, 1988.

When you discuss sexual behaviors, you may hear themes of loss or sadness. These themes are part of the grieving process. Many of our clients will be mourning the loss of specific sexual behaviors: the way sex used to be, spontaneous and without protection. These themes may also emerge with feelings of fear, denial, and anger about the "whys" and "why nows." Acknowledge the loss and encourage the verbalization of feelings. By encouraging the grief process, we help clients work through the feelings to reach acceptance of risk reduction behaviors in their lives. Table 14.6 outlines the stages of sexual behavior change, the developmental steps necessary for incorporating safer sex into one's lifestyle. These stages can happen in any particular order or simultaneously, depending on the individual (Palacios-Jimenez & Shernoff, 1986).

What the well dressed man is wearing to bed.

SO YOU THINK YOU KNOW HOW TO USE A CONDOM?

Since condoms leak or break, they aren't a sure guarantee against transmission of the "AIDS virus". However, they do reduce your risk, and, <u>used properly,</u> they rarely break. Some simple do's and don't's of condom usage are:

DO Put the condom on BEFORE you enter your partner.
DO Make sure there is no air in the condom, including the tip.
DO Use plenty of <u>water-based</u> lubricant. (Examples: K-Y jelly, For-Play, PrePair, and Probe) NEVER USE SALIVA!
DO Hold on to the base of the condom when you're pulling out after intercourse to prevent it from coming off inside your partner.
DO Use a fresh condom each time you have sex.

DON'T Use oil- or petroleum-based lubricants. (Examples: Baby Oil, Vaseline, Vaseline Intensive Care, Elbow Grease, Crisco)
DON'T Use old or misused condoms. (For example, condoms you've kept in your wallet.)
DON'T Wait until halfway after you begin sex to put a condom on.
DON'T Blow a condom up to test it. This weakens them.
DON'T Re-use condoms EVER!

THE A-B-C'S OF PUTTING ON A CONDOM

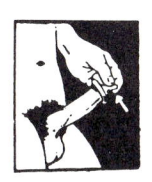

←A Gently squeeze the tip of the condom with one hand, making sure there is no air in the tip. (This leaves room for the semen when you ejaculate [cum], and forces out any air bubbles, which are a major reason condoms break.)

→B While you continue to squeeze the tip of the condom, forcing out any air, begin to unroll the condom down the length of your penis...

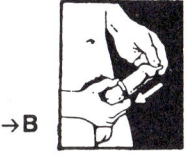

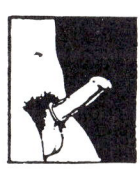

←C ...carefully unrolling it all the way down to the base of your penis to the hair.

Figure 14.1 Example of Patient-Teaching Handout

Table 14.6 *Stages of Safer Sexual Behavior Change*

1. *Grief:* feeling the loss of sexual expression as it used to be.
2. *Affirmation:* acknowledging the need to change sexual practices.
3. *Knowledge:* learning how to practice safer sex.
4. *Eroticizing:* imagining safer sex as stimulating and satisfying.
5. *Negotiating:* arranging with sexual partner to practice safer methods.
6. *Implementation:* using safer sex practices.

SOURCE: Adapted from Palacios-Jimenez & Shernoff, 1986.

Teaching safer sex is not simply telling people what not to do. Since sexual expression strikes a deep chord in self-concept and self-expression, we need to allow our clients to express their feelings regarding changes in their sexual behaviors. Our goal in discussing safer sex techniques is to facilitate satisfactory sexual relationships within the context of risk reduction behavior. Information alone will not necessarily lead to behavior change. We need to deal with the feelings. Unless clients feel good about themselves and their sexuality, they will have difficulty making the choice to practice risk reduction behavior with their partners. For many, safer sex practices need to be presented in a manner that promotes sensuality and erotic feelings. Rather than simply stressing what clients should avoid, equally emphasize what practices are permissible. Elaborate on the interpersonal, intimate aspects of safer sex practices, which promote satisfaction in feelings of closeness to another person. Many community agencies offer programs for eroticizing safer sex, which can be used for referral.

Barriers to Safer Sex Practices

1. Fear of Rejection

People may perceive that their partners will refuse to follow safer sex guidelines or refuse to have sex with them. These fears may exist regardless of the context of the sexual relationship, long-standing or short-term. Teaching safer sex includes helping people feel important enough to deserve protection from infection as well as vulnerable enough to need it. Depending on the obstacles indicated by the client, role-playing a conversation may help clients to initiate more readily safer sex methods with their partners.

2. Denying Vulnerability

Often, people need to feel they can trust their intimates. Safer sex implies a lack of trust and, therefore, contradicts values associated with intimate sexual relationships. Another component to denying vulnerability includes refusing to acknowledge any association with a high-risk group. "I'm not a drug addict! I've only shot up a couple times!" One way to counter this obstacle is to point out that everyone who is sexually active with more than one partner is vulnerable. Decreasing associations with "risk groups" and emphasizing risk *behaviors,* such as sexual activity, tends to decrease the stigma associated with using safer sex.

3. Fatalistic Attitudes

Some people feel "It's too late for me. I'm already infected. Why should I worry about anyone infecting me?" Even clients who have tested positive for HIV should protect themselves against reinfection, as well as protecting their partners. Multiple exposures to the HIV virus or exposure to other sexually transmitted diseases are thought to be two factors that contribute to the development of symptoms.

4. Failure to Eroticize

"Safer sex is dull and unexciting." Explore with these clients what sex means to them: the excitement of risk-taking, the affirmation of an identity, or sexual desirability. Try to find out what is really being threatened by using safer sex methods, as well as speaking to the expressed concern on eroticism.

5. Lack of Faith in Intervention

Clients may refuse to use safer sex methods due to disbelief that they work. Explain that latex condoms have been shown effective at blocking the virus, and that populations using safer sex methods show less incidence of acquiring the infection (Friedland & Klein, 1987). This obstacle to behavior change may be more than simply ignorance or lack of trust in scientific evidence. For the client who is sexually active, it may be partially denial of vulnerability. For the client choosing celibacy, it may be coming to terms with mortality or sexual orientation. Encourage clients to verbalize and listen carefully to help them identify associated issues. Offer the option of sexual counseling with a supportive therapist.

Summary

Risk reduction depends on the individual's decisions. We provide our clients with all the information to make knowledgeable decisions. We affirm their self-esteem and self-awareness to enable them to negotiate with their sexual partners. By encouraging our clients to discuss sexual issues in an accepting atmosphere, we equip them to protect themselves and their partners against HIV transmission. The rest is up to them.

References

AIDS Action Education (1986). So you think you know how to use a condom? Available from AIDS Action Committee, 661 Boylston Street, Boston, MA 02116.

Bay Area Physicians for Human Rights. (1985, June). *AIDS safe-sex guidelines.* Available from San Francisco AIDS Foundation, 333 Valencia Street, Fourth Floor, San Francisco, CA 94103.

Bjorklund, E. (1987). Prevention: Reducing the risk of AIDS. In J.D. Durham and F.L. Cohen (Eds.), *The person with AIDS: Nursing prospectives,* (pp. 178-191). New York: Springer.

Elmassian, B.J., & Wilson, R.W. (1982). Assessment and diagnosis of sexual problems. *Nurse Practitioner, 7,* 13-22.

Friedland, G.H., & Klein, R.S. (1987). Transmission of the human immunodeficiency virus. *New England Journal of Medicine, 317,* 1125-1135.

Gordon, M. (1982). *Nursing diagnosis: Process and application.* New York: McGraw-Hill.

Hogan, R. (1985). *Human sexuality: A nursing perspective.* Norwalk, CT: Appleton-Century-Crofts.

Krozy, R. (1978). Becoming comfortable with sexual assessment. *American Journal of Nursing, 78,* 1036-1038.

Mandel, A. (1982). Getting the most from patient interviews. *Nursing '82, 12*(11), 46-49.

Palacios-Jimenez, L., & Shernoff, M. (1986). *Facilitator's guide to hot, horny and healthy: Eroticizing safer sex.* Available from Department of Education, Gay Men's Health Crisis, Box 274, 132 W. 24 Street, New York, NY 10011.

Shaw, N., & Paleo, L. (1986). Women and AIDS. In L. McKusick (Ed.), *What to do about AIDS* (pp. 142-154). Berkeley, CA: University of California Press.

Strawn, J. (1987). The psychosocial consequences of AIDS. In J.D. Durham and F.L. Cohen (Eds.), *The person with AIDS: Nursing prospectives,* (pp. 126-149). New York: Springer.

Part IV

Different Ways of Comforting

Chapter 15

Complementary Therapies: Maximizing the Mind-Body Connection

Jill M. Strawn

A diagnosis of AIDS is not necessarily a death sentence, but transforming that diagnosis into an opportunity for healing demands total commitment. The decision to live must be total, involving every thought, cell, habit, and belief.
—Jason Serinus

Many people with HIV infection are rapidly turning to complementary therapies, such as acupuncture, meditation, massage, guided imagery, and spiritual healing. Consisting of a wide variety of approaches, complementary therapies are characterized by: (a) existing outside the Western allopathic repertoire, (b) requiring a relatively active participation on the part of the consumer, and (c) taking into account the whole person as the context for the illness being treated. They have been widely used to treat cancer and other chronic illnesses. The medical establishment by and large dismisses the whole idea *and* those well-educated researchers who think there may be something to it (Robbins, 1988). Are these complementary therapies quackery or the secret to understanding how individuals can actively participate in their own healing process?

The lack of effective, safe, and affordable treatments for HIV infection sets the stage for self-help approaches, under-the-counter medications, and even greedy opportunists who take advantage of desperate people. As nurses, we know that clients look to us for guidance in health areas that are complex and unfamiliar. What will you say if your HIV-positive client asks you for your opinion of the multitudes of complementary therapies? How can you be knowledgeable about all the rapidly growing approaches? What if *you* don't believe they are worth pursuing? How would you suggest people get started if they are sure about wanting to try something more than the doctor has ordered? This chapter will provide you with an understanding of how complementary therapies might work, what they are, who might benefit from them, and how to find resources for individuals no matter where they live.

Mind-Body Connections

As a group, nurses have long believed that human beings are more than just their physical parts (Blattner, 1981; Ehrenreich & English, 1973; Krieger, 1981; Nightingale, 1969). Nursing stresses the total person—mind, body, and spirit—and attempts to assess individual states of health and illness from that perspective. While the medical model focuses on disease and reductionism, nursing models tend to be integrative and holistic. This difference in viewing people and illness creates much misunderstanding and tension between nursing and medicine (Melosh, 1982). Belief in mind-body unity is at least as old as the written word. It wasn't until Descartes espoused the separation of mind and body function (1637) that this separatist belief took hold so widely.

Centuries later, Western medicine developed in a reductionist manner, creating specialty after specialty that looked only at one particular organ system or part of the body. The extreme consequence of this approach is the belief that people's feelings, life experiences, support systems, and environments have no significant influence on their physical well-being. Single factors such as viruses, bacteria, or genetics are believed to be the sole cause of disease. This is a male, militaristic view of an identified enemy that can be targeted with a heavy-artillery approach or "magic bullet" (Reuben, 1986).

Recent advances in the sciences support the mind-body connection. Pathogens carry only the *potential* for illness. The host environment determines the extent of their impact or damage. If someone is experiencing physical exhaustion, malnutrition, clinical depression, or an interpersonal crisis of some kind, illness is more likely to manifest itself (Justice, 1987).

An exciting new research field, psychoneuroimmunology (PNI), explores the interconnectedness of the mind (consciousness) and central nervous system with immune function. Many health professionals and researchers believe that stress, grief, and depression cause immunosuppression and have been associated with the onset of various diseases (Ader, 1981; Pelletier & Herzing, 1988; Pert, 1986; Solomon, 1985). If negative thoughts and emotions can decrease immune response, can positive ones increase it? Can individuals actually improve their immune status through attitude change, positive emotional states, and other behavioral and psychological modifications? So far, research suggests that several complementary therapies can be effective in some instances: clinical biofeedback, meditation, autogenic training, Jacobson's progressive relaxation, hypnosis, general relaxation, behavioral modification, and visualization techniques (Pelletier & Herzing, 1988).

Some theorists propose that there lies a yet undetected healing system in the human body that manifests itself only when challenged (Cousins, 1982; O'Regan, 1987). Complementary therapies attempt to tap human resources for healing that are often ignored by conventional medicine. Based on a philosophy of holistic health, complementary therapies view the whole person in context with the environment.

Practitioners of most complementary therapies stress that all healing takes place from within the individual. The therapies are intended to restore the clients' equilibrium so that their own healing processes can take over. Healing does not necessarily equal cure, though one may certainly lead to the other. Clients pursuing complementary therapies should know that their quality of life is likely to improve, but that cure is not guaranteed and perhaps should not always be the primary goal.

Complementary therapies were formally called alternative therapies, implying a different option for treatment from traditional medicine. Practitioners are increasingly considering complementary therapy as a helpful counterpart or balance to medication.

Complementary health care/therapies fall into the following categories:

1. Accepted medical techniques applied in a new manner, e.g., hypnosis for weight control.

2. New techniques for old problems, e.g., biofeedback pain control.

3. Nonmedical techniques for health problems, e.g., polarity therapy, massage, visualization, and imagery in the treatment of cancer.

4. Non-Western unscientific techniques: highly organized health systems, concepts, and practices that exist apart from Western scientific medicine, e.g., Chinese acupuncture, Native American healing systems (Blattner, 1981).

Long-Term Survivors of AIDS

We are now aware that there are success stories related to persons with HIV infection (Badgley, 1986; Bolen, 1985; Callen, 1987; Jacobs & Serinus, 1987; Reuben, 1986). Not all HIV-infected persons are dying within a year or two of diagnosis. Some people have survived more than five years. Some are doing wonderfully well, living active and productive lives. The influence of all the negative media surrounding the deaths and pain caused by the epidemic creates "negative programming" in health care workers, the general public, and HIV-infected individuals. We cannot allow an HIV-positive confirmation, AIDS, or ARC diagnosis to be interpreted as an automatic death sentence. There is much to be hopeful about, and nurses must convey this news.

George Solomon, a researcher in psychoneuroimmunology, recently studied long-term survivors of AIDS. His most famous client was diagnosed with ARC in 1983 and, shortly thereafter, with AIDS. This man developed PCP twice, cryptococcus once, and lymphoma, for which he underwent chemotherapy. He is now free of any signs of cancer or infection. His physician described this client's attitude:

> He is feisty as hell. He seeks out treatments. He takes charge of his own care. He doesn't put up with anything. He has the fiercest determination to live I have ever seen. He has projects; he is involved. He is now teaching in college and his helper cell count is 28. (Normal count is between 500 and 1500.) This also shows that with 28 helper cells, which 'ain't too good,' you can still live, which shows you can't just go by the lab workup. Of course, he is on treatment, too, AZT (Solomon, 1988, p. 10).

Cancer as a Rehearsal for AIDS

If the above sounds familiar, it is because this resembles the profile that has emerged from years of studying survivors of cancer. A strong will to live and particular personality characteristics are major contributing factors in the treatment results of some kinds of cancer. A Type C coping pattern consisting of conformity, compliance, self-sacrifice, and suppression of emotion, particularly anger, has been described by Temoshok and others as leading to an unfavorable prognosis of cancer, and possibly to susceptibility to cancer initially (Locke & Colligan, 1988; Solomon, 1988).

Because cancer is ultimately a problem of immune function, there are similarities in the approaches to self-healing for cancer and AIDS. People with cancer have long sought out the gamut of nonmedical therapy approaches. As a result of their experiences, this field has matured in a way that benefits people with HIV infection. Seasoned practitioners of complementary therapies who have been working with seriously ill individuals for many years are now working with people who have HIV infection. Many reference books about self-healing are available for clinicians and laypeople. There is scientific data on some of the self-help modalities. In short, we are not starting from the beginning. For those who choose to educate themselves and seek out experienced practitioners, the risk of quackery is minimal.

Common Complementary Therapies

Visualization and Imagery

As the holistic health movement was burgeoning in the late seventies, Carl and Stephanie Simonton (1978) proposed visualization and imagery for self-healing. Emphasizing active participation, they describe a daily meditation that involved visualizing one's cancer in some symbolic form and picturing a victory over the unwanted cells. Reports on success of imagery have been largely word-of-mouth and through clinical observation. The popularity of the method grew, however, and became assimilated into many self-help programs for people with cancer. More recently, a similar approach advocated by a charismatic surgeon in his book, *Love, Medicine, and Miracles,* has caused a resurgence of interest (Siegel, 1986).

Attitudinal Healing

Louise Hay healed herself of vaginal cancer without medical intervention (1984). She believes that since all "disease" has a spiritual origin of not loving oneself, individuals can heal themselves through a program of self-love. She recommends the use of meditation, forgiving others and oneself for past behaviors, and positive affirmations to create a new positive mindset, along with taking care of one's body. Her message of hope and acceptance has won strong acceptance among people with HIV infection, who report an enhanced quality of life and better health (Hay, 1986).

Healing Groups

People with HIV infection who have a spiritual orientation toward healing have formed healing groups or circles: various-sized groups who meet on a regular basis for personal support in one's efforts to be healed. Some of the groups are based solely on Louise Hay's philosophy, modeled after her weekly sessions of 400-600 persons. Other groups draw on a variety of spiritual traditions—utilizing prayer, laying on of hands, meditation, and chanting, as well as discussion. Many are associated with organized churches. Some groups are HIV-specific, others include any concern, treating both the ill and the healthy.

Diet Therapies

Proponents of various diets often make appealing claims about the positive consequences of following their approach. Some diets are only one aspect of a lifestyle or philosophical or spiritual world views. One such diet perspective is macrobiotics, based on the Oriental belief that disease is caused by imbalances in yin and yang energy. At the base of all diets is a belief that the right foods can help heal mental and physical problems. The role of good nutrition and a balanced diet for optimal health is well-accepted across both traditional and nontraditional lines of belief. General dietary recommendations reflect these beliefs, calling for decreases in the amount of calories that come from fatty foods and refined sugars, and increases in the intake of whole-grained products and fresh fruits and vegetables. More recently, diets that purportedly boost the immune system have appeared, clearly focusing on the HIV threat.

Thymus Gland Stimulation

Treatments focused on stimulating or renewing thymus function are being pursued by the complementary therapies approach, as well as through formal research. The thymus gland is located at the top of the breastbone above the heart. It is most active in the first seven years of life and is 50 percent atrophied by adulthood. A critical component of the immune system, the thymus imprints T-lymphocytes with their characteristic surface antigens. T-lymphocytes (T-cells) form antibodies and attack foreign invaders, but are also the specific target of HIV. It is believed that the thymus gland can be stimulated through use of organically bound iodine, iron and mineral substances, chlorophyll, wheat grass juice, barley greens, homeopathic thymus extract, and thymosis (Serinus, 1986). By stimulating the thymus gland, T-lymphocyte production might be increased.

Releasing Energy of Life

Ancient cultures had a recognition and explanation for the life energy that courses through all organisms. It was called by different names—*kopavi, ch'i,* or *prana*—and its flow was considered crucial for the well-being of all living things. Illness was believed to result from the blockage of this energy. Some of the complementary therapies that reflect this philosophy are included in Table 15.1, such as acupressure, acupuncture, crystals, and reiki.

Many modern holistic remedies recognize a similar basis for understanding symptoms and choosing treatment. In 1935, Harold Saxton Burr published his Electrodynamic Theory of Life, which stated that all living forms—humans, animals, trees, plants, and lower forms of life—possess and are controlled by electromagnetic fields. These organizing fields of life, or L-fields, can be measured and mapped with great precision (Russell, 1978). Recent technology known as magnetic resonance imaging (MRI) depicts the inside of the human body using magnetic energy. Possibly, this progression of sophisticated technology may be able to explain the basis for the ancient cultures' beliefs.

Table 15.1 *Bodywork and Oral Therapies*

Bodywork Therapies

Modality	Definition	Other Information
Acupressure	Deep massage at the sites of acupoints to stimulate or sedate the flow of *ch'i*.	Life energy, *ch'i*, flows continuously through the universe and humans; this flow occurs through particular conduits known as meridians, within which lie a series of localizations called acupoints, through which *ch'i* may be intercepted (Krieger, 1981).
Acupuncture	The insertion and twirling of very fine needles into acupoints to stimulate or sedate the flow of *ch'i*.	

Modality	Definition	Other Information
Chiropractic	The process of normalizing the structural and functional integrity of the nervous system through manipulation of the bones and joints.	A biomechanical approach to health that emphasizes the study of body mechanics, applied kinesiology, postural stability, vertebral adjustments, and the dynamic self-regulation control system of the body. Chiropractors have four years of training and are licensed in all states; they may offer general health and nutrition counseling; some states allow third-party reimbursement (Dintenfass, 1978).
Crystals	Quartz crystals are used during healing techniques to potentiate the energy of the healing source that is being directed into the client. Crystals can be used as an adjunct to meditation, focusing and purifying thoughts and intentions.	Crystal enthusiasts claim that the properties relevant to the scientific uses of quartz can be carried over to the human potential or spiritual movement—i.e., that its piezoelectric properties can be used to enhance personal growth (Duhamel, 1988).
Guided Imagery and Creative Visualization	The use of mental images to facilitate relaxation, healing, or desired behavior changes.	In guided imagery, the images are suggested by a therapist or narrator on an audio tape, while in creative visualization the individual draws upon his or her imagination.
Hatha Yoga	The use of various body positions and stretching in coordination with deep breathing to achieve a sense of awakening, balance, and stamina.	Hatha yoga is the beginning level of a system of physical, mental, and spiritual approaches to achieve unity with the supreme consciousness (Blattner, 1981).

Table 15.1 *Bodywork and Oral Therapies* (continued)

Modality	Definition	Other Information
Polarity Therapy	Manipulation practices using pressure points, stretching exercises, a diet that includes herbs, and studies of the flow and balance of energy in daily life.	Developed by Randolph Stone as a synthesis of Eastern and Western medicine and philosophy (Krieger, 1981).
Progressive Relaxation	An organized series of verbal suggestions of relaxation administered by a therapist, audio tape, or by oneself for the purpose of identifying and eliminating areas of tension.	Can be used alone or in conjunction with hypnosis, guided imagery, and visualization; music is often used as an adjunct.
Reiki	Universal energy is focused through the hands and applied in a systematic treatment to the body; the seven major *chakras,* or energy centers, of the body are balanced during a treatment.	The origins of Reiki are found in ancient Tibet and were rediscovered by Mikao Usui of Japan; Barbara Weber Ray founded the American Reiki Association in 1980.
Therapeutic Massage	Stimulation of muscle groups by stroking, pinching, vibration, shaking, and striking in a controlled manner; acupoints may be massaged.	The purpose of therapeutic massage is to help make the clients aware of their bodies in a positive way and reduce feelings of isolation through tactile affirmation; to improve cardiovascular and lymphatic circulation; to relieve constricted and congested tissues; to reduce effects of atrophy; to promote relaxation (McCormick & Riederer, 1986).

Modality	Definition	Other Information
Therapeutic Touch	An act of healing or helping that involves the use of hands to assess and intervene with the client's energy system; the client sits or lies comfortably while the practitioner works in a meditative state.	Therapeutic touch derives from, but is not the same as, laying on of hands; there is no religious belief involved or necessary; the client generally experiences relaxation, sometimes warmth; some conditions are helped by one treatment, while others require periodic attention; developed by Delores Krieger, Ph.D., R.N.

Oral Therapies

Algae		
Blue Green Manna	Aphana Klamathomenon flosaque, single-cell algae that grow in Klamath Lake in Oregon; an elemental and complete food substance rich in chlorophyll, eight essential amino acids, vitamins, lipids, and glycoproteins.	It is claimed to rejuvenate the thymus gland, stimulate the spleen, increase energy to the brain; detoxify the liver.
Spirulima	Contains high levels of beta carotene, gamma linoleic acid (GLA), iron, vitamin B 12.	Grows so fast it can produce 20 times more protein/acre than soybeans; it is claimed to decrease cholesterol, have anticancer properties, enhance iron and trace mineral absorption; immune system stimulator.
Flower Essences Bach Flower Remedies	Bach developed 38 remedies from flowers that are best understood as homeopathic dilutions, which help balance the mental, emotional, physical, and spiritual aspects of the individual.	He believed that the basis of disease is found in disharmony between the spiritual and mental aspects of a human being.

Table 15.1 *Bodywork and Oral Therapies* (continued)

Modality	Definition	Other Information
Herbal Remedies	Each plant has its own unique chemicals including alkaloids, polysaccharides, alcohol, and steroids. These chemicals can be extracted and used as medicines in the form of teas and powders.	Herbal medicine has a long history: Almost every ancient civilization used herbs as medicine; Oriental herbs are different from those common in the United States and are often prescribed in conjunction with acupuncture.
Homeopathy	A natural pharmaceutical science that uses various plant, mineral, or animal materials in very small doses to stimulate natural defenses.	The basis for this approach is the belief that a substance that produces symptoms in overdose in a healthy person cures these symptoms in microdose in an ill person. Practitioners of homeopathy were accepted in this country as a respected part of medicine until the AMA formed to oppose them; most other countries fully accept homeopathy.

The Underground Network

Given the lack of medical treatment options for HIV infection, clients display considerable interest in any experimental drugs that seem promising. Unfortunately, the Federal Drug Administration process for approving experimental drugs for use on human beings is long and costly. Many clients realize that they could be dead long before most drugs in the pipeline are approved. In the mid-1980s, people with HIV infection commonly traveled to Mexico for treatments not approved in the United States. In 1986, when rumors began to circulate about the hopefulness of ribavarian, a person with HIV infection in San Francisco set up an organization to purchase the drug in Mexico, distributing it at a discount in the U.S. This "buying club" became the model of organizations later started in New York City and other heavily HIV-infected areas. Other experimental drugs were added to the inventory, as were cut-rate AZT and generic pentamidine.

The classes of drugs most widely sought are antivirals and immune enhancers.

AL-721 and dextran sulfate are currently among the most popular. In addition to the buying clubs, there are also so-called "guerrilla clinics" where clients go to receive drugs they cannot administer themselves, such as dinitrochlorobenzene (DNCB). Newsletters detail information on all these drugs and how to obtain them. Project Inform in San Francisco operates an informational phone service and provides written materials on the drugs and some guidance on how to decide about getting involved. Martin Delaney, Project Inform's co-director, has stated that whether or not the drugs should prove efficacious, the sense of empowerment and participation on one's own care produces much healing (Kolata, 1988).

Under-the-counter experimental drugs are not considered holistic. They are included in this chapter only because they are linked in consumers' minds with all therapies not sanctioned by the medical community.

Responsibility Versus Blame

One of the thorniest issues in relaying the concept that people participate in their states of health is that of blame and guilt. Many critics of the idea of self-healing claim that expecting people to help and heal themselves sets them up for failure and self-blame if they fail to meet their goals for healing. This viewpoint confuses the focus of responsibility for participation versus responsibility for outcome.

The philosophical basis for complementary therapies emphasizes the clients' responsibility for active participation in therapy. It calls for people to choose therapies and actions, giving them a sense of control over their treatment. This control over treatment does *not* equal responsibility or control over outcome. We need to be aware that clients sometimes misinterpret this emphasis on self-help to think that they did something wrong if they are not healed: not believing enough, not practicing enough, not doing enough.

The client is responsible for applying the therapies, not making them work. Healing is up to the body (spirit). People add to the confusion of responsibility versus blame when they equate *healing* with *cure*. Most people who participate in complementary methods will probably experience some healing. They will not necessarily be cured. Those with a certain level of spiritual understanding can comprehend that healing can occur, and the client may still eventually die.

The Nurse's Role in Complementary Therapies

Assess the Client's Learning Needs

The following are some guidelines that can be used to assess a client's interest and readiness to explore alternative therapies:

- Client's physical status is stable or improving.
- Client's mental functioning is not sufficiently impaired by delirium, dementia, or depression.

- Does the client know about complementary therapies in general? for HIV infection?
- Is the client emotionally/spiritually prepared to hear about therapy that may heal without curing?
- Has the client thought about trying any particular methods?
- Nurses should evaluate what modality is best to start with: video tape, audio tape, article, book, or personal testimony, depending on client's reading ability, vision, and particular area of interest.

Offer Information

Clients have the right to know all the treatment modalities available to them. Since complementary therapies offer a sense of control and hope that traditional medicine lacks, people with HIV infection have found them a helpful addition to standard therapy. In offering information, always give clients a choice. Emphasize that complementary therapy does *not* eliminate the need for traditional approaches, but may be used to augment the effect of medication.

Be sensitive to the clients' needs. Some clients with undying faith in their physician may not tolerate hearing about complementary therapies. Respect whatever your clients' needs may be. Conversely, some clients may be looking for a miracle cure and misinterpret your information. Have clients explain back what they have heard you say and check for accuracy. An outline of the basic learning content is shown in Table 15.2.

Table 15.2 *Learning Content*

The progression of learning if one is starting from the basics:

1. People's lifestyle and mental health can contribute to vulnerability to illness.
2. People with physical and mental illness can influence their experience in a positive manner.
3. People with HIV infection are actively seeking treatment in addition to, or instead of, medical therapies to facilitate healing.
4. These approaches include:

nutritional supplements	hypnosis
diet therapies	guided imgery and creative visualization
herbal remedies	therapeutic touch
yoga	Reiki
acupuncture	polarity therapy
therapeutic massage	spiritual approaches to healing
progressive relaxation	

Remain Neutral

If you have difficulty believing in a therapeutic value to complementary treatments, consider the positive effects of hope and active participation in a chosen modality of care. Conversely, some people will choose to avoid complementary therapies due to a reluctance to change lifelong lifestyle habits, a disbelief in their own ability to change their fate, or the high cost of some of the therapies. The majority of the persons who have supported complementary therapies are middle- and upper-class white men. Unless these therapies are modified to be available and sensitive to the needs of people of various cultural, ethnic, or socioeconomic backgrounds, complementary therapies will probably remain a luxury item for an elite segment of those infected.

What if the attending physician is opposed to complementary therapies? As professional nurses, we always have a legal right to give our professional opinion, stating it as such (Benner, 1984). We also have the responsibility to avoid pressuring clients into our point of view. Just as we have the right to a different opinion from the physician's, our clients have the right to a different opinion from ours.

Advocate for the Client

Clients need to be open and honest with their physician about the complementary therapies they are using. Physicians should know the client's whole program in order to collect data accurately on new medications. Otherwise, changes in condition may be attributed solely to a medication when the client is also having acupuncture, meditating, and taking Chinese herbs. People often feel uncomfortable discussing complementary therapies with their doctors or divulging the use of under-the-counter medications. Ideally, clients would negotiate their use of complementary therapies when entering a relationship with a physician (Woods, 1988). Unfortunately, clients may initially meet physicians in the midst of an acute episode, or otherwise feel intimidated and dependent on their care, making such frank discussion impossible. As nurses, we may be more privy to complete information, helping clients to strategize and role-play approaches to a particular physician. Also, we may be able to recommend those care givers who are more likely to be open-minded regarding complementary therapies.

Help Clients Get Started

If the client has lifestyle behaviors that are clearly detrimental to health, starting with improving them makes sense. For example, a cigarette smoker, heavy drinker, or drug user should focus on eliminating that habit. In addition to whatever formal programs are available (AA, SmokeEnders, or drug treatment), some of the body-mind modalities may be useful in decreasing tension and symptoms of withdrawal: acupuncture, hypnosis, progressive relaxation with guided imagery. If a client's dietary habits have been poor, promoting change in that area may be the best place to start. If anxiety is an overriding problem, decreasing that symptom is a priority, since other learning will be difficult until anxiety is brought under control.

If there is no obvious place to start, try introducing the idea of a positive influence on the immune system through a combination of diet, visualization, and imagery. This, of course, can be done simultaneously with any other treatment modality, but care should be taken not to overwhelm the clients with new behaviors that lead them to feel unable to succeed in any. If a client has limited energy or reading ability, an audio tape is a good first step.

Locating Resources

Communities vary on the availability of local sources of complementary therapies. Here are some hints for finding them:

- Subscribe to one of the newsletters listed in the resource section at the end of this chapter; this will provide the latest information and mail-order accessibility of some products.
- Contact the local community-based AIDS organization to determine what resources they have available; ask if they have a referral list for practitioners of complementary therapies; have they gotten feedback on the people on the list?
- Determine which bookstore in the area carries the widest selection on holistic health/alternative therapies; review the inventory and make suggestions for additional stock, especially for AIDS-focused literature.
- Ask your employer to purchase appropriate books and newsletters for the nursing library.
- Take the resource list to your local library and ask if some or all of these volumes can be purchased.

The Bottom Line: Keeping Hope Alive

People with HIV infection need to be offered hope for increased quality of life as well as survival. Complementary therapies offer that hope. While it is not yet possible to say exactly how each therapy helps people, or to predict the likelihood of success for each approach, there are enough testimonies and positive clinical observations to justify making clients aware of their availability. Nurturing someone's will to live is a privilege that nurses must embrace. It can be done without ignoring the reality of the disease and in an individualized manner respectful of the person in our care.

Resources

Books

Badgley, L. (1986). *Healing AIDS Naturally*. San Bruno, CA: Human Energy Press.

Callen, M. (Ed.) (1987). *Surviving and Thriving with AIDS: Hints for the Newly Diagnosed.* New York: People With AIDS Coalition.
Hay, L. (1984). *You Can Heal Your Life.* Farmingdale, NY: Coleman Publishing.
Moffatt, B. (1986). *When Someone You Love Has AIDS: A Book of Hope for Family and Friends.* Santa Monica: IBS Press.
Moffatt, B., Spiegel, J., Parrish, S., & Helquist, M. (1987). *AIDS: A Self-Care Manual.* Santa Monica: IBS Press.
O'Connor, T. (1986). *Living with AIDS: Reaching Out.* San Francisco: Corwin Press.
Rossman, M. (1987). *Healing Yourself: A Step by Step Program for Better Health through Imagery.* New York: Walker & Co.
Serinus, J. (Ed.) (1986). *Psychoimmunity and the Healing Process: A Holistic Approach to Immunity and AIDS.* Berkeley: Celestial Arts.
Shames, R., & Sterin, C. (1978). *Healing with Mind Power.* Emmaus, PA: Rodale Press.
Siegel, B. (1986). *Love, Medicine, and Miracles.* New York: Harper & Row.
Simonton, C., & Simonton, S. (1978). *Getting Well Again.* New York: Bantam Books.

Articles

Bolen, J. (1985). William Calderon's triumph over AIDS brings new hope. *New Realities, 6*(5), 8-15.
Jacobs, S. (1987). Living with AIDS. *Yoga Journal, 75,* 30-36.
Reuben, C. (1986, September). AIDS: The promise of alternative treatments. *East/West,* 52-69.
South, J. (1987). Power-boosting your immune system: Immuno stimulant nutrients. *Health World, 2*(1), 37-40.

Audio Tapes

AIDS: Passageway to Transformation. Caroline Myss. Available from Stillpoint, P.O. Box 640, Walpole, NH 03608.
AIDS: A Positive Approach. Louise L. Hay. Available from Hay House, 3029 Wilshire Blvd., Suite 206, Santa Monica, CA 90404.
Relaxation and Visualization. AIDS Health Project. Available from AIDS Health Project, Box 0884, San Francisco, CA 94143.
A Strong Immune System. Dick Sutphen. Free to those testing positive to HIV antibody. Available from Valley of the Sun Publishing, Box 3004, Agoura Hills, CA 91301.
Tapping Deeper Resources: Visualization and AIDS. Margo Adair & Lynn Johnson. (Two cassettes and two meditations with four meditations for people with

AIDS, one cassette and two meditations for the worried well.) Available from Tools for Change, P.O. Box 14141, San Francisco, CA 94114.

Video Tapes

Doors Opening: A Positive Approach to AIDS. Louise Hay. Available from Hay House, 3029 Wilshire Blvd., Suite 206, Santa Monica, CA 90404.
Hope and a Prayer. Attitudinal Healing. An Interview with Bernie Siegel, M.D. Available from Hay House (see above).

Newsletters and Organizations

AIDS Treatment News. ATN Publications, P.O. Box 411256, San Francisco, CA 94141.
Healing AIDS: A Newsletter of Healing Tools, Resources and AIDS. 3835 20th Street, San Francisco, CA 94114.
Love Heals Newsletter: A Guide with Tools and Information for People Interested in a Holistic Approach to Improving Their Lives. (contribution requested) 548 Tremont Street, Boston, MA 02116.
Positive Direction News. 304 Newbury Street, Suite 203, Boston, MA 02115
Project Inform (donations accepted) 347 Dolores Street, Suite 301, San Francisco, CA 94110; Information Line about Experimental Drugs: 1-800-822-7422.
PWA Coalition Newsline. Holistic Healthcare for AIDS (free to PWAs; $20/year for others) 263A West 19th Street, New York, NY 10011.
Treatment Issues: The GMHC Newsletter of Experimental AIDS Therapies. GMHC, Department of Medical Information, 132 West 24th Street, Box 274, New York, NY 10011.

References

Ader, R. (1981). *Psychoneuroimmunology.* New York: Academic Press.
Badgley, L. (1986). *Healing AIDS naturally: Natural therapies for the immune system.* San Bruno, CA: Human Energy Press.
Benner, P. (1984). *From novice to expert: Excellence and power in clinical nursing practice.* Menlo Park, CA: Addison-Wesley.
Blattner, B. (1981). *Holistic nursing.* Englewood Cliffs, NJ: Prentice-Hall, Inc.
Bolen, J. (1985). William Calderon: Incredible triumph over AIDS brings new hope. *New Realities, 6*(5), 8-17.
Callen, M. (Ed.) (1987). *Surviving and thriving with AIDS: Hints for the newly diagnosed.* New York: People with AIDS Coalition.
Cousins, N. (1982). *Human options.* South Yarmouth, MA: J. Cusley.
Descartes, R. (1960). *Discourse on method and meditations.* (translated by J. Lafleur) New York: Bobbs Merrill (original works published 1637 and 1641).

Dintenfass, J. (1978). Chiropractic today. In Kaslof, L. (Ed.), *Wholistic dimensions in healing: A resource guide* (pp. 64-66). Garden City, NY: Doubleday & Co., Inc.

Duhamel, M. (1988). Crystal consciousness in the eighties: What's the craze all about? *New Realities, 8*(6), 30-34.

Ehrenreich, B., & English, D. (1973). *Witches, midwives and nurses: A history of women healers.* Old Westbury, NY: The Feminist Press.

Hay, L. (1984). *You Can Heal Your Life.* Farmingdale, NY: Coleman Publishing.

Hay, L. (1986) Doors opening: A positive approach to AIDS. (Available from Hay House, 3029 Wilshire Blvd., Suite 206, Santa Monica, CA 90404.)

Jacobs, S., & Serinus, J. (1987, July/August). Living with AIDS. *Yoga Journal, 75,* 30-36, 76-77.

Justice, B. (1987). *Who gets sick: Thinking and health.* Houston: Peak Press.

Kolata, G. (1988, July 10). A market for drugs: AIDS patients and their aboveground underground. *New York Times,* E32.

Krieger, D. (1981). *Foundations of holistic health nursing practices: The renaissance nurse.* Philadelphia: J.B. Lippincott.

Locke, S., & Colligan, D. (1988, January/February). Is the cure for cancer in the mind? *New Age Journal,* 23-27.

McCormick, M., & Riederer, M. (1986). Massage therapy for patients with acquired immune deficiency syndrome. *The Massage Journal,* Spring, 9-10.

Melosh, B. (1982). *The physician's hand: Work culture and conflict in American nursing.* Philadelphia: Temple University Press.

Nightingale, F. (1969). *Notes on nursing: What it is and what it is not.* New York: Dover Publications. (originally published in 1860).

O'Regan, B. (1987, May). Healing, remission and miracle cures. *Institute of Noetic Sciences Special Report,* 3-14.

Pelletier, K., & Herzing, D. (1988). Psychoneuroimmunology: Toward a mind-body model. *Journal of the Institute for the Advancement of Health, 5*(1), 26-56.

Pert, C. (1986). The wisdom of the receptors: Neuropeptides, the emotions and the bodymind. *Journal of the Institute for the Advancement of Health, 3*(3), 8-16.

Reuben, C. (1986, September). Chipping away at AIDS: The promise of alternative treatments. *East/West,* 52-69.

Robbins, W. (1988, March 16). Doctors urge campaign against AIDS quackery. *New York Times,* A21.

Russell, E. (1978). The fields of life. In Kaslof, L. (Ed.), *Wholistic Dimensions in Healing: A Resource Guide.* Garden City, NY: Doubleday & Co., Inc.

Serinus, J. (Ed.) (1986). *Psychoimmunity and the healing process: A holistic approach to immunity and AIDS.* Berkeley: Celestial Arts.

Siegel, B. (1986). *Love, medicine, and miracles.* New York: Harper & Row.

Simonton, C., & Simonton, S. (1978). *Getting well again.* New York: Bantam Books.

Solomon, G. (1985). The emerging field of psychoneuroimmunology—with a special note on AIDS. *Journal of the Institute for the Advancement of Health, 2*(1), 6-19.

Solomon, G. (1988). Mind, brain, and the immune system: The healthy elderly and long-term survivors of AIDS: Psychoimmune connections. *Advances, 5*(1), 6-14.

Woods, W. (1988). Whether to take experimental drugs: Counseling issues. *Focus: A Guide to AIDS Research, 3*(6), 1-3.

Chapter 16

Nurturing the Spirit

Jennifer Phillips

Nurturing the spirit involves accepting and comforting clients through the emotional battles brought on by catastrophic illness: shock, denial, grief, anger, fear, helplessness, and distrust. Caring for these clients also entails dealing with the existential questions of life: Why did this happen? What does this mean? What can I believe? This chapter offers some guidance on responding therapeutically to these challenging emotions and reactions. The discussion will help you to provide a comforting presence with spiritual insight into the needs of the person with HIV infection.

Loss and Change as Spiritual Stressors

Change is the one constant in our lives; no two days are alike. Even positive changes require that we adjust, accept that things will never be exactly the same, grieve what has been lost in the process of moving on, and take stock of our new circumstances. For the person with HIV-related illness, change may be experienced as a gradual and uneven decline of health, or as a sudden and dramatic upsetting of the world.

Robert, a thirty-two-year-old graphic designer, liked to work out three times a week at a Nautilus center. He had been promoted at work and was financing his lover Steve's dental school tuition. They had been together for seven years. Although both had families in the Southwest, neither family knew their son was gay. Robert woke one morning feeling flu coming on. Two days later, his respiratory distress increased alarmingly. Steve brought him into the emergency room where he was admitted and placed on mechanical ventilation in the intensive care unit. After a series of invasive tests, a diagnosis of pneumocystis carinii pneumonia came, and with it the label of AIDS. Scratching notes on a pad because he was unable to speak with the respirator in place, Robert conversed with Steve about whether they should call his parents and break the news: Not only was Robert critically ill; he had AIDS and was gay, and this was his lover of seven years, whom they had never met, calling. Robert and Steve had to consider a "do not resuscitate" decision in the event his heart should stop. Steve realized that no durable power of attorney had been drawn up. If Robert should be unable to voice his wishes, Steve had no rights to make decisions. Robert's parents would be legal next of kin. The world changed completely in the course of three days for these two men.

The next few weeks saw Robert improving and off ventilation but weakened. He wondered whether he could return to work and what he should tell his boss and friends. When the chaplain called, Robert said, "I can't believe that a few weeks ago I was hiking in the Rockies and today I can't walk to the bathroom! I don't know whether to tell my boss I'll be at work on the first of the month, or buy a cemetery plot."

Such a drastic change has its impact on the inner life as well as on every aspect of the outer life. A client often wonders, "If my whole life can change so quickly, what can be trusted? What use are plans? What can I hold on to?"

The individual's course through the stages of HIV infection is unpredictable. Statistics on average life expectancy, average latency period before onset of symptoms, and so on, bring no clear indication of what will come. At some point in coping with illness, clients find hope in the uncertainty, feeling that they can beat the odds, or anticipate the most favorable course. At other times, the idiosyncrasy of HIV-related disease may bring unbearable anxiety and stress. Coupled with the fear of the unknown is the distress of waiting: waiting for a diagnosis, waiting for test results, waiting for the next new symptom, waiting for death itself. When we come to empathize deeply with clients, we may feel ourselves riding this roller coaster of uncertainty with them.

We need to be clear and calm in delivering information and in hearing questions and feelings, recognizing the shock of change for all concerned. Most clients and families value full information given gradually in simple language, with some sense of the parameters of what can be expected. Care givers are often reluctant to reveal a poor prognosis for fear they are taking away hope. We can allow clients room for realistic hopes by sketching a worst- and best-case scenario, explaining that most clients fall between extremes. If people hope for the best and make plans to deal with the worst, then they can ride out what comes with a maximum sense of peacefulness. When what has to be done to provide for oneself and others has been done, then fears can be laid aside to focus on wellness.

Denial

Consider the immense difference between these two responses. One client says, "This is all a mistake. I'm perfectly well and I intend to live my life exactly as usual.

I don't want or need medical care." Contrast this with another who, despite being critically ill, says, "I'm feeling better today and hoping to get home sometime next week if all goes well." The first response constitutes an unhelpful attitude of denial that prevents responsible behavior for self-care and refuses to allow for truth-telling in relationships. It is a rigid defense with no room for modification or new information. The second, while it may not appear realistic to us, is an adaptive way of maintaining optimism in a difficult circumstance. When next week comes with no improvement, the second client is likely to be able to verbalize, "Well, I'm disappointed. But I am still very weak and perhaps next week I'll be ready."

Even when clients know death is approaching, make necessary plans, and have occasional conversations about dying, they may not want to think about that reality constantly or with every person. Since we tend to prepare for our dying a little at a time, it helps to have those around us respond flexibly as that agenda comes and goes. The best intervention is to make sure the client has heard accurate information and carried out the necessary business to deal with it. Then simply be ready to talk about dying when the client seems to indicate the need. At other times, share the hopes and wishes for improvement.

Sometimes when a diagnosis of ARC or AIDS is given, the person receiving the information may not be the least surprised. The matter-of-fact response may be interpreted as "denial" by a care giver who is more distressed than the patient. Many people with HIV infection, particularly in the gay community, have been living with the threat of AIDS hanging over their heads for years. Some have had vague symptoms that have been dismissed by their physicians. A diagnosis can come as relief from the long tension of the unknown, or simply a confirming of the person's long-familiar inner awareness of illness. It is helpful if we as care givers keep our distress separate from our clients' feelings and refrain from battering them with the truth once it has been spoken. The human spirit is resilient and finds surprising ways of adapting to painful reality, given time.

Grief and Rage

With the complex losses that AIDS brings comes the need to grieve. Grief is not a stage, but an ongoing process of allowing change and healing. It often comes in waves with intervals between. People with HIV infection and those close to them have much to grieve. There are the changes of the body that may leave some unrecognizable even to themselves: massive weight loss, Kaposi's or herpes lesions and other skin infections, swelling, pigment changes, hair loss, weakness, and disability. There are changes of mind and personality: loss of memory, communication impairment, mood alteration, confusion, withdrawal from addictive chemicals, regression related to dependency, and outright dementia. There are role changes in family and work. There may be relationship losses. Hopes and dreams for the future are also casualties of the disease. All must be grieved.

Grief and rage can be opposite sides of a single coin, one inward-looking, the other facing outward. Both are manifestations of a single sorrow for immense loss. We best facilitate the process of grieving and raging by maintaining a constant presence that gently holds the person (whether physically or metaphorically), so that he knows he will not be abandoned or condemned or shamed because of the power of the emotion being released. We have much common ground with persons affected by HIV as they grieve and rage, for their plight touches our own losses and angers. Thus, our own experiences of grief and rage will be our best teachers of how to help.

At its deepest point, grief feels as if it is inconsolable: There is no comfort anywhere. Even for the religious person, God may seem utterly absent. Devoted friends may be perceived as being far-off and useless. A touch from a care giver who simply sits close by may bring more consolation than any words. Grief cannot be talked away but it abates in its own time, usually followed by exhaustion and healing sleep. The grieving process honors what is precious and being lost; grief does not need to be fixed or diverted but simply traveled through.

Rage may be harder to sit with, since we may be tempted to take the anger as a personal assault, and indeed it may be expressed as an attack. It will help if we remember that rage is a global feeling with no shades of gray; it allows no allies. Rage often creates an enormous anxiety about being abandoned. While the care giver may need to move back a step or two from the raging patient or family member, it is important to maintain a presence or at least to assure the person we will return and continue to care. However, the care giver has no responsibility to suffer injury at the hands of a raging person and can set limits when behavior is out of control. For the raging person, God, if seen at all, is seen as the enemy and persecutor. It is neither necessary nor helpful for us as care givers to defend God. We can best communicate a sense of God's constancy of the universe's beneficence simply by constantly caring despite raging behavior and acknowledging the need to rage and the injustice of illness and suffering.

When the passion of grief and rage is spent, some people may settle into depression, either lasting or transient. If depression persists, the nurse may wish to arrange a psychiatric assessment. However, some depression may be a fitting response to debilitating and progressive illness in a young person. When all the usual pieces of living have been disrupted, it takes time to organize the new segments into a comprehensible and acceptable reality. The person with long-term HIV infection may have severely limited energy and possibly limited cognitive ability for this task. It is helpful to differentiate among sadness, exhaustion, and depression. As a spiritual state, depression is characterized by an inability to receive love and comfort and a general experience of meaninglessness and feeling stuck. For us as care givers, sitting with a depressed person can feel like swimming too long underwater. There can be a strong urge to escape either by leaving or avoiding the person or by trying to cheer the person up. Again, simple, caring constancy is most helpful.

Fear as a Spiritual Condition

The patient and family coping with HIV infection have many areas of fear. Many clients who have friends with AIDS fear developing the symptoms they have seen in others. Most commonly, these fears may center around dying in pain, losing control of the body, and losing one's mind. Care givers can help by reminding clients that their course will not necessarily follow anyone else's, and by explaining that clients can control their symptoms. If pain is the primary fear, review medication options in detail, especially those for the end of life. For example, explain how a morphine drip can be finely adjusted to balance the desire for alertness and the desire for analgesia. Also suggest alternative pain management techniques such as relaxation exercises, guided imagery, centering meditation, and self-hypnosis. Such techniques can also be learned by loved ones for managing their anxiety and for assisting the client. Most importantly, these approaches give clients some sense of control over their pain and, therefore, their destiny.

The fear of loss of control of the body and loss of the mind has no easy remedies. Part of coming to terms with the fear involves grieving the actual losses of capacity over time. Since anticipating losses that have not happened can become overwhelming, a focus on the present may be more helpful. The more we can communicate to people with HIV infection that their acceptability and worth does not depend on how well they function, look, or communicate, the more comfort will be conveyed. These fears have not only to do with loss of function but with loss of identity itself. We may wish to suggest to our clients that who they are is never lost to God or to the people who love them most.

Greg, a young man who eventually died of invasive Kaposi's sarcoma, once said to the chaplain: "When I look in the mirror, I don't know the person I see any more!" Another man had lost half his weight and all his hair to HIV infection and its treatments. When I recognized a photograph of him as he had formerly been, he said, "Thank goodness someone recognized me; the last person who looked at this thought it was my brother!" As the body becomes foreign and alien in appearance and feeling, there can be a deep terror of becoming lost to others, to oneself, and even to God.

Loss of control and identity and the fears concomitant with these losses raise issues of shame for many clients, which add to the sense of being stricken with a "dirty" or "untouchable" disease. When we touch and call by name without repugnance, we reassure the suffering person that he is still the person he always was, worthy of love and care.

People with HIV infection and their loved ones also commonly struggle with fears of transmission that may or may not be rooted in reality. A sexual or drug-sharing partner, or a baby, may have been infected before the client became sick or before that person knew of the infection. In such a situation, the care giver may helpfully raise the question to the guilt-ridden client or family member: "Do you believe that it is possible to be forgiven for your role in this?" It may also fall within the care giver's own structure of belief to suggest that God is often more forgiving of us than we are of ourselves. Even without such a belief system, a care giver may acknowledge the painfulness of guilt. We can raise the possibilities of seeking reconciliation in relationships and of trying to live as well as possible in the future, knowing the past cannot be undone.

Fear of future transmission may persist despite education about transmission-reduction behaviors. One man with HIV-related cancer feared going home from the hospital because he had an infant. Though he had been told that casual transmission of HIV had never been documented, he continued to fear that the child could catch AIDS if he handled her or coughed on her. A general practitioner who also was an anxious new father had said to him, "Frankly, if it were I, I wouldn't risk it." The fear was magnified.

As with care givers' fears of contracting AIDS from a patient, the patient's fears of transmitting HIV infection may be largely irrational and cannot be talked or educated away. A choice must be made to move on in relationships despite the unreasonable fears. Once this decision has been made, the fears tend to subside gradually. Acknowledging the fears and their painfulness, whether rational or irrational, is a good first step. To choose not to be paralyzed by fear is a spiritual discipline, an act of trust in one's own ideal potential self as well as in the goodness of the universe.

Fear of abandonment is pervasive in people with HIV infection. Many clients are, in fact, abandoned by someone they love or, at times, by everyone dear to them. The stigma of AIDS creates a fear of abandonment even where loved ones have formerly been perceived as reliable. The decline clients perceive in their own lovability, productivity, and energy to invest in relationships all leads to an increase in abandonment fear.

For those who have received early wounds of nurture, whether from parents who were ill, deceased, alcoholic, addicted, abusive, depressed, or otherwise unreliable, the fear of being abandoned is likely to be overwhelming. Those who have had few lasting relationships in their lives may develop patterns of driving others away so that they do not need to endure the pain and helplessness of being left. We as care givers should look past hostile and alienating behavior to see whether there is an underlying expectation that we too will abandon. We can work to maintain some level of caring contact that over time may allow trust to build.

Building Community in the Face of Fear

Persons with HIV infection may call upon nurses to assist in the process of community building in ways that other clients seldom do. Since fear is magnified by loneliness, the strengthening of a community of caring is an ideal way to counteract many of the besetting fears of clients and their loved ones. AIDS service organizations, support groups, and other helping resources in the community provide essential services and support. Clients and families seem to cope best when they have not just one faithful person, but a whole network of committed friends and care givers at home.

For the newly diagnosed person with HIV infection, there may be questions of what to tell whom and when. It may be safest for clients to "test the water" by first telling a few friends who are less essential to their support network. Once a person or two have responded affirmatively, then clients may be ready to risk telling a few more-important others. One client strategized to tell an AA sponsor first. After that person had promised support, he worked up the courage to tell his mother and father. The relief after the first few people respond well can be so tremendous that the client wants to tell everyone. The care giver may do well to recommend going slowly for a while, as not everyone will want to hear. The newly diagnosed person already has enough with which to cope without having to give attention to shocked or angry acquaintances.

Sometimes as a diagnosis becomes known, clients find themselves quite alone. Some clients lack support networks from the beginning. For such people, the nurses, social workers, chaplains, and others on the care team may be a surrogate community at the end of life. We may find ourselves stepping far beyond our usual professional boundaries. This can result in a wonderful mutuality of growth and care, as long as we are careful to respect the limits of our time and energy, making only commitments that can be honored.

As a spiritual crisis, the fear of being abandoned may be brought toward healing through reflection on the ways in which the individual feels connected on some level with all other people and with life in general. If the person is so inclined, meditation upon the inner place of connection with the Divine, with humanity, and with one's own deepest, most unchanging self may allay fear and panic.

Autonomy, Dependence, and Control: Reenvisioning Relationships

From a spiritual perspective, the span of life contains a balance and flow from dependence to autonomy and often back again, traveling from childhood to adulthood and into late life and dying. Full humanity requires an ability to move from one to the other and back with some flexibility; this is not an easy discipline to attain.

People with HIV infection experience various changes of role in relationships. They may have been family breadwinners who are now forced to receive financial support from friends, relatives, or the state. They may have been parents or independent adults and now suddenly are unable to care for their children; they may even be childlike in the need to have basic care given by parents again. They may have been spouses who suddenly become recipients in the patient-nurse relationship with a lover. The loss of relationship roles is a profound one and must be grieved.

It can be an act of love to allow oneself to relinquish control in a relationship and accept dependency with equanimity. It may be helpful to clients to reflect upon how they might be willing to be care givers if their loved ones were ill, since love requires both the willingness to give and to receive. Being "a burden" to loved ones is a fear of many patients. Sometimes it has to do with underlying fears that care givers will grow weary and leave. For these people, reassurance from loved ones—strengthening the emotional bonds and extent of the support network—may bring comfort. At other times, it has to do with an unwillingness to experience the dependent side of loving relationships and can be presented as a spiritual task. Sometimes it has to do with deep, sad feelings of helplessness. Comfort may come from a reminder that our worth does not come from what we can do but from who we are.

In a society that values productivity so highly, the individual disabled by illness may be challenged to build a whole new image of self-worth at a time when resources are at an ebb. Maintaining self-esteem and peacefulness when employment is lost or relinquishing the caretaking role in relation to others that is particularly stressful. As nurses, we are in a special position to help in role transition because we have learned to cherish and value strangers in their time of least productivity and greatest dependency. We can reflect to our clients what *we* see and value in them at this moment, building their self-concept in their relational, emotional, or spiritual skills. Yet, as care givers we will be even more of a resource through this painful change if we have experienced being dependent adults ourselves. Our own experiences may help us understand the process of letting go of this part of life. Few people take to the dependent role comfortably. Our own discomfort can sensitize us to the magnitude of our clients' distress.

Trust

HIV infection brings a massive insult to the trustworthiness of life. The breakdown of the immune system and subsequent invasive opportunistic infections may be experienced as betrayal by one's own body. Confrontation with the very limited resources of the medical system to heal or protect may be experienced as a parallel outer betrayal. If loved ones flee or the surrounding community expresses hostility, then the sense of betrayal may become global. In such circumstances, God also is seen as a betrayer who has failed to protect, love, and mend. The loss of hopes and dreams early in adult life may also feel like a cruel trick of fate.

Perhaps the greatest insult to trust comes for persons who contracted HIV infection through blood products in the health care system, for they may perceive that they were betrayed by those who promised healing. Clients with iatrogenic disease may face either: 1) two illnesses concurrently if their primary illness has continued after HIV infection, or 2) having just been healed of one ailment, being stricken with a second, more deadly one. The hope for healing from the medical system may be corroded beyond repair for such a person and, consciously or unconsciously, health care providers may be greeted with suspicion and mistrust.

Some clients with iatrogenic HIV infection express a strong need to blame, but may not feel safe blaming the physicians on whom they are still reliant for care. It can be easier to blame the anonymous donor, the blood bank staff, or some blanket category of people such as homosexuals or IV drug addicts. Behind the blame is an acute vulnerability that we may recognize and honor with the utmost gentleness and honesty in care giving.

Many of the people with HIV infection who are long-term IV street drug users may also have profound difficulties trusting their care givers. The world that centers around drug sales and use lacks a regard for truth or a capacity for care or empathy, since even group drug-using events are dominated by individuals' need to supply their addiction. The sense of cultural alienation between clients and care givers to this population is profound from the start and is increased when color, national origin, and/or language also differ.

We as care givers must bear in mind how foreign a world the hospital is even for us who belong to the prevailing cultural and economic community of the institution. Clients who invest their trust in care givers despite differences of color, neighborhood, language, sexual orientation, or behavior bestow a precious gift upon us. Expect trust-building to take time and constancy. Resist the temptation to categorize people who cannot trust us as unlovable or noncompliant. Maintaining a lively human interest in clients, their loved ones, and their way of making meaning from, and coping with, illness will gradually communicate trustworthiness, as will consistent truth-telling.

Emerging Spiritual Questions

There are a great variety of spiritual questions and concerns for people affected by HIV. Many of these do not need the attention of a professional pastor, rabbi, chaplain, or priest, but can be shared helpfully among any individuals who find themselves journeying in the spirit. As nurses, we have a constant presence and a potential depth of relationship with clients and families, which often render us ideal companions to share faith questions. When asked, we do not need to supply an answer, since the only valid answers are those that individuals develop for themselves. Often, we need only to hear in order to relieve the loneliness of the asking.

Very commonly, an ill person may wonder whether suffering is a punishment or judgment for past behavior or an underlying character flaw. This question may arise from a sense of being an overall bad person, from being an acceptable person who has done some bad things that must be paid for, or simply from the need to have the suffering make sense and fulfill some sort of logic. The care giver could try to sound out which of these underlying positions is being voiced. People with HIV infection, particularly those who have perceived their sexual behaviors or drug-using behaviors as in violation of the norms of their family, religious values, or conscience, may have deep, lifelong feelings of shame. Shame finds its best healing as the true self is disclosed in a trustworthy relationship, discovering unconditional love with nothing hidden. Where the illness has an actual basis in chosen behavior, the issue may be less one of shame than of guilt and remorse for having made damaging choices.

Guilt may need forgiveness: from other people who have been injured by the behaviors, from oneself (often the most difficult) and from the Divine, possibly through a formal religious ritual of reconciliation. Self-forgiveness begins with allowing oneself to be imperfect and limited, and in loving the pained self who has chosen poorly. One way we come to terms with our limitations is by recognizing that we choose some aspects of self, while others are beyond choice, as is sexual orientation for many. Alienation may call for reconciliation on all levels: with others, with self, and with God. This takes some labor to accomplish, yet it can be the most important work of a life-threatening illness. When people suffering shame or guilt ask, "Am I being punished?" they are also asking, "Can I be loved and forgiven?" The Divine is that reality with which reconciliation and forgiveness are always possible.

A question voiced by many people with HIV infection, especially those who came from a religious family of origin, is, "Who will be my community of faith?" Churches and synagogues differ in their openness and welcome to those with AIDS as well as to addicts and gay and lesbian individuals. The community of origin may not be the community that can or will serve the person now. The family pastor may or may not be a help to the person with HIV infection, depending on sensitivity, acceptance, and broadness of theological understanding. Care givers should be alert to religious visitors who increase the distress of the patient. The signs of distress are not tears, which may be needed for the grieving and healing of the spirit, but rather increased feelings of rage, shame, guilt, and alienation.

Even persons without any previous religious affiliation may wish to be connected to a spiritual adviser at the end of life, perhaps to work through questions of faith, or perhaps simply to make arrangements for a funeral, burial, or memorial service. Even those long alienated from the religious establishment may yearn for a point of connection before death: a prayer, a pastoral visit, receiving the sacraments of the church, or being memorialized according to their tradition. There are both traditional and nontraditional communities of faith to support people with HIV infection in many areas. Care givers may consult sensitive chaplains or pastors or the community AIDS service organization to find out which ones can be most supportive.

"What if I die?" is a spiritual question that may begin at the time of a positive HIV test and recur at intervals until the end of life. We could respond simply, "What do you think will happen when you die?" to allow a person to review hopes, beliefs, and expectations. We may listen to the response while asking ourselves, "Does this person's expectation satisfy him and bring him peace?" Sharing our own expectations may be a warm and mutual response as long as there is no assumption that the client will be able to adopt our own set of beliefs.

My impression as a chaplain is that "What if I die?" is a universal question of people who are ill, even when it is not voiced. The least hopeful response is, "Well, you're not going to die; you're doing better," because ultimately it is untrue as well as fear-laden. If death seems to be a burdensome issue for the client or family, the care giver can sound out where the fear actually lies. Some people simply fear nonexistence or the process of leaving the world; others fear the pain of dying, or being left alone, or being in the dark, or the unknownness of it. Fears may be very specific, and some can be allayed. Dying is, after all, as natural a process as being born, and it may be that there are arms to catch us as we slide from this world just as there were arms to catch us when we slid into it.

As with other terminally ill clients, suicide may become an issue at times; it is one that raises much anxiety for care givers. In my four years of working with 150 or so people with HIV-related illness, suicides have been very rare (see Chapter 17 for statistics on suicide in HIV-infected populations and guidelines for assessment). It may be that the danger of actual suicide is greater at the point of receiving a positive test result than at or after being diagnosed with AIDS. The guidelines that apply for nurses in evaluating suicidal ideation in other clients pertain also to those with HIV infection. Similarly, when people with HIV infection discuss suicide with care givers, they are struggling to maintain some sense of control in the face of their feelings of helplessness. For most, it is enough to know that they do have an "out" if they ever need it.

Suicide may be raised as a spiritual question: "If I kill myself, will God forgive me?" To say no is to say between the lines, "The feelings you are having and, therefore, you, the person who is feeling them, are unacceptable and unlovable." There is nothing in Christian or Jewish scriptures that says that suicide is unforgivable to God. Whether family members could forgive is a more concrete question; indeed, they may not. If the question of suicide and God's forgiveness is raised, it may need a careful hearing and discussion. A spiritual adviser with some experience may be a valuable resource. From my own religious tradition (Judeo-Christian), I would never consider suicide the best spiritual option, but the judgment of God should not be summoned as an argument in the debate. The most helpful response may not be a debate at all, but an assurance that care will continue, that pain can be relieved, that the individual is cherished, that his suffering is known, that the need for some sense of control is human and legitimate, and that the client is not alone or without hope.

As death nears, questions often arise of "What has my life meant?" and "What does my suffering mean?" Such a question may be an invitation to the care giver to sit down and hear the story of that life, receiving it as a legacy, perhaps from a client who has no one else to whom to entrust it. It is a great privilege to receive the gift of another human being's story as he prepares to die. The receiving is itself a healing act and belongs as much to the nurse's domain as to that of any other care giver or friend.

There are no better or worse ways of meaning-making. One person may assess the value of life very concretely: in terms of children raised, a business built, money in the bank, numbers of friends, tasks completed. Another may evaluate life on the basis of spiritual growth, depth of relationships, or fidelity to some sense of vocation and purpose. People may value life based on how much and varied their experience has been. At times, people evaluate their lives in very passive ways: "I never did anyone an intentional injury," "I've always followed the rules." We comfort when we listen, celebrate the successes as that person measures them, and empathize with the disappointments. After all has been heard, respect the mystery of that life and express appreciation for having been invited to hear it. Sometimes, a person cannot let go of life until he has told his story to someone. The desire to be known is a deep common thread of our humanity.

"Why is life so unfair?" cry some persons with HIV infection. Care givers may find themselves asking the same question. HIV often strikes those whose lives are just beginning: babies, young adults who have emerged from the disorder of adolescence into settled lives and careers and relationships, or those whose whole lives have suffered deprivation and alienation. AIDS is unfair. The ability to accept the unfairness varies. Many of us carry a belief that life should work on a "tit-for-tat" basis: If we're good, we should reap a reward, and if we've suffered a lot, we deserve a break. Illness respects none of these values. A response of "Yes, this is unfair" or "Yes, you do deserve better" expresses support for our common plight in unfair lives. There may be no answer to the why of it. Like so many spiritual questions, "Why is life unfair" asks less for an answer than for someone to stand in solidarity with the questioner.

Spiritual concerns may be related to ethnic origins, so the care giver will be wise to avoid answering questions in favor of listening to them. In particular, the role of religion in healing varies among cultures. The North American medical system assists the healing of individuals best when it works in harmony with the healing energy of the person's own culture. It is my own belief that you cannot cure the body if you are doing violence to the spirit; compelling treatment on individuals that violates their sense of relationship with their Transcendent Reality will not produce healing. Ethnic healing practices and standard health care practice may not fit together easily, but clients will be helped best when their care givers can listen patiently to the wisdom of that person's culture, then clearly and reasonably make a case for the best treatment options science offers, allowing the person to take responsibility for choosing the method of healing. The same holds true for clients who have an interest in adding holistic therapies to their healing regimens. Many of these therapies can dovetail with standard treatments. Where there is conflict, carefully educate and allow the client to choose, recognizing that there is a spirit as well as a body to be healed. Spiritual healing does not always appear to "make sense" to others.

The time of illness can bring a crisis in prayer for the person to whom prayer is important. The alienation that often accompanies HIV infection may be translated into a sense of being blocked in prayer. The changes of routine, energy, role, body image, privacy, and dependency can disrupt usual ways of praying, along with all the exigencies of the hospital environment and the central nervous system that affect some clients. The care giver does not need to be an expert in prayer to be helpful to clients who voice distress in this area. Simply encourage people to pray in any way they can, in any way that brings comfort.

In a time of crisis, the prayer ways of childhood may bring extraordinary comfort: a recited bedtime prayer, the Our Father, a psalm, the Rosary, or a mantra prayer. Conversational prayer, simply "talking to God," is the most used sort for many Americans. Anxiety, panic, and the yearning for a cure can cause this kind of praying to degenerate into a desperate begging that can feel like being a prisoner rattling the bars of a cell. As a cure doesn't come, God may be perceived as being further and further away and not listening or loving. One suggestion for a person feeling desperately unheard is to change to a nondialogical way of prayer. Suggest that the client use a mantra or centering prayer technique: the simple repetition of a word or phrase or sound allowing thoughts to simply float away. The calm repetition of a comforting sound may help the spirit to be still and peaceful. Just sitting in quiet awareness of one's breath coming in and going out from the chest, abdomen, or nostrils produces a similar inner quietness in which the connection to the Eternal Dimension may be renewed.

The loss of one's usual community of prayer may make prayer more difficult. We can bring comfort by praying with a client or even keeping quiet company while that person prays. For those whose energy is depleted and whose cognition is severely impaired, expression of the self seeking the Divine may renew the sense of prayerfulness, even by a single word, thought, or sigh. We provide a community as we accept and encourage whatever prayer expression a client may offer, reassuring our clients that the Infinite is not limited in hearing, connecting, receiving.

Being a spiritual friend to people affected by HIV infection does not require special credentials. We as care givers need only take time to listen from our hearts, with great respect for human diversity and attentiveness to our spiritual journeys. Although we think of spirituality as being private, it is a shared dimension of humanness, enhanced by the supportive presence of others.

Chapter 17

The Psychosocial Impact of HIV Infection: Minimizing the Losses

Ann M. Locke

As with any chronic or incurable illness, one of the most critical nursing contribution is the psychosocial interventions. Our role in care of clients with HIV infection is one of counter-coper: to maximize clients' coping capacity and ability to solve specific illness-related problems (Weisman, 1984). The following chapter highlights some of the common responses to living with HIV infection, as well as the families' reactions. Both the text and tables show specific nursing interventions for comforting the client with HIV infection.

The Expressed Concerns

Fear

Fear of death is a realistic reaction to HIV infection, as the person faces the ultimate loss of control. The goal of nursing care for all fearful people is to help them confront their fears and feel the emotions in order to allow them to subside. Once confronted, fear of death is best countered with hope for the future. Table 17.1 outlines specific interventions for dealing with all the emotions associated with AIDS.

Psychological stamina, the ability to maintain hope in the face of an uncertain future, is a critical ingredient to one's well-being (Miller, 1983). People gather hope in a number of ways, such as focusing on the advancement of treatments or the promise of complementary therapies. Hope is often defined as the estimation of achieving goals. Since HIV infection affects people at the life stage of producing or creating (Erikson, 1963), people maintain hope in their goals for careers or

Table 17.1 *General Interventions for People With HIV Infection*

1. *Communicate Acceptance and Concern:*
   - Touch: make physical contact when greeting, talking, or caring for client.
   - Eye contact: shows acceptance and increases trust.
   - Physical proximity: stand close to the client.
   - Body language: gestures that show openness, desire to connect, such as leaning forward, arms open.
   - Avoid judgmental-sounding language. Terms such as "high-risk behavior" or "homosexual" can sound condemning within some contexts. Speak openly about a gay lifestyle, sexual contacts, or drug use.

2. *Establish a Trusting Relationship:*
   - Take all concerns seriously, such as pain, guilt, fatigue.
   - Follow through on everything that you say you will do.
   - Do everything possible to relieve concerns, including physical interventions for comfort and psychological ones.

3. *Encourage Verbalization of Emotions:*
   - Avoid the temptation to dismiss fears as unrealistic. All negative emotions (fear, anger, grief) must be felt and expressed in order for them to be resolved and fade.
   - Help the client determine how to vent the emotions: making an audio or video tape, writing a journal, making a quilt panel, organizing a self-help group, volunteering for legislative work for persons with AIDS, talking to a friend, counselor, or nurse.

4. *Give the Client Control:*
   - Keep clients and families fully informed.
   - Encourage clients to make all decisions possible, ranging from the type of treatment to the time of day for bathing.
   - Encourage clients to do everything they can for themselves, and maintain as "normal" a life as possible, even within the hospital (i.e., hobbies, seeing friends, working, spiritual activities).
   - Introduce the concept of complementary therapies as a way of gaining control over one's treatment and well-being, such as relaxation techniques, guided imagery, and hypnosis (see Chapter 15).

5. *Reinforce a Positive Self-Concept:*
   - Give positive feedback for all accomplishments, such as reaching the goal of getting out of bed.
   - Ask clients, and encourage them to focus on, what they like about themselves, or what they do/did well.

Table 17.1 *General Interventions for People With HIV Infection*

6. *Help Clients Continue Roles and Relationships:*
   - Encourage them to continue their work as much as possible, or to undertake any task that is important to them.
   - Help clients see new ways to continue relationships such as:
     1) even if they cannot physically care for their children, they can provide essential affection, counsel, and reinforcement.
     2) even if they cannot provide physical intimacy, they can give emotional intimacy to a spouse.
   - Provide privacy for clients when visiting with all others in order to invite the expression of affection with friends and family.

7. *Facilitate a Positive Body Image:*
   - Facilitate exercise programs.
   - Minimize the display of invasive intervention such as IV lines.
   - Encourage clients to dress in street clothes.
   - Encourage and facilitate the client's usual grooming habits, such as seeing a hairdresser or manicurist.
   - Facilitate the use of attitudinal healing methods (i.e., affirmation, meditation, positive thinking) to fortify self-concept and self-image.

---

families. People may not only cling to existing developmental goals of intimacy and work achievement, but may also develop new short-term goals as a source of hope, such as living to see a family event (Campbell, 1987). Thus, once the shock of the diagnosis has faded, people begin to think of themselves as living with AIDS instead of dying with AIDS.

In addition to death, people fear the losses associated with death: pain, disfigurement, dementia. For people with HIV infection, these fears are realistic. Most people will develop some symptoms of neurological impairment during the course of the illness (Levy, Bredesen, & Rosenblum, 1985). Pain (and discomfort) is common, if not from the opportunistic infections or HIV symptoms, then from the invasive interventions. These fears need to be acknowledged, voiced, *accepted,* as all negative emotions need acceptance. Educate clients about the options for therapy that will be available to them (see Table 17.2). As always, assure them of your continuing efforts to do all you can for them, regardless of their level of functioning.

Denial

Denial is an often misused term. True denial is the refusal to acknowledge some dreaded reality, such as denying the presence of HIV infection when diagnosed with

Table 17.2 *Physical Problems Requiring Psychosocial Interventions*

1. **Pain**

   Cause:
   - Peripheral neuropathy
   - Abdominal cramps from intense, chronic diarrhea
   - Mouth soreness from candida
   - Skin sensitivity from lesions of Kaposi's sarcoma
   - Chest pain associated with pneumonia
   - Pain and bruising from multiple invasive procedures, such as lumbar punctures, multiple intravenous line insertions

   Factors Increasing Pain Sensitivity:
   - Anxiety: anxiety over pain and whether pain can/will be relieved heightens the brain's sensitivity to perceive pain.
   - Drug Use: intravenous drug use also lowers the person's pain threshold, decreasing tolerance for discomfort.

   Interventions:
   - Treat all pain, regardless of source or level.
   - Medicate as prescribed by physician. Avoid narcotic analgesics that may alter level of consciousness and heighten anxiety associated with loss of control.
   - Decrease anxiety by establishing trust (see Table 17.1).
   - Decrease psychological pain of fear, rejection, self-esteem, as outlined in Table 17.1.
   - Use complementary therapy: relaxation exercises, guided imagery, meditation.

2. **Dementia**

   Definition:
   - Irreversible, chronic organic brain syndrome resulting in impairment of intellectual functioning (Plutzky, 1974).

   Symptoms:
   - Mild to moderate impairment: client may be aware of these deficits, responding with anxiety, depression, psychosomatic complaints, or psychosis.
   - Advanced impairment: poor judgment, or impulsive, agitative, or aggressive behavior.

   Treatment:

   Goal: Facilitate maximum functioning as long as possible by:
   - Interpersonal contact with nurses and visitors is often most effective in maintaining intellectual functioning.
   - Interventions to enhance self-esteem and control, as outlined in Table 17.1.
   - Psychotropic drugs

AIDS (Forchuk & Westwell, 1987). This differs from the people who acknowledge the presence of HIV infection, but are convinced that positive thinking will cure them. Such people are restructuring their perspective of the dreaded reality in order to find hope for living, a positive coping mechanism. Thus, the first nursing task is to distinguish between true denial versus a reluctance to disclose one's feelings or a coping mechanism of seeing positive elements in the face of a difficult situation. All sources of hope need encouragement, even if they seem unrealistic to us.

True denial is a protective mechanism. Confronting the denial only increases the person's anxiety, thereby increasing the need for denial. Instead, help people verbalize their feelings about *related* issues, which gently facilitates awareness of the emotions that trigger the denial. Avoid reinforcing denial; instead, agree with the part of the denial based in reality, which allows clients time to come to terms with the future in their own way (Forchuk & Westwell, 1987). For example, we can teach safer sex methods to clients and their partners without confronting them with a hard diagnosis. We can simply state that anyone who has been sexually active with more than one partner in the past ten years should use safer sex practices. This approach helps clients to learn to live with AIDS while still struggling to face the diagnosis.

Although true denial of AIDS is rare, it causes great concern for health care workers. The fear of a client's infecting others due to denial is a common, if unrealistic, fear of nurses. We are responsible for equipping our clients and their families with necessary information in a therapeutic way. We are not responsible for "making" them accept their diagnosis or any lifestyle changes. Our anxiety over denial will decrease as we see our role as facilitator and helper of the healing and coping processes. The outcome is up to our clients.

Anger

Once confronted with the diagnosis, many people feel anger—anger at being struck down in the prime of life, anger at the helplessness and hopelessness, anger at the lack of a cure, the sluggish process of research, the social apathy and rejection. Unlike many other terminal illnesses, HIV infection can be prevented. Anger is lashed out at the perceived cause of the pain: the lover, the spouse, the addict, oneself. Anger looking to blame, to explain the catastrophe, causes serious disruption of the family relationships. When both the client and the spouse have AIDS, they may vent their anger at each other, a who-did-this-to-whom struggle to relieve oneself of guilt. Many persons with AIDS feel angry at themselves: angry at the addiction, angry at having accepted a blood transfusion, angry at their own sexuality, angry at having trusted lovers who lied about their past.

The client with HIV infection has many valid reasons to be angry. Sometimes the anger is directed at anyone entering the room, including nurses. Often, this feels to us like a lack of appreciation or a personal rejection of us as care givers. Misdirected anger further alienates and isolates people with HIV infection, increasing their fear of rejection and helplessness, often increasing their anger. Expect and accept the anger, understanding the origin as separate from us or our nursing care. Direct the anger positively: letters to a legislator, working with an AIDS community group (see Table 17.1). The more we can tolerate intense emotions without feeling the need to "fix" them, the more effective we will be at listening therapeutically.

Guilt

Guilt arises when clients fear or perceive that they have infected others, or have engaged in behavior that was "wrong." Unresolved conflicts associated with sexual identity can resurface at the time of diagnosis. Since Western society often portrays a negative view of homosexuality, many people internalize this perspective, making it difficult for them to accept their natural tendencies or feelings. The association of AIDS as a "gay plague" or "judgment from God" illustrates not only the lack of acceptance of homosexuality in our society, but also the persecution of people with HIV infection. Separating one's self-concept from such a negative environment demands a strong ego, which can be easily shattered with the diagnosis of a devastating illness. When individuals apply society's negative view to themselves, they often interpret AIDS as a retribution for wrongdoings or bad behavior. The perceived "bad self" is condemned for lacking self-control over sexual needs. The guilt may be so intense that people may even try to relieve it with self-punitive actions (Abrams, Dilley, Maxey, & Volberding, 1986). Similar guilt, self-hatred, and self-blame arise with others who blame themselves for the contact with HIV, such as intravenous drug users. Guilt also arises with anxiety or knowledge of spreading the disease to a loved one, either sexually or perinatally.

When giving comfort, help clients see HIV as an indiscriminate microbe rather than a deliberate punishment from society or a Supreme Being. The first people infected in the United States *happened* to be gay. Had the initial contacts been heterosexual, the gay population might be the low-risk segment of our society. This type of discussion helps clients distinguish between the disease being associated with sexuality versus being caused by sexuality. Guilt eats away at the person's self-esteem, will to live, ability to feel worthy of relationships. All of the nursing interventions listed on Table 17.1 are critical. These clients need all the comfort we have to give.

Isolation

People with HIV infection report being treated as having a socially unacceptable disease (Longo, Spross, & Locke, 1988). The cultural taboos of sexuality and death are attached to AIDS, creating the connotation of a despised and contemptible disease (see Chapter 1). The stigma of AIDS exaggerates the feelings of abandonment, ostracism, and isolation already associated with having a contagious and deadly illness.

The loss of sexual activity, due to either body-image disturbance or physical symptoms, precipitates isolation by the loss of a significant form of intimate communication as well as the loss of feeling lovable (Flaskerud, 1987). People sometimes withdraw from a lover because they cannot tolerate being so dependent within the relationship. Other times, the separation of lovers happens as the family of origin takes over the physical care, often transporting the client back to the home town. Clients can feel guilty about leaving a lover in favor of the care of a parent as well as the pain of separating from the primary relationship.

Many clients struggle with the dilemma of whether or not to share their diagnosis with others. Some families of origin may be unaware of their son's sexual orientation, making the revelation of the diagnosis a loaded issue. Other clients feel they have let their children down by contracting the disease through intravenous drug use. They want to protect their children from knowing about their drug habit and maintain a positive concept in the children's minds. Maintaining such a secret becomes a source of tremendous distress to clients, who isolate themselves by withholding information, yet fear rejection and pain if they disclose the diagnosis.

As nurses, our responsibility is to listen, to accept the decisions of the client. We can ask questions: "How do you think they will respond?" "What would happen if ...?" We can help clients see alternatives, identify the advantages and disadvantages of each alternative, and support whatever decision they make. In the case where the nurse is asked to further the deception by telling the family a different diagnosis, the most prudent response is to refrain from telling anyone anything. Simply refer inquiries back to the client. Let clients know they must handle the situation in the way they think best.

Abandonment may be a reality in some cases. Although most people with AIDS are supported by someone (parents, lovers, friends), many experience rejection by others: siblings, children, spouses, friends, roommates (Forstein, 1984). Feelings of isolation are reinforced by avoidance behavior of health care workers due to fear of contagion (Rogers, 1988). The use of precautions further isolates clients from others, reinforcing their feelings of being untouchable.

The pain of being labeled with this disease calls for all of our skill at making contact. The interventions on Table 17.1 consist of many basic nursing activities—touching, listening, reinforcing—but they are so critical to people in the pain of isolation. Facilitate the families and friends to feel comfortable being close to the client by giving accurate information on contagion and encouraging all close contact. Provide privacy and maximize the opportunity for intimate interaction with all close relationships.

Depression

When anger and guilt are turned inward, people feel depressed. The multiple losses of roles and relationships, loss of financial resources, loss of work identity, loss of adult independence, loss of bodily function and integrity deplete the psychological stamina of the person with HIV infection. One of the characteristics of depression is a low self-esteem. For the person with HIV infection, self-esteem diminishes as body image and integrity disintegrate.

Body image, the image of physical self, acts as a standard frame of reference for how we "should" look and function. Our body image develops slowly during the growth and development process, depending on how we think others respond to our appearance (Norris, 1978). Perceived social acceptance, feeling acceptable and lovable, depends largely on a positive body image. Changes in body image threaten the very core of our self-concept, our worth and self-esteem. The visible skin lesions of Kaposi's sarcoma may feel like a red letter *A,* such an obvious sign of AIDS. The weight loss also signals HIV infection, invites questions, and may symbolize a visible loss of self. The chronic diarrhea often accompanying AIDS represents loss of control, unattractiveness, uncleanliness, and unacceptability. The invasive procedures, such as Hickman lines, feel like a bodily assault to clients. Each bodily disfigurement threatens the person's social acceptability, sexuality, productivity, independence, financial security, and self-esteem. People respond to threats to self-concept, the multiple losses of HIV infection, with grief, anger, and depression.

We can build clients' self-esteem not only through therapeutic interaction (see Table 17.1), but also with our physical care. Symptom management of weight loss and diarrhea, as outlined in Chapter 11, improves self-concept as well as physical self. Invasive therapies can be minimized. For example, instead of an unsightly Hickman catheter, offer the client the choice of a central catheter with an implanted port, one totally covered by the skin (i.e., Portacath). Although the subcutaneous puncture site of the implanted catheter requires a needlestick, such minor discomfort might be worthwhile to the client grieving loss of body image. Some cancer rehabilitation programs offer cosmetic advice for minimizing disfiguring symptoms, such as the "Look Good—Feel Better" program associated with the American Cancer Society.

Severe depression can result in suicide ideation. Men with AIDS have a suicide risk 36 percent greater than men of the same age group (between 20 and 59), and 66 percent greater than the general population (Marzuk, 1988). Assess clients' behavior, extent of social support, life stresses, current physical and mental status, and past history. Table 17.3 offers an assessment tool for determining the severity of depression. Clinical depression is a more serious disorder than a situational depression, which usually responds to therapeutic interaction without medication. If you suspect someone is at risk for suicide, consult a psychiatrist. It is better to err in the direction of protecting the client.

Suicide, for some, may be a way of taking control, of avoiding putting loved ones through the pain of discovering the AIDS diagnosis or lifestyle issues. Taking one's own life, or "self-delivery," allows people to choose how and when to die. As nurses, our responsibility is to protect our clients and keep them safe while in our care. We are not responsible for what they might do after discharge. We need to do our best to offer comfort and hope, accepting whatever choices they make that are beyond our control.

Table 17.3 *Assessment of Clinical Depression*

Clinical depression is characterized by the presence of four or more of the following symptoms for one month or longer, indicating the need for psychiatric evaluation and possible medication.

S - Sleep disturbance (increase or decrease)

I - Interest (increase or decrease)

G - Guilt (increase)

E - Energy (decrease)

C - Concentration (decrease)

A - Appetite (increase or decrease)

P - Psychomotor activity (increase or decrease)

S - Suicidal ideation (increase)

Cassem, 1978.

The Family's Experience

The family plays a critical role for the client with HIV infection. People often turn to family and friends for expressing their concerns, needs, anxieties, and grief, rather than to health care professionals. People maintain a "healthy" self-concept by confiding in those who know them as well people rather than as sick people (Longo et al., 1988). Thus, a critical nursing intervention is to facilitate the families' and friends' support. For the HIV-infected client, maintaining an intact and functioning family may be a challenge.

Family Interactions

A family is an intimate cognitive, emotional, and communicative system. A change in one person in the family causes an imbalance in the system, requiring all others to reorganize (Bahnson, 1975). For many people with HIV infection, the imbalance affects not just one family, but two. The gay client's primary support and loyalty may well be his family of choice, rather than his family of origin. Yet, once diagnosed with a serious illness, his family of origin may suddenly enter his life after being somewhat removed for years. The family of origin often holds the legal right as next of kin, even though the gay family may be more aware of the client's expressed wishes and needs (see Chapter 5).

As nurses, we may find ourselves interacting with two families, both in crisis, and possibly in conflict, and sometimes strangers to each other. Our role is to facilitate meeting the client's needs. We need to take our cues from our client as to who is most critical and competent to meet which needs, gathering support from all sources available. When caring so intensely for another, it's difficult for us to watch discharge plans evolve that we feel compromise the client's needs, regardless of which family we may favor. We need sensitivity to all concerned. In the course of a long, draining illness, we strive to maintain a balance of care demands between families. Both families may become emotionally and physically exhausted, so that the client's final days may be in an institution. Families sometimes feel they have failed when their loved one needs to be hospitalized, or dies in a hospital. However, a hospital death can be best for all concerned and may be the client's wish. We need to allow the client to determine the needs, providing support and affirming the family in meeting these needs as best they can.

Guilt

The family's reaction to the diagnosis may parallel the client's: denial, anger, depression, and guilt. Guilt for the family arises with "What did I do wrong?" or "What could I have done better?" Families blame stress in the family as the source of illness, or the lack of family attention in diagnosing the infection too late. The client's parents often wonder if they failed their son by some mistake in his upbringing that caused his sexual orientation. Lovers feel guilt at the thought that they might have been the source of the HIV exposure (Wolcott, 1985). Guilt is magnified when family members experience a "survivor"s response": shame that they are still living when the loved one is dying.

In families previously torn by conflict, guilt emerges from having "wished the client dead." Such guilt may generate open demonstrations of love and care that are often unreal. In other cases, family members may avoid contact with the client because it increases their feelings of guilt (Bahnson, 1975).

Anger, Rejection, and Withdrawal

The family, like the client, may fear social rejection and ostracism by those outside the immediate family because of the diagnosis of AIDS. In order to avoid the stigma and loss of jobs, friends, and community reputation, the family may withdraw from the client in order to preserve their own relationships with others.

When family members separate from the client to preserve their own self-image, we need to find alternative supports from the hospital staff and community at large. We may become the primary support, both emotional and physical, during the client's final days. Local AIDS community organizations often provide "buddies" who devote extraordinary time over the entire course of the illness to meeting a client's needs in much the way a family does. Psychiatric, spiritual, and social work professionals can add to our support. We need sensitivity to our own needs as well as those of the client, structuring our services so that both client needs and nursing needs are respected. This may mean more than one primary nurse or some kind of rotation system among a few key nurses, as well as a support group of some kind for the nurses involved.

Grief

Families are simultaneously confronted with caring for their ill family member and wondering who will care for them when that person is gone. While being stressed with intense physical and emotional demands of a terminally ill loved one, they are threatened with the permanent loss of one of the most important people in their lives. They are riddled with anxiety and self-doubt about the competency of their care for the person and the emptiness of their lives once the person is gone. This is often the point of anticipatory grieving, a time when families give up false hope and come to terms with the cause of death (Gelcer, 1983). Gay families may also experience a cumulative grief reaction: an unresolved grief response triggered by multiple, successive losses of loved ones to HIV infection. Family members who seem to be in shock, unable to eat, work, or concentrate, or are in any way dysfunctional may be experiencing an incapacitating grief reaction and may benefit from professional psychiatric counseling.

Our role in helping families work through their emotions mirrors our role with clients: Listen, encourage verbalization, and accept the feelings. We cannot change the family's feelings and experience, but we can provide a comforting presence. Give positive feedback to all helpful interactions, physical and verbal, that the family gives to the client. Guide the family on how to help the client, emphasize the importance of their presence and involvement, encourage open and honest communication.

People with HIV infection may be our most emotionally demanding client population due to the devastating nature and alienating stigma of the disease. They need all of our skills and compassion in both providing direct comfort and facilitating families' and friends' support through the emotional and social battles of HIV infection.

References

Abrams, D., Dilley, J., Maxey, L., & Volberding, P. (1986). Routine care and psychosocial support of the patient with the acquired immunodeficiency syndrome. *Medical Clinics of North America, 70*(3), 707-721.

Bahnson, C.B. (1975). Psychologic and emotional issues in cancer: The psychotherapeutic care of the cancer patient. *Seminars in Oncology, 2*(4), 293-309.

Campbell, L. (1987). Hopelessness: A concept analysis. *Journal of Psychosocial Nursing, 25*(2), 18-22.

Cassem, N. (1978). Depression. In T. Hackett & N. Cassem (Eds.), *MGH handbook of general hospital psychiatry* (pp. 209-225), St. Louis: C.V. Mosby Co.

Erikson, E. (1963). *Childhood and society*. New York: W.W. Norton and Co., Inc.

Flaskerud, J. H. (1987). AIDS: Psychosocial aspects. *Journal of Psychosocial Nursing, 25*(12), 9-16.

Forchuk, C., & Westwell, J. (1987). Denial. *Journal of Psychosocial Nursing, 25*(6), 9-13.

Forstein, M. (1984). The psychosocial impact of the acquired immunodeficiency syndrome. *Seminars in Oncology, 11*(1), 77-82.

Gelcer, E. (1983). Mourning is a family affair. *Family Process, 22,* 501-516.

Levy, R., Bredesen, D., & Rosenblum, M. (1985). Neurological manifestations of the acquired immunodeficiency syndrome (AIDS): Experience at UCSF and review of the literature. *Journal of Neurosurgery, 62,* 475-495.

Longo, M., Spross, J., & Locke, A. (1988). Identifying major concerns of persons with AIDS: Report on research. Working paper.

Marzuk, P., Tierney, H., Tardoff, K., Gross, E.M., Morgan, E.B., Hsu, M., & Mann, J.J. (1988, March 4). Increased risk of suicide in persons with AIDS; and, AIDS and suicide. *Journal of the American Medical Association, 259*(9), 1333-1337 and 1369-1370.

Miller, J. (1983). Patient power resources. In J. Miller (Ed.), *Coping with chronic illness: Overcoming powerlessness* (pp. 3-10), Philadelphia: F.A. Davis Co.

Norris, C. (1978). Body image. In C. Carlson & B. Blackwell (Eds.), *Behavioral concepts and nursing intervention* (pp. 5-36), New York: J.B. Lippincott Co.

Plutzky, M. (1974). Principles of psychiatric management of chronic brain syndrome. *Geriatrics, 29*(8), 120-127.

Rogers, D. (1988). Caring for the patient with AIDS. *Journal of the American Medical Association, 259*(9), 1368.

Weisman, A. (1984). *The coping capacity: On the nature of being human.* New York: Human Sciences Press, Inc.

Wolcott, D.L., Fawzy, F.I., & Pasnau, R.O. (1985). Acquired immune deficiency syndrome (AIDS) and consultation-liaison psychiatry. *General Hospital Psychiatry, 7,* 280-293.

Chapter 18

Patient Teaching: Empowering for Self-Care

Ruth Muller

Without a vaccine or a cure, our most effective weapon against HIV infection is education. As nurses, we hold the best position to educate by: 1) our knowledge of health and illness, 2) our skill in applying principles of learning, and 3) our access to clients. Education is an essential ingredient for empowering people and their loved ones for self-care, for control, for maximum independence.

This chapter covers the "how to's" for teaching persons and families with HIV infection: both the process and the content. The learning needs of this population are briefly outlined along with guidelines for getting the material across in the midst of a bustling inpatient setting. Four tables provide specific content from which to select and develop your teaching plan. All of the tables are designed as teaching tools and handouts for your clients and/or those caring for them, either families of choice (friends and lovers) or families of origin.

Individualize for Effective Teaching

Since our clients vary in their learning ability and needs, our teaching plans must vary. Some general principles to keep in mind as you set the stage for learning include:

1. Provide a quiet, private, and uninterrupted environment.
2. Find out what clients *need to know:* what they already know, what they *want* to know, and what they have to know for self-care at home, if applicable.

3. Take advantage of the "teachable" moment; feed them the information when they are ready and willing to receive it.

4. Treat learners as adults by giving them control of the learning situation.

5. Expect clients to take responsibility for their learning and decision making regarding their care.

We can spot a teachable moment by finding the person free from any barriers to learning. The diagnosis of HIV infection, AIDS, or ARC may evoke anxiety, anger, depression, or denial. Any strong emotion to the disease could block clients' ability to learn. When you encounter an emotional block, hold your teaching plans for the moment and try to help the client deal with the feelings. Often this means just listening and accepting. Then come back another time for presenting the content.

Other barriers to learning for people with HIV infection entail the physical discomforts or disabilities of the illness: pain, fatigue, or memory and cognitive deficits. Wait for a time of relief or partial relief from pain and fatigue, letting the client determine the best time for learning. Keep the information simple and brief, given in small doses. Written information provides follow-up for all clients, but it is essential for people with cognitive or memory loss. Lastly, avoid the frustration of trying to teach in the presence of one of these barriers. If clients fail to indicate a willingness and readiness to learn, wait for a better chance, or in the event of imminent discharge, teach the person who will be delivering the care at home instead.

Maximizing the Teaching Time

Right Learning Style

When thinking about how to approach your clients, consider the methods as well as the content. Since people learn differently, try to present information so that clients can use it. You can introduce your teaching plan by explaining to your clients that you would like to teach them to do things that will help them care for themselves. Ask them what methods have worked in the past when they wanted to learn new things. Some teaching-learning strategies include:

- listening to lectures or dialogue with a professional;
- reading written materials independently;
- doing a return demonstration on a specific task;
- watching a video or listening to a tape.

All of these methods can be used separately or in combination, depending on the content and on the individual's needs.

Right Time

Try to plan your teaching according to the person's biorhythms. Find out whether your client is a "morning" or "afternoon" person. If necessary, plan teaching times for evening and night shifts in order to accommodate individual client preferences.

Focus teaching sessions as well as physical care in between frequent rest periods. For best results, time your teaching when the client is most rested, comfortable, and alert.

Right Social Support

Try to enlist the aid of the family of origin or of choice in your teaching. Let the client decide who should be included and to what extent. Clients often feel less isolated and institutionalized when their chosen loved ones continue to give care in the hospital. Such involvement can be tremendously therapeutic for the family, who often feel helpless and isolated. Invite family members to participate in the client's care, if both they and the client seem eager to do so. Since families tend to be easily intimidated by a hospital environment and health care professionals, extend the invitation to them. By involving family members early in the care, you can teach much of the home care content long before discharge.

Since family members are likely to feel self-conscious and nervous in front of a professional nurse, they will need your patience, reassurance, encouragement, and kindness. Present new information in small increments, give them a chance to demonstrate the learning, and praise each accomplishment. For example, involve them in the client's hygiene by demonstrating how to bathe one arm, while they repeat the bathing on the other arm. By incorporating teaching in the process of giving care, you simultaneously accomplish several goals: present content of bathing, provide physical care, observe a return demonstration, evaluate the learning, and give the family a concrete way of helping their loved one.

Right Communication

Document in the client's chart your patient-teaching interaction. Briefly state what content was covered, the client's readiness and demonstrated comprehension, and any plans for future teaching still needed. Just as we always record vital signs, our recording of patient-teaching informs other members of the health care team about the client's cognitive/emotional status and needs, allows others to build on our work, and gives us credit for a critical nursing role. Share the outcome of your teaching with home health agencies either by phone or by a written referral, so that they can reinforce your instruction.

The Content: What Clients Need to Know

In preparing for this chapter, I interviewed both hospitalized and community-based persons with HIV infection and their families to find out what they wanted to know. The most overwhelming response from all those interviewed was to *write everything down for when we go home!* While hospitalized, people had access to health professionals. They could ask for clarification, reiteration, or explanations whenever needed. Problems arose when they returned to home or work and tried to explain issues to friends, coworkers, or other family members. Thus, the following teaching tools and those at the end of this chapter were created to accompany the nurse's interaction.

All clients and/or those caring for them need the essential information listed on Table 18.1: disease process, symptom management, reportable signs and symptoms, medications, plans for follow-up, and infection control. Table 18.1 can be used as a guideline or checklist for preparing clients/families for discharge.

Table 18.1 *Essential Teaching Content for Discharge*

I. Disease Process

- Provide simple, short definitions of all diagnoses, including all opportunistic infections currently experienced by client.

Outcome Criterion:

Client and/or family can explain in their own words each of the client's medical diagnoses.

II. Symptom Management

- Fever:
    A. Teach clients/families how to take a temperature. If they have difficulty reading a mercury thermometer, suggest they buy a digital thermometer and bring it in for a demonstration.
    B. Explain that any medication for fever (antipyretic) should be prescribed by the physician. Caution against aspirin, which can contribute to bleeding (especially if the client is thrombocytopenic), and against Tylenol (acetaminophen may sometimes interact with zidovudine, formerly AZT, to cause side effects).
    C. Equip clients/families with self-care diary for recording fevers and emphasize the importance of accurate records for symptom treatment (see Table 18.4).

Outcome Criteria:

A. Clients/families demonstrate temperature taking on their home thermometer.
B. Clients/families verbalize the need to use the medication prescribed by their doctor for fever control.
C. Clients/families explain the importance of self-care diary and demonstrate how to fill it out.

- Fatigue:

Explain to clients/families methods for energy conservation.

Table 18.1 *Essential Teaching Content for Discharge*

Outcome Criteria:

Clients/families will be able to describe the following energy conservation measures:
- A. Pace activities in between frequent rest periods.
- B. Perform activities seated whenever possible.
- C. Use a terry cloth robe to dry oneself after bath/shower.
- D. Avoid extremes of temperature.
- E. Rest for an hour after meals.
- F. Use assistive devices as needed, i.e., shower chair, bedside commode, etc.

- Diarrhea:

  Explain fluid replacement and nutritional therapy as discussed in Chapter 11, as well as anti-diarrhea medication.

Outcome Criteria:
- A. Clients/families identify the amount and type of fluid needed for replacement therapy.
- B. Clients/families list foods needed and foods to avoid.
- C. Clients/families explain when and how to take anti-diarrhea medication.

- Weight Loss:
  - A. Explain high-protein, high-caloric foods (see Chapter 11).
  - B. Assess if the client is experiencing any particular barriers to eating (mouth soreness, taste changes, nausea, etc.) and review ways to overcome existing problems (see Chapter 11).

Outcome Criteria:
- A. Clients/families list foods of choice for weight gain.
- B. Clients/families identify strategies for overcoming barriers to eating.

III. Reportable Signs and Symptoms

- Before discharge, obtain from the physician parameters for reporting fever (how high a temperature, for how long) and diarrhea (how many stools per day). These parameters differ depending on the client's known symptoms and the primary care provider. Equip your client/family with the information regarding early warning signals on Table 18.3. Provide the self-care diary (Table 18.4) for recording problems accurately, as explained above.

Outcome Criterion:
- A. Clients/families will verbalize importance of reporting signs and symptoms, and when to call their physician.

Table 18.1 continued on page 230

Table 18.1 *Essential Teaching Content for Discharge* (continued)

IV. Medications

- Since people with HIV infection tend to experience more side effects, such as rashes and fevers, than other clients, they need detailed explanations of the major side effects for each medication. Include and explain a written description of the medication, action, and side effects as well as a written schedule.

Outcome Criteria:

A. Clients/families will describe in their own words what each medication does and what side effects are possible.
B. Clients/families will repeat how and when to take each medication.

V. Plans for Follow-Up

- Make sure every client/family has a definite appointment with the physician/primary care provider before leaving hospital. Provide clients with written information and verbal explanations of the information below.

Outcome Criteria:

A. Clients/families have physician's name, phone number, and appointment time, date, and place.
B. Clients/families have names of agencies, person to contact, and phone numbers of any home care providers being used.
C. Clients/families have list of local AIDS community resources, what they provide, and how to reach them.

VI. Infection Control

- All clients need to know how to practice safer sex, as outlined in Chapter 14. They also need to know how to protect themselves from infection from causative organisms and how to protect the household members from HIV transmission. Appendix 18.9 at the end of this chapter provide home care and personal care measures.

Outcome Criteria:

A. Clients/families will describe safer sex methods.
B. Clients/families will identify basic infection control measures in household activities of daily living.

In answer to the question "What do you need to know about the disease?" people identified five areas:

- What is AIDS?

- What does ARC mean?
- What does HIV mean?
- What if my test is positive for HIV?
- Exactly what tests do they do on blood samples?

Some brief answers to these questions listed in Table 18.2 provide easy handout information for people to take home.

Table 18.2 *AIDS-related Terms*

AIDS: These initials stand for acquired immune deficiency syndrome, a disease caused by the HIV, which infects the white blood cells of your body's immune system. This breakdown of your immune system is what makes you less resistant to infections that are commonly found in people with AIDS.

ARC: When your body has been exposed to the HIV but has responded in a less severe manner, you may have ARC, AIDS related complex.

HIV: These initials stand for human immunodeficiency virus. It is the specific name given to the viral organism that causes the malfunction of the immune system.

HIV Testing: a way to determine, by having your blood drawn and examined, if you have been exposed to the HIV. The test looks for the presence in your blood of an *antibody* to the HIV. If the antibody is found to be present (that is, the test is positive), it means you have come in contact with the HIV. Two tests are being used presently to look at blood samples. One is called the *ELISA* (enzyme linked immunoabsorbent assay). The other is called the *Western Blot* and is done as a confirmatory test to avoid false positives with use of ELISA alone.

HIV ELISA Test: blood test that indicates the presence of antibodies to the HIV. It does not detect or diagnose the disease AIDS. It only indicates that viral infection has occurred.

Western Blot Test: confirmatory blood test used to detect the presence of antibodies to the HIV. Compared to the ELISA test, the Western Blot is more specific and more expensive. It is used when there is reason to confirm a positive ELISA test.

Antibody: a substance formed by the body's immune system in reaction to a foreign substance (in this case, the HIV). It is the body's attempt to form a substance to protect itself.

Used by permission of Brigham and Women's Hospital.

People need to know how to manage the discomfort and distress of their symptoms. Table 18.1 includes teaching content for home treatment of fever, fatigue, diarrhea, and weight loss. Chapter 11 reviews diarrhea, weight loss, and associated symptom management. Persons infected with HIV need to know the danger signals of infection and when to call their primary care provider for help or information. Since clients can easily mistake some of the early symptoms of HIV infection for a common illness like the flu, they need specific guidelines even if they are currently asymptomatic. Be sure to obtain parameters for fever, diarrhea, and weight loss from the physician before the client's discharge. Table 18.3 provides a teaching tool for when to call the health care provider.

Table 18.3 *Early Warning Signals*

Call your primary care provider/physician at the first sign of any of the following:

- persistent *tiredness* for no reason
- night sweats, chills, *fevers* that keep coming back
- *weight loss* of more than 10 pounds over a short period of time
- *swollen glands* (lymph nodes) in the neck, armpits, groin that never seem to go away
- *sore throat* that is persistent, or white patches/spots in the mouth
- a persistent *cough* that you have not had before
- tendency to *bruise* or *bleed easily* from any part of the body
- persistent *diarrhea* (mild or severe)
- pink or purple *blotches* or bumps on the skin
- decrease in memory, ability to concentrate, alertness, or any *confusion*
- changes or difficulty *moving:* walking, keeping your balance, performing self-care tasks

With the current emphasis on home care, primary providers rely *heavily* on accurate information about signs and symptoms that occur at home. Self-care diaries provide vital information on temperature fluctuation, fluid and nutritional intake, weight changes, and symptoms such as sweats, chills, fatigue, diarrhea, or decreased urine output. Table 18.4 provides an example of such a self-care diary, to be completed by clients or by those responsible for their care. The health care provider will need to review this diary at each appointment in order to assess indicators of opportunistic infections and strategize ways of coping with the discomforts of HIV infection.

Table 18.4 *Self-Care Diary*

Date_____   A.M. Weight_____

Time:					
Temperature					
106					
105					
104					
103					
102					
101					
100					
99					
98					
97					
Medications					
Diarrhea					
Sweats					
Chills					
Confusion					
Fluid Intake					
Food Intake					
Urine Output					

Contact With Provider   Instruction Received

_____   _____

_____   _____

_____   _____

_____   _____

Other information needed and sought after includes explanations of diagnoses and medications. Appendixes 18.1 and 18.2 (at the end of this chapter) describe the common conditions of pneumocystis carinii pneumonia and Kaposi's sarcoma. Appendixes 18.3 through 18.8 (at the end of this chapter) are handouts on medications frequently used in the treatment of people with HIV infection. You can select which teaching tool will be most helpful for each individual client. Be sure to include clear instructions in lay terms on frequency of each medication, such as three times a day, or with meals. Plan with the client the best times of day for each treatment.

Clients and families identified preparation and delivery of home care as their most pressing concern. A major concern of home care is infection control. Since HIV transmission occurs only through blood, semen, and vaginal secretions, the main focus of infection control is keeping clients safe from opportunistic infection. In order to protect family members from HIV infection, provide specific information on safer sex methods, as explained in Chapter 14. Appendix 18.9 includes complete guidelines for protecting both clients and their household members from causative organisms, including personal hygiene, household chores, nutritional and cooking hints, pet care, and trash disposal. This handout can be used to initiate discussion about family roles in home care. Emphasize what is safe, such as casual and social contact, as well as what is unsafe, such as sexual intercourse without a condom. By providing concrete actions for infection control in a clear, calm way, we help to eliminate unrealistic fears of contagion for the family and fears of opportunistic infection for the clients. Both families and clients feel more in control and ready for going home when they have a chance to plan, organize, and learn in advance.

The clients and families interviewed also indentified items that they needed at home. They suggested that the nurse tell people in advance to equip their homes with the items listed in Appendix 18.10, "Checklist for PWAs: Items to Have on Hand." In addition to *objects* that they needed, there are also *services* that they needed to do for themselves while they were able. Appendix 18.11, a "To-Do List," outlines the self-care tasks they identified as important. It provides a useful tool to help clients anticipate their needs and plan for them.

Developing Additional Learning Tools

As client needs change, you may need written handout information beyond that contained in this chapter. Before you start writing, first consult all the resources and colleagues possible, locally and nationally, to see if a tool has already been developed. Often, we duplicate each other's work out of a reluctance to ask for assistance or information. Yet as nurses, we are most responsive to a request for help and most willing to share. If, after searching widely, you still need to develop your own resource, consider the following guidelines.
  1. Thoroughly review the literature on your topic.
  2. Format the information carefully. Keep it simple, with large, legible print.

Allow enough space between content so that the reader can separate sections readily and follow the train of thought easily.

3. Write your materials for a sixth-grade level. Use simple words, short sentences, and plain language. Explain any technical or medical terms with simple, clear definitions. Pilot your draft on a few laypeople to check for comprehension.

4. Be straightforward and factual in your content. Clear, explicit information helps to eliminate uncertainty or misunderstanding.

5. Have one or more experts review the completed product. Some institutions have an interdisciplinary Patient Education Committee to review such materials.

Comprehensive, sensitive teaching helps to equip people for self-care: maximum independence, comfort, and wellness. By knowing disease process and symptom management, they can maintain some physical comfort and symptom control. By knowing how and when to contact their primary care provider, they can deal with problems at an earlier and more treatable state. By knowing infection control, they can maintain social support. With education, clients can go home feeling prepared, equipped, in control, and comfortable.

Appendix 18.1

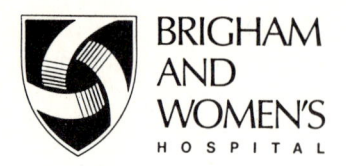

Definition: Pneumocystis Carinii Pneumonia (PCP)

Pneumocystis carinii pneumonia is a disease of the lungs caused by a virus. It is one of the opportunistic infections found in persons with AIDS. It can be very severe and you may need to be hospitalized to get special medications.

Even though you may have been previously hospitalized and given IV medications (trimethoprim/sulfamethoxacole or pentamidine) for your pneumonia, the recurrence of *fever, dry cough,* and perhaps some *shortness of breath* are symptoms to which you should be alert. If you become aware of one or several of these, especially a temperature of 101 degrees or greater for 24 hours that you can't explain any other way, call your health care provider. This pneumonia can recur and needs to be treated right away. When you call, be sure to be able to tell your care giver:

- the sequence of events;
- what your temperature has been at what time;
- whether you are coughing up sputum (phlegm) or not;
- whether you have taken any medicines.

To help yourself, you should:

- Drink as much fluid as possible. This will help bring your fever down. It can also make it easier for you to cough up sputum. Try to move around so your lungs can expand better. Do not sit or lie in one position for long periods of time. Your provider will probably tell you to take an anti-fever medicine. Do so regularly.
- Take your temperature every four hours and write down the results and the time you took your temperature on your self-care diary sheet. Have this handy when you call your doctor or nurse. Bring it with you on your appointments.

Used by permission of Brigham and Women's Hospital.

Appendix 18.2

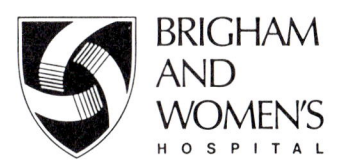

BRIGHAM AND WOMEN'S HOSPITAL

Definition: Kaposi's Sarcoma (KS)

Kaposi's sarcoma (KS) is a malignancy commonly seen in AIDS patients. KS may occur at any time during the course of your illness. You may note the appearance of pink or purple blotchy areas on your skin. These lesions, as they are called, generally do not cause pain, but may become painful if they grow rapidly. You should make an appointment to see a dermatologist who has been recommended by your health care provider. The physician will perform a skin biopsy to determine if the rash is KS. Treatment of KS consists of radiation therapy (X-ray therapy) and administration of chemotherapy (anti-cancer drugs). These treatments can cause certain side effects, which usually can be managed. Consult your care giver or local AIDS support community for information on the causes and management of these side effects as well as for hints to help understand what is happening and why.

Used by permission of Brigham and Women's Hospital.

Appendix 18.3

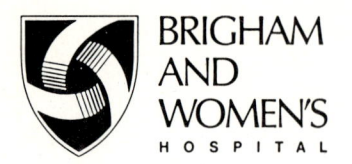

BRIGHAM AND WOMEN'S HOSPITAL

Medication: Trimethoprim/ Sulfamethoxazole (Bactrim, Bactrim DS, Septra)

What It Does

Bactrim fights bacteria and is used to treat urinary tract infections and certain types of pneumonia and ear and bloodstream infections.

Special Instructions

- Drink a full glass of water with each dose. Drink plenty of water during the day. It is critical to keep the kidneys flushed.
- "DS" means double strength.
- It is best to take Bactrim on an empty stomach, one hour before or two hours after meals.
- Take Bactrim as prescribed, even after you begin to feel well. Failure to do so could allow the infection to return.
- If you miss a dose of Bactrim, take the missed dose as soon as you remember or take a double dose the next time you are scheduled to take a dose.

Be Alert To:

- Headache, loss of appetite, abdominal pain, sleeplessness, listlessness, skin *rash*, sore throat, *chills or fever*, mouth sores or pain, nausea or vomiting, diarrhea.

If any of these symptoms become bothersome and interfere with your usual activities, notify your health care provider.

Directions

Dosage:

Frequency:

Times:

Used by permission of Brigham and Women's Hospital.

Patient Teaching: Empowering for Self-Care

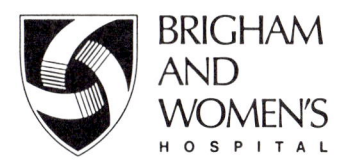

Appendix 18.4

BRIGHAM AND WOMEN'S HOSPITAL

Medication: Ketoconazole (Nizoral)

What It Does

Ketoconazole is a drug used to fight yeast (candida) and fungal infections of the skin, mouth, lungs, and brain.

Special Instructions

- It is important to take this medicine for the whole length of time your doctor prescribed, even if your infection appears to have gone away.
- This medicine can cause dizziness or drowsiness. Until you have taken it for a few days to know its effect on you, do not drive or do other things that require you to be very alert.
- Wait at least two hours after taking antacids (Mylanta, Amphogel, Maalox) or these other drugs: Zantec, Pepcid, Cimetidine.
- Avoid using alcohol.
- Use sunglasses and avoid long periods of exposure to bright light.

Be Alert To:

- Redness, swelling, or irritation in your mouth; nausea, vomiting, diarrhea, or constipation; yellowing of the skin or itching.

If any of these symptoms become bothersome and interfere with your usual activities, notify your health care provider.

Directions

Dosage:

Frequency:

Times:

Used by permission of Brigham and Women's Hospital.

Appendix 18.5

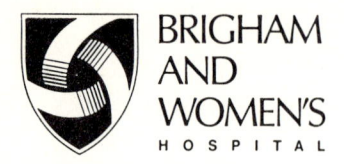

BRIGHAM AND WOMEN'S HOSPITAL

Medication: Acyclovir (Zovirax)

What It Does

Acyclovir is a drug used to treat the viruses that cause herpes simplex and genital herpes. It is a medicine that is helpful in managing the disease but does not eliminate or cure it.

Special Instructions

- Using Acyclovir will not prevent your spreading the infection to others.
- If an ointment form is prescribed by your doctor, apply enough to cover all your sores well.
- Wear gloves when you apply it and wash your hands carefully after applying ointment to prevent spreading the virus to other parts of your body or to other people.
- DO NOT USE other over-the-counter creams, lotions, or ointments. This can delay healing and may cause spreading of the sores.
- If you have genital herpes, condoms should always be worn during sexual contact. This means that you must put on the condom before foreplay. It is even better to avoid sexual contact while sores are present and not healed.
- Drink plenty of fluids.

Be Alert To:

- Headache, dizziness, nausea, vomiting, diarrhea, rash, itching, bloody urine, or decrease in urination.

If you develop tingling, itching, or pain, call your health care provider. These may be signs that a new area of sores is developing.

If any of these symptoms become bothersome and interfere with your usual activities, notify your health care provider.

Used by permission of Brigham and Women's Hospital.

Directions

Dosage:

Frequency:

Times:

Appendix 18.6

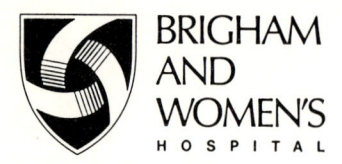

BRIGHAM AND WOMEN'S HOSPITAL

Medication: Nystatin Suspension (Mycostatin, Nilstat, Nadostine)

What It Does

Nystatin is an antibiotic used to fight yeast and fungi infections of the skin and mouth. The most common one is candida (thrush).

Special Instructions

- It is very important that you use Nystatin rinses daily as often as prescribed.
- Continue to take Nystatin for the prescribed length of time, even if your infection appears to have gone away.
- Before mouth administration, your mouth should be clear of food and you should brush your teeth.
- Keep medication in your mouth for several minutes and swish it around before swallowing.
- Avoid use of any other over-the-counter mouth washes or rinses while on this medication.

Be Alert To:

- Increased redness, swelling, or irritation in the mouth; nausea, vomiting, or (rarely) diarrhea.

If any of these symptoms become bothersome and interfere with your usual activities, notify your health care provider.

Directions

Dosage:

Frequency:

Times:

Used by permission of Brigham and Women's Hospital.

Appendix 18.7

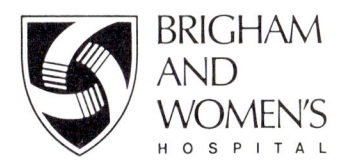

BRIGHAM AND WOMEN'S HOSPITAL

Medication: Pentamidine Isethionate (Pentam 300)

What It Does

Pentamidine is a medicine that has been found to be effective in the treatment of pneumocystis carinii pneumonia. It works against the organism, called a "protozoan," that causes the pneumonia.

Special Instructions

- This drug can cause sudden and severe drops in your blood pressure. If you have been lying down and receiving IV pentamidine, be very careful getting up to a standing position. Sit for a few moments on the edge of the bed where you were resting before rising to your feet. Your health care provider will have been checking your blood pressure during the slow IV infusion.
- This drug can cause hypoglycemia (low blood sugar). This may not occur until several days after you start receiving the drug. Your health care provider will check your blood sugar level and help make arrangements or teach you how to do this yourself when you get home.
- If you are using a nebulizer to take this medication:
  - Unscrew the two pieces of the nebulizer and hold upright while you put dissolved medicine in bowl.
  - Set regulator or air compressor at 6 liters (6 l on gauge) to start mist, or as prescribed.
  - Close your mouth over the mouthpiece, and take *slow*, deep breaths.
  - Make sure others do not stand directly where mist is escaping as you use the nebulizer, or they may receive the medication, too, depending upon the nebulizer.
  - Use nebulizer until all medicine is gone, or for 20 minutes.

Used by permission of Brigham and Women's Hospital.

Be Alert To:

- Feelings of dizziness, light-headedness, fever, nausea, confusion, lack of appetite, metallic taste. You will usually experience these sensations to some degree during your therapy course. You need to report them if they are new for you, different from before, or if you have not discussed them with your health care provider. If you experience wheezing, a bronchodilator medication may help. Check with your physician.
- Call your health care provider right away if you develop a rash, very itchy skin, or facial flushing while on this medicine or if your fever has been at 100 degrees or higher for 24 hours.

Directions

Dosage:

Frequency:

Times:

Appendix 18.8

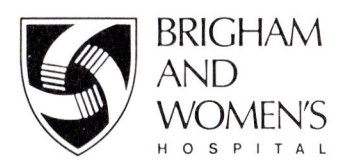

BRIGHAM AND WOMEN'S HOSPITAL

Zidovudine (Retrovir, formerly AZT)

What is zidovudine?

Zidovudine is a drug that inhibits the growth of the virus that causes AIDS, the human immunodeficiency virus (HIV). Zidovudine is not a cure for AIDS, but it may prolong life and decrease the number of infections that occur with AIDS and ARC. It may also help with weight gain and strength. The long-term effects of this drug are unknown because it is such a new drug. Zidovudine is now available by doctor's prescription to all individuals with AIDS and ARC. Prescriptions of zidovudine can be filled by most hospital and commercial pharmacies, just as any other medication. A number of individuals experience side effects from zidovudine, so it is important that you see your physician regularly for checkups.

What are the major side effects?

The major side effect of zidovudine is a decrease in red and white blood cells. A decrease in red blood cells leads to anemia. You may feel increasingly fatigued or short of breath when you are anemic. People on zidovudine sometimes need blood transfusions to correct the anemia. If your white blood cell count decreases, you may become even more vulnerable to infection. Your doctor or nurse practitioner will need to draw blood at regular and frequent intervals to determine the effects that the zidovudine is having on these important blood components. A decrease in the dosage or stopping the zidovudine may be necessary to protect you from dangerous side effects. For some people, the drug may be restarted at a lower dose if the red and white blood cell counts improve. Other side effects include nausea and vomiting, muscle aches, difficulty sleeping, headaches, and increased fatigue.

How long will it take to work?

Decreases in the number of infections have been reported after six weeks of taking zidovudine. Weight gain has been noted in patients in zidovudine therapy as early

From Christopher L. LaCharite and Janice Bell Meisenhelder, *Zidovudine: New Hope for AIDS.* Unpublished paper, 1988.

as four weeks into therapy. The greatest weight gain has been observed between twelve and sixteen weeks after beginning the medication. Your ability to perform activities of daily living may improve in four weeks and peak between the eighth and sixteenth week.

How do I take zidovudine?

Zidovudine comes in 100-mg capsules. The usual beginning dosage is 200 mg (two capsules) every four hours around the clock. Doses may be different depending upon the results of your blood tests, so it is important to follow the medication instructions exactly. Do not make any changes in times or amounts without your doctor's advice. Because you need to take zidovudine around the clock, set your alarm clock to wake you for your nighttime dose. Prepare the dose and set a glass of water nearby at bedtime so that your amount of waking time is limited.

How much does zidovudine cost?

Zidovudine generally costs between $600 and $800 per month. Information regarding assistance for payment of zidovudine can be obtained through an AIDS social worker or a community AIDS organization.

Can I take other medications with zidovudine?

Many of the medications you are now on will be able to be continued. Tylenol (acetaminophen) may increase the chance of having side effects from zidovudine and should only be taken with your doctor's permission. To be safe, consult your physician or primary care provider before taking any over-the-counter medications.

What else do I need to know?

It's always important to keep your physician or nurse appointments, but even more important when you are on zidovudine. Your physician/nurse practitioner will want to monitor your laboratory values, weight, and functional performance status. It is important that you keep in contact with them and report any shortness of breath, feelings of fatigue, chills, fever, nausea, or any other unusual symptoms.

Most important, zidovudine will not cure AIDS. Since you can still spread the AIDS infection to others even while you are taking zidovudine, you need to continue with safer sex practices.

Appendix 18.9

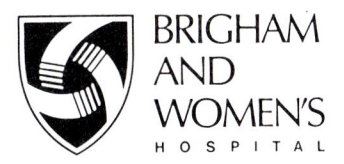

BRIGHAM AND WOMEN'S HOSPITAL

Home Care Guidelines for People With AIDS, ARC, and HIV Infection

Following are a number of important guidelines that persons with HIV infection should follow in order to maintain their own level of health and to protect others from being infected with the virus. There is no reason why persons with HIV, ARC, or AIDS should not continue to have the usual social contacts with people that they have had in the past. However, care should be taken not to share body secretions, particularly blood or semen. In order for body secretions to be shared, there must be a point of entry into another person's body. Preventing this transfer of body secretions while still maintaining one's sexuality requires foresight and common sense.

Personal Hygiene

Maintaining a state of personal cleanliness is essential to both the person with AIDS and others. This includes bathing regularly; washing hands after the use of bathroom facilities or contact with one's own body fluids such as semen, mucus, or blood; and washing hands before preparing food. A daily regimen of cleanliness in the area of skin, nail, hair, dental, rectal, and vaginal care is important for maintaining health and observing and managing possible symptoms.

Handwashing

- Wash hands before and after contact with contaminated materials, use of bathroom, before eating, and before cooking.
- If not washed, keep hands away from eyes, nose, and mouth.
- Use cool water to prevent skin from chapping.
- Use liquid soap instead of bar soap to prevent spread of germs.

Nail Care

- Keep fingernails and toenails clean and cut to prevent fungal infections.

Adapted from material prepared by AIDS Action Committee, Boston, MA

Hair Care

- Avoid excessive washing.
- Use only gentle shampoos, such as baby shampoo or castile soap.
- Use a hair and scalp conditioner.
- Cover your head in bed to reduce hair loss due to friction.
- Give your scalp a good treatment using mayonnaise. Apply mayonnaise, then apply a warm, wet towel for 15-20 minutes, then shampoo as usual.

Skin Care

- Use body lotions or creams to restore moisture to dry skin.
- Bathe using only a mild soap; rinse well.
- Take showers rather than baths, if capable, especially if you have foot or skin fungus.

Dental Regimen

- Brush after meals using a soft toothbrush.
- Floss at least once a day.
- Inform dentist about condition.
- Schedule regular dental checkups.
- Use rinses made up of diluted hydrogen peroxide to kill bacterial infections and promote healing (1 part peroxide to 10 parts water).

Rectal and Vaginal Care

- Use sitz baths, witch hazel wipes, or other soothing ointments when irritation occurs.
- Avoid excessive use of cleansing enemas; if used, make sure they are disposable.
- Use disposable vaginal douches for irritation.

Self-Care Symptom Management Guide

Patients should watch for changes in:

- breathing;
- temperature;
- weight;
- bowel habits;
- water loss (dehydration);
- energy levels (fatigue);
- mood, personality, behavior, speech, or memory.

What to Do

- Record any changes daily.
- Consult your health care provider (physician, nurse, etc.).
- Maintain good personal hygiene (fluid and nutritional intake).
- Keep all medical appointments.
- Maintain communications with family, lover, friends, and health care provider.

Disposable Masks

- Use masks only once; purchase new ones at drug stores or surgical supply stores.
- Have visitors with respiratory infections wear masks while in your presence to protect you from infection.
- Persons with AIDS who are coughing should cover their mouth with tissue or handkerchiefs. Persons visiting or living with a person with AIDS should do the same.

Household Chores

Kitchen and bathroom facilities may be shared with others. Normal sanitary practices will prevent the growth of fungi and bacteria that may potentially cause illness to both immunocompromised and immunocompetent people. These practices include:

- Wash dishes and silverware in hot, soapy water; rinse dishes and let air dry, or use dishwasher.
- Clean kitchen counters with scouring powder to remove food particles. Sponges used to clean in the kitchen where food is prepared should not be the same sponges used to clean up bathroom-type spills. Dirty-looking sponges should not be used to wash dishes or clean food preparation areas.
- Clean inside of refrigerator with soap and water to control molds.
- Mop up spills of body fluids or waste immediately with paper towels and dispose of properly; wash affected area with a 1:10-strength chlorine bleach solution (1 part bleach to 10 parts water). This solution may also be used to disinfect kitchen and bathroom floors, shower, floor (bleach will kill the fungus responsible for athlete's foot), sinks, and toilet bowls.
- Mop kitchen floor at least once a week.
- Mop bathroom floor at least once a week.
- Towels and washcloths should not be shared without laundering. Toothbrushes, razors, enema equipment, and sexual toys should never be shared.
- Keep living quarters well ventilated. Airborne diseases are less likely to be a problem when diluted by air.
- Sponges used to clean the floor or any body fluid spills should not be used to

wash dishes or clean food preparation areas. Mop water should not be poured down sink where food is prepared. Sponges used to clean up spills should not be washed out at sinks where food preparation occurs. Sponges and mops can be disinfected by soaking in 1:10 bleach for 5 minutes (longer may disintegrate sponge).
- Clean spills on carpets using soap and water.
- Clothes and bed linens can be washed in usual manner unless soiled with body fluids, in which case they should be bleached; clothes can be washed with those of other family members.
- Trash disposal should be the same as for any household. Body wastes are flushed down the toilet. Other trash may be adequately handled by normal means (weekly trash pickups from cans lined with a plastic bag and topped with a tight-fitting lid to keep out rodents). In the event of large amounts of sputum or wound drainage, etc., on facial tissues or dressings, it is a good idea to collect them in a lined trash can in the house.
- Sanitary napkins and tampons should be wrapped in a small plastic bag and then placed in a plastic-lined, tightly covered trash can in the house.

Nutritional and Cooking Hints

- Take a good vitamin and mineral supplement to ensure proper nutrition when dietary habits are poor.
- Maintain an intake of 2,000 to 2,700 calories and 45 to 55 grams of protein a day.
- Select four servings each from the fruits-and-vegetable and grain groups; three servings from the meat group; and two servings from the dairy group each day.
- Avoid high-lactose foods such as milk and yogurt, if they cause diarrhea.
- Your dishes and eating utensils may be shared provided they are washed in soapy water between uses. A disinfectant is not necessary.
- People with AIDS can safely cook for others provided hands are washed thoroughly before beginning. It's also a good idea not to lick the fingers or taste from the mixing spoon while cooking (advice for everyone).
- Because unpasteurized milk and milk products have been associated with salmonella infections in the past, these should not be included in the diet. Salmonella infections are not well tolerated by people with AIDS.
- If organically grown food is used (composted with human or animal feces), food should be cooked and fruits should be peeled. "Organic" lettuce is not safe.

Pets

- Gloves should be used when cleaning bird cages and cat litter boxes to avoid risk of contracting illnesses such as psittacosis and toxoplasmosis. Tropical fish tanks may contain organisms in the mycobacterium family that are not well tolerated by persons with AIDS. Get someone else to clean your tank.

Other

Decisions on group housing or sharing apartments with another PWA need to be made on an individual basis.

Persons with AIDS living together can do so safely by observing the same common-sense hygiene practices discussed above. The opportunistic infections acquired by persons with AIDS are caused by organisms commonly found in the environment. The risk of becoming sick from one of these infections is based on the amount of immune system impairment, not on casual household contact.

Appendix 18.10

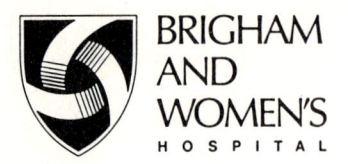

BRIGHAM AND WOMEN'S HOSPITAL

Checklist for PWAs: Items To Have on Hand

Since each individual has different needs, some of the items you *might* need are:

- extra sheets, bright pillowcases;
- large plastic bags (for use as protection under sheet);
- small plastic bags (for sanitary napkin, tampon, condom disposal);
- liquid soap (bars can harbor germs dangerous to PWAs);
- bleach (for laundry and spill cleanup);
- hydrogen peroxide (for mouth rinse);
- dental floss/soft toothbrush;
- thermometer;
- urinal, bedpan, plastic basin (ask nurse to give you patient's from hospital);
- disposable gloves and masks;
- extra sponge and mop (for cleanup);
- room deodorizer or potpourri;
- rubbing alcohol (cooling massage, bring down temperature);
- small fan if no air conditioner;
- cardboard carton to make into over-bed table if available;
- used coffee can (for needle disposal).

Also:

- Stock up on favorite foods, good books, videos.
- Think about moving bed close to bathroom.
- Rent needed medical equipment and have ready (oxygen, commode, hospital bed).

Used by permission of Brigham and Women's Hospital.

Appendix 18.11

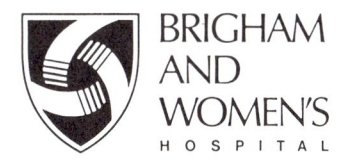

BRIGHAM AND WOMEN'S HOSPITAL

"To Do List": Suggestions for PWA or PWARC to Consider

These are some things you might want to think about, discuss with those close to you, or do during periods when you feel reasonably well. They are offered to help you decrease your feelings of stress and uncertainty and to help you plan ahead. They give you a variety of hints but allow you the flexibility to make decisions about their use according to your own coping style.

- Consider carefully *whom* to tell of your illness and *how* to tell them.
- Check on what your insurance does and does not cover. Write down what is explained to you.
- Make a list of hotline numbers to have handy so you can call and get quick answers, helpful information, and suggestions. Include the telephone numbers of health care providers.
- Investigate the existence of support groups in your area. Ask a friend to accompany you to a meeting for support.
- Start learning about holistic therapies if you feel they could be helpful to you.
- Make out a food preference list, a "wish list" of all the first things you grab when you haven't felt well in the past. Include your all-time favorites.
- Make an appointment with your lawyer. If you don't have one, call the local bar association or, better yet, the AIDS community organization in your area for referral. You may want to discuss:
  - making out a will to determine who will receive your possessions;
  - guardianship or adoption of your children;
  - power of attorney detailing the specific right to make medical treatment decisions should you become unable to speak for yourself;
  - possibly a living will document, which, although not "legal," will still clearly indicate your desires and feelings.
- Make sure you have an anti-fever medicine in the house and fill whatever other prescriptions have been written for you. Investigate to see if you can find a pharmacy that will deliver medicine to your home when the physician calls in

Used by permission of Brigham and Women's Hospital.

a prescription. This is extremely helpful if you're not feeling well enough to go out.
- At some point, you may want to think about what kind of funeral or memorial service you would like to have. Discussing this with someone close to you or talking it over with your spiritual adviser can be an empowering experience, since it allows you to control another part of your life.

Appendix A.1

Recommendations for Prevention of HIV Transmission in Health-Care Settings

Introduction

Human immunodeficiency virus (HIV), the virus that causes acquired immunodeficiency syndrome (AIDS), is transmitted through sexual contact and exposure to infected blood or blood components and perinatally from mother to neonate. HIV has been isolated from blood, semen, vaginal secretions, saliva, tears, breast milk, cerebrospinal fluid, amniotic fluid, and urine and is likely to be isolated from other body fluids, secretions, and excretions. However, epidemiologic evidence has implicated only blood, semen, vaginal secretions, and possibly breast milk in transmission.

The increasing prevalence of HIV increases the risk that health-care workers will be exposed to blood from patients infected with HIV, especially when blood and body-fluid precautions are not followed for all patients. Thus, this document emphasizes the need for health-care workers to consider **all** patients as potentially infected with HIV and/or other blood-borne pathogens and to adhere rigorously to infection-control precautions for minimizing the risk of exposure to blood and body fluids of all patients.

The recommendations contained in this document consolidate and update CDC recommendations published earlier for preventing HIV transmission in health-care settings: precautions for clinical and laboratory staffs (1) and precautions for health-care workers and allied professionals (2); recommendations for preventing HIV transmission in the workplace (3) and during invasive procedures (4); recommendations for preventing possible transmission of HIV from tears (5); and recommendations for providing dialysis treatment for HIV-infected patients (6). These recommendations also update portions of the "Guideline for Isolation Precautions in Hospitals" (7) and reemphasize some of the recommendations contained in "Infection Control Practices for Dentistry" (8). The recommendations contained in this document have been developed for use in health-care settings and emphasize the need to treat blood and other body fluids from **all** patients as potentially infective. These same prudent precautions also should be taken in other settings in which persons may be exposed to blood or other body fluids.

Definition of Health-Care Workers

Health-care workers are defined as persons, including students and trainees, whose activities involve contact with patients or with blood or other body fluids from patients in a health-care setting.

SOURCE: Centers for Disease Control. Recommendations for prevention of HIV transmission in health-care settings. *MMWR* 1987:36 (suppl. no. 2S) :[1–18].

Health-Care Workers with AIDS

As of July 10, 1987, a total of 1,875 (5.8%) of 32,395 adults with AIDS, who had been reported to the CDC national surveillance system and for whom occupational information was available, reported being employed in a health-care or clinical laboratory setting. In comparison, 6.8 million persons — representing 5.6% of the U.S. labor force — were employed in health services. Of the health-care workers with AIDS, 95% have been reported to exhibit high-risk behavior; for the remaining 5%, the means of HIV acquisition was undetermined. Health-care workers with AIDS were significantly more likely than other workers to have an undetermined risk (5% versus 3%, respectively). For both health-care workers and non-health-care workers with AIDS, the proportion with an undetermined risk has not increased since 1982.

AIDS patients initially reported as not belonging to recognized risk groups are investigated by state and local health departments to determine whether possible risk factors exist. Of all health-care workers with AIDS reported to CDC who were initially characterized as not having an identified risk and for whom follow-up information was available, 66% have been reclassified because risk factors were identified or because the patient was found not to meet the surveillance case definition for AIDS. Of the 87 health-care workers currently categorized as having no identifiable risk, information is incomplete on 16 (18%) because of death or refusal to be interviewed; 38 (44%) are still being investigated. The remaining 33 (38%) health-care workers were interviewed or had other follow-up information available. The occupations of these 33 were as follows: five physicians (15%), three of whom were surgeons; one dentist (3%); three nurses (9%); nine nursing assistants (27%); seven housekeeping or maintenance workers (21%); three clinical laboratory technicians (9%); one therapist (3%); and four others who did not have contact with patients (12%). Although 15 of these 33 health-care workers reported parenteral and/or other non-needlestick exposure to blood or body fluids from patients in the 10 years preceding their diagnosis of AIDS, none of these exposures involved a patient with AIDS or known HIV infection.

Risk to Health-Care Workers of Acquiring HIV in Health-Care Settings

Health-care workers with documented percutaneous or mucous-membrane exposures to blood or body fluids of HIV-infected patients have been prospectively evaluated to determine the risk of infection after such exposures. As of June 30, 1987, 883 health-care workers have been tested for antibody to HIV in an ongoing surveillance project conducted by CDC (*9*). Of these, 708 (80%) had percutaneous exposures to blood, and 175 (20%) had a mucous membrane or an open wound contaminated by blood or body fluid. Of 396 health-care workers, each of whom had only a convalescent-phase serum sample obtained and tested ≥90 days post-exposure, one — for whom heterosexual transmission could not be ruled out — was seropositive for HIV antibody. For 425 additional health-care workers, both acute- and convalescent-phase serum samples were obtained and tested; none of 74 health-care workers with nonpercutaneous exposures seroconverted, and three (0.9%) of 351 with percutaneous exposures seroconverted. None of these three health-care workers had other documented risk factors for infection.

Two other prospective studies to assess the risk of nosocomial acquisition of HIV infection for health-care workers are ongoing in the United States. As of April 30, 1987, 332 health-care workers with a total of 453 needlestick or mucous-membrane exposures to the blood or other body fluids of HIV-infected patients were tested for HIV antibody at the National Institutes of Health (10). These exposed workers included 103 with needlestick injuries and 229 with mucous-membrane exposures; none had seroconverted. A similar study at the University of California of 129 health-care workers with documented needlestick injuries or mucous-membrane exposures to blood or other body fluids from patients with HIV infection has not identified any seroconversions (11). Results of a prospective study in the United Kingdom identified no evidence of transmission among 150 health-care workers with parenteral or mucous-membrane exposures to blood or other body fluids, secretions, or excretions from patients with HIV infection (12).

In addition to health-care workers enrolled in prospective studies, eight persons who provided care to infected patients and denied other risk factors have been reported to have acquired HIV infection. Three of these health-care workers had needlestick exposures to blood from infected patients (13-15). Two were persons who provided nursing care to infected persons; although neither sustained a needlestick, both had extensive contact with blood or other body fluids, and neither observed recommended barrier precautions (16,17). The other three were health-care workers with non-needlestick exposures to blood from infected patients (18). Although the exact route of transmission for these last three infections is not known, all three persons had direct contact of their skin with blood from infected patients, all had skin lesions that may have been contaminated by blood, and one also had a mucous-membrane exposure.

A total of 1,231 dentists and hygienists, many of whom practiced in areas with many AIDS cases, participated in a study to determine the prevalence of antibody to HIV; one dentist (0.1%) had HIV antibody. Although no exposure to a known HIV-infected person could be documented, epidemiologic investigation did not identify any other risk factor for infection. The infected dentist, who also had a history of sustaining needlestick injuries and trauma to his hands, did not routinely wear gloves when providing dental care (19).

Precautions To Prevent Transmission of HIV

Universal Precautions

Since medical history and examination cannot reliably identify all patients infected with HIV or other blood-borne pathogens, blood and body-fluid precautions should be consistently used for **all** patients. This approach, previously recommended by CDC (3,4), and referred to as "universal blood and body-fluid precautions" or "universal precautions," should be used in the care of **all** patients, especially including those in emergency-care settings in which the risk of blood exposure is increased and the infection status of the patient is usually unknown (20).

1. All health-care workers should routinely use appropriate barrier precautions to prevent skin and mucous-membrane exposure when contact with blood or other body fluids of any patient is anticipated. Gloves should be worn for touching blood and body fluids, mucous membranes, or non-intact skin of all patients, for handling items or surfaces soiled with blood or body fluids, and for performing venipuncture and other vascular access procedures. Gloves should be changed after contact with each patient. Masks and protective eyewear or face shields should be worn during procedures that are likely to generate droplets of blood or other body fluids to prevent exposure of mucous membranes of the mouth, nose, and eyes. Gowns or aprons should be worn during procedures that are likely to generate splashes of blood or other body fluids.
2. Hands and other skin surfaces should be washed immediately and thoroughly if contaminated with blood or other body fluids. Hands should be washed immediately after gloves are removed.
3. All health-care workers should take precautions to prevent injuries caused by needles, scalpels, and other sharp instruments or devices during procedures; when cleaning used instruments; during disposal of used needles; and when handling sharp instruments after procedures. To prevent needlestick injuries, needles should not be recapped, purposely bent or broken by hand, removed from disposable syringes, or otherwise manipulated by hand. After they are used, disposable syringes and needles, scalpel blades, and other sharp items should be placed in puncture-resistant containers for disposal; the puncture-resistant containers should be located as close as practical to the use area. Large-bore reusable needles should be placed in a puncture-resistant container for transport to the reprocessing area.
4. Although saliva has not been implicated in HIV transmission, to minimize the need for emergency mouth-to-mouth resuscitation, mouthpieces, resuscitation bags, or other ventilation devices should be available for use in areas in which the need for resuscitation is predictable.
5. Health-care workers who have exudative lesions or weeping dermatitis should refrain from all direct patient care and from handling patient-care equipment until the condition resolves.
6. Pregnant health-care workers are not known to be at greater risk of contracting HIV infection than health-care workers who are not pregnant; however, if a health-care worker develops HIV infection during pregnancy, the infant is at risk of infection resulting from perinatal transmission. Because of this risk, pregnant health-care workers should be especially familiar with and strictly adhere to precautions to minimize the risk of HIV transmission.

Implementation of universal blood and body-fluid precautions for **all** patients eliminates the need for use of the isolation category of "Blood and Body Fluid Precautions" previously recommended by CDC (7) for patients known or suspected to be infected with blood-borne pathogens. Isolation precautions (e.g., enteric, "AFB" [7]) should be used as necessary if associated conditions, such as infectious diarrhea or tuberculosis, are diagnosed or suspected.

Precautions for Invasive Procedures

In this document, an invasive procedure is defined as surgical entry into tissues, cavities, or organs or repair of major traumatic injuries 1) in an operating or delivery room, emergency department, or outpatient setting, including both physicians' and dentists' offices; 2) cardiac catheterization and angiographic procedures; 3) a vaginal or cesarean delivery or other invasive obstetric procedure during which bleeding may occur; or 4) the manipulation, cutting, or removal of any oral or perioral tissues, including tooth structure, during which bleeding occurs or the potential for bleeding exists. The universal blood and body-fluid precautions listed above, combined with the precautions listed below, should be the minimum precautions for **all** such invasive procedures.

1. All health-care workers who participate in invasive procedures must routinely use appropriate barrier precautions to prevent skin and mucous-membrane contact with blood and other body fluids of all patients. Gloves and surgical masks must be worn for all invasive procedures. Protective eyewear or face shields should be worn for procedures that commonly result in the generation of droplets, splashing of blood or other body fluids, or the generation of bone chips. Gowns or aprons made of materials that provide an effective barrier should be worn during invasive procedures that are likely to result in the splashing of blood or other body fluids. All health-care workers who perform or assist in vaginal or cesarean deliveries should wear gloves and gowns when handling the placenta or the infant until blood and amniotic fluid have been removed from the infant's skin and should wear gloves during post-delivery care of the umbilical cord.
2. If a glove is torn or a needlestick or other injury occurs, the glove should be removed and a new glove used as promptly as patient safety permits; the needle or instrument involved in the incident should also be removed from the sterile field.

Precautions for Dentistry*

Blood, saliva, and gingival fluid from **all** dental patients should be considered infective. Special emphasis should be placed on the following precautions for preventing transmission of blood-borne pathogens in dental practice in both institutional and non-institutional settings.

1. In addition to wearing gloves for contact with oral mucous membranes of all patients, all dental workers should wear surgical masks and protective eyewear or chin-length plastic face shields during dental procedures in which splashing or spattering of blood, saliva, or gingival fluids is likely. Rubber dams, high-speed evacuation, and proper patient positioning, when appropriate, should be utilized to minimize generation of droplets and spatter.
2. Handpieces should be sterilized after use with each patient, since blood, saliva, or gingival fluid of patients may be aspirated into the handpiece or waterline. Handpieces that cannot be sterilized should at least be flushed, the outside surface cleaned and wiped with a suitable chemical germicide, and then rinsed. Handpieces should be flushed at the beginning of the day and after use with each patient. Manufacturers' recommendations should be followed for use and maintenance of waterlines and check valves and for flushing of handpieces. The same precautions should be used for ultrasonic scalers and air/water syringes.

*General infection-control precautions are more specifically addressed in previous recommendations for infection-control practices for dentistry (8).

3. Blood and saliva should be thoroughly and carefully cleaned from material that has been used in the mouth (e.g., impression materials, bite registration), especially before polishing and grinding intra-oral devices. Contaminated materials, impressions, and intra-oral devices should also be cleaned and disinfected before being handled in the dental laboratory and before they are placed in the patient's mouth. Because of the increasing variety of dental materials used intra-orally, dental workers should consult with manufacturers as to the stability of specific materials when using disinfection procedures.
4. Dental equipment and surfaces that are difficult to disinfect (e.g., light handles or X-ray-unit heads) and that may become contaminated should be wrapped with impervious-backed paper, aluminum foil, or clear plastic wrap. The coverings should be removed and discarded, and clean coverings should be put in place after use with each patient.

Precautions for Autopsies or Morticians' Services

In addition to the universal blood and body-fluid precautions listed above, the following precautions should be used by persons performing postmortem procedures:
1. All persons performing or assisting in postmortem procedures should wear gloves, masks, protective eyewear, gowns, and waterproof aprons.
2. Instruments and surfaces contaminated during postmortem procedures should be decontaminated with an appropriate chemical germicide.

Precautions for Dialysis

Patients with end-stage renal disease who are undergoing maintenance dialysis and who have HIV infection can be dialyzed in hospital-based or free-standing dialysis units using conventional infection-control precautions (21). Universal blood and body-fluid precautions should be used when dialyzing **all** patients.

Strategies for disinfecting the dialysis fluid pathways of the hemodialysis machine are targeted to control bacterial contamination and generally consist of using 500-750 parts per million (ppm) of sodium hypochlorite (household bleach) for 30-40 minutes or 1.5%-2.0% formaldehyde overnight. In addition, several chemical germicides formulated to disinfect dialysis machines are commercially available. None of these protocols or procedures need to be changed for dialyzing patients infected with HIV.

Patients infected with HIV can be dialyzed by either hemodialysis or peritoneal dialysis and do not need to be isolated from other patients. The type of dialysis treatment (i.e., hemodialysis or peritoneal dialysis) should be based on the needs of the patient. The dialyzer may be discarded after each use. Alternatively, centers that reuse dialyzers—i.e., a specific single-use dialyzer is issued to a specific patient, removed, cleaned, disinfected, and reused several times on the same patient only— may include HIV-infected patients in the dialyzer-reuse program. An individual dialyzer must never be used on more than one patient.

Precautions for Laboratories[†]

Blood and other body fluids from **all** patients should be considered infective. To supplement the universal blood and body-fluid precautions listed above, the following precautions are recommended for health-care workers in clinical laboratories.

[†]Additional precautions for research and industrial laboratories are addressed elsewhere (22,23).

1. All specimens of blood and body fluids should be put in a well-constructed container with a secure lid to prevent leaking during transport. Care should be taken when collecting each specimen to avoid contaminating the outside of the container and of the laboratory form accompanying the specimen.
2. All persons processing blood and body-fluid specimens (e.g., removing tops from vacuum tubes) should wear gloves. Masks and protective eyewear should be worn if mucous-membrane contact with blood or body fluids is anticipated. Gloves should be changed and hands washed after completion of specimen processing.
3. For routine procedures, such as histologic and pathologic studies or microbiologic culturing, a biological safety cabinet is not necessary. However, biological safety cabinets (Class I or II) should be used whenever procedures are conducted that have a high potential for generating droplets. These include activities such as blending, sonicating, and vigorous mixing.
4. Mechanical pipetting devices should be used for manipulating all liquids in the laboratory. Mouth pipetting must not be done.
5. Use of needles and syringes should be limited to situations in which there is no alternative, and the recommendations for preventing injuries with needles outlined under universal precautions should be followed.
6. Laboratory work surfaces should be decontaminated with an appropriate chemical germicide after a spill of blood or other body fluids and when work activities are completed.
7. Contaminated materials used in laboratory tests should be decontaminated before reprocessing or be placed in bags and disposed of in accordance with institutional policies for disposal of infective waste (24).
8. Scientific equipment that has been contaminated with blood or other body fluids should be decontaminated and cleaned before being repaired in the laboratory or transported to the manufacturer.
9. All persons should wash their hands after completing laboratory activities and should remove protective clothing before leaving the laboratory.

Implementation of universal blood and body-fluid precautions for **all** patients eliminates the need for warning labels on specimens since blood and other body fluids from all patients should be considered infective.

Environmental Considerations for HIV Transmission

No environmentally mediated mode of HIV transmission has been documented. Nevertheless, the precautions described below should be taken routinely in the care of **all** patients.

Sterilization and Disinfection

Standard sterilization and disinfection procedures for patient-care equipment currently recommended for use (25,26) in a variety of health-care settings—including hospitals, medical and dental clinics and offices, hemodialysis centers, emergency-care facilities, and long-term nursing-care facilities—are adequate to sterilize or disinfect instruments, devices, or other items contaminated with blood or other body fluids from persons infected with blood-borne pathogens including HIV (21,23).

Instruments or devices that enter sterile tissue or the vascular system of any patient or through which blood flows should be sterilized before reuse. Devices or items that contact intact mucous membranes should be sterilized or receive high-level disinfection, a procedure that kills vegetative organisms and viruses but not necessarily large numbers of bacterial spores. Chemical germicides that are registered with the U.S. Environmental Protection Agency (EPA) as "sterilants" may be used either for sterilization or for high-level disinfection depending on contact time.

Contact lenses used in trial fittings should be disinfected after each fitting by using a hydrogen peroxide contact lens disinfecting system or, if compatible, with heat (78 C-80 C [172.4 F-176.0 F]) for 10 minutes.

Medical devices or instruments that require sterilization or disinfection should be thoroughly cleaned before being exposed to the germicide, and the manufacturer's instructions for the use of the germicide should be followed. Further, it is important that the manufacturer's specifications for compatibility of the medical device with chemical germicides be closely followed. Information on specific label claims of commercial germicides can be obtained by writing to the Disinfectants Branch, Office of Pesticides, Environmental Protection Agency, 401 M Street, SW, Washington, D.C. 20460.

Studies have shown that HIV is inactivated rapidly after being exposed to commonly used chemical germicides at concentrations that are much lower than used in practice (27-30). Embalming fluids are similar to the types of chemical germicides that have been tested and found to completely inactivate HIV. In addition to commercially available chemical germicides, a solution of sodium hypochlorite (household bleach) prepared daily is an inexpensive and effective germicide. Concentrations ranging from approximately 500 ppm (1:100 dilution of household bleach) sodium hypochlorite to 5,000 ppm (1:10 dilution of household bleach) are effective depending on the amount of organic material (e.g., blood, mucus) present on the surface to be cleaned and disinfected. Commercially available chemical germicides may be more compatible with certain medical devices that might be corroded by repeated exposure to sodium hypochlorite, especially to the 1:10 dilution.

Survival of HIV in the Environment

The most extensive study on the survival of HIV after drying involved greatly concentrated HIV samples, i.e., 10 million tissue-culture infectious doses per milliliter (31). This concentration is at least 100,000 times greater than that typically found in the blood or serum of patients with HIV infection. HIV was detectable by tissue-culture techniques 1-3 days after drying, but the rate of inactivation was rapid. Studies performed at CDC have also shown that drying HIV causes a rapid (within several hours) 1-2 log (90%-99%) reduction in HIV concentration. In tissue-culture fluid, cell-free HIV could be detected up to 15 days at room temperature; up to 11 days at 37 C (98.6 F), and up to 1 day if the HIV was cell-associated.

When considered in the context of environmental conditions in health-care facilities, these results do not require any changes in currently recommended sterilization, disinfection, or housekeeping strategies. When medical devices are contaminated with blood or other body fluids, existing recommendations include the cleaning of these instruments, followed by disinfection or sterilization, depending on the type of medical device. These protocols assume "worst-case" conditions of extreme virologic and microbiologic contamination, and whether viruses have been inactivated after drying plays no role in formulating these strategies. Consequently, no changes in published procedures for cleaning, disinfecting, or sterilizing need to be made.

Housekeeping

Environmental surfaces such as walls, floors, and other surfaces are not associated with transmission of infections to patients or health-care workers. Therefore, extraordinary attempts to disinfect or sterilize these environmental surfaces are not necessary. However, cleaning and removal of soil should be done routinely.

Cleaning schedules and methods vary according to the area of the hospital or institution, type of surface to be cleaned, and the amount and type of soil present. Horizontal surfaces (e.g., bedside tables and hard-surfaced flooring) in patient-care areas are usually cleaned on a regular basis, when soiling or spills occur, and when a patient is discharged. Cleaning of walls, blinds, and curtains is recommended only if they are visibly soiled. Disinfectant fogging is an unsatisfactory method of decontaminating air and surfaces and is not recommended.

Disinfectant-detergent formulations registered by EPA can be used for cleaning environmental surfaces, but the actual physical removal of microorganisms by scrubbing is probably at least as important as any antimicrobial effect of the cleaning agent used. Therefore, cost, safety, and acceptability by housekeepers can be the main criteria for selecting any such registered agent. The manufacturers' instructions for appropriate use should be followed.

Cleaning and Decontaminating Spills of Blood or Other Body Fluids

Chemical germicides that are approved for use as "hospital disinfectants" and are tuberculocidal when used at recommended dilutions can be used to decontaminate spills of blood and other body fluids. Strategies for decontaminating spills of blood and other body fluids in a patient-care setting are different than for spills of cultures or other materials in clinical, public health, or research laboratories. In patient-care areas, visible material should first be removed and then the area should be decontaminated. With large spills of cultured or concentrated infectious agents in the laboratory, the contaminated area should be flooded with a liquid germicide before cleaning, then decontaminated with fresh germicidal chemical. In both settings, gloves should be worn during the cleaning and decontaminating procedures.

Laundry

Although soiled linen has been identified as a source of large numbers of certain pathogenic microorganisms, the risk of actual disease transmission is negligible. Rather than rigid procedures and specifications, hygienic and common-sense storage and processing of clean and soiled linen are recommended (26). Soiled linen should be handled as little as possible and with minimum agitation to prevent gross microbial contamination of the air and of persons handling the linen. All soiled linen should be bagged at the location where it was used; it should not be sorted or rinsed in patient-care areas. Linen soiled with blood or body fluids should be placed and transported in bags that prevent leakage. If hot water is used, linen should be washed with detergent in water at least 71 C (160 F) for 25 minutes. If low-temperature(≤70 C [158 F]) laundry cycles are used, chemicals suitable for low-temperature washing at proper use concentration should be used.

Infective Waste

There is no epidemiologic evidence to suggest that most hospital waste is any more infective than residential waste. Moreover, there is no epidemiologic evidence that hospital waste has caused disease in the community as a result of improper disposal. Therefore, identifying wastes for which special precautions are indicated is largely a matter of judgment about the relative risk of disease transmission. The most practical approach to the management of infective waste is to identify those wastes with the potential for causing infection during handling and disposal and for which some special precautions appear prudent. Hospital wastes for which special precautions appear prudent include microbiology laboratory waste, pathology waste, and blood specimens or blood products. While any item that has had contact with blood, exudates, or secretions may be potentially infective, it is not usually considered practical or necessary to treat all such waste as infective (*23,26*). Infective waste, in general, should either be incinerated or should be autoclaved before disposal in a sanitary landfill. Bulk blood, suctioned fluids, excretions, and secretions may be carefully poured down a drain connected to a sanitary sewer. Sanitary sewers may also be used to dispose of other infectious wastes capable of being ground and flushed into the sewer.

Implementation of Recommended Precautions

Employers of health-care workers should ensure that policies exist for:
1. Initial orientation and continuing education and training of all health-care workers—including students and trainees—on the epidemiology, modes of transmission, and prevention of HIV and other blood-borne infections and the need for routine use of universal blood and body-fluid precautions for **all** patients.
2. Provision of equipment and supplies necessary to minimize the risk of infection with HIV and other blood-borne pathogens.
3. Monitoring adherence to recommended protective measures. When monitoring reveals a failure to follow recommended precautions, counseling, education, and/or re-training should be provided, and, if necessary, appropriate disciplinary action should be considered.

Professional associations and labor organizations, through continuing education efforts, should emphasize the need for health-care workers to follow recommended precautions.

Serologic Testing for HIV Infection

Background

A person is identified as infected with HIV when a sequence of tests, starting with repeated enzyme immunoassays (EIA) and including a Western blot or similar, more specific assay, are repeatedly reactive. Persons infected with HIV usually develop antibody against the virus within 6-12 weeks after infection.

The sensitivity of the currently licensed EIA tests is at least 99% when they are performed under optimal laboratory conditions on serum specimens from persons infected for ≥12 weeks. Optimal laboratory conditions include the use of reliable reagents, provision of continuing education of personnel, quality control of procedures, and participation in performance-evaluation programs. Given this performance, the probability of a false-negative test is remote except during the first several weeks after infection, before detectable antibody is present. The proportion of infected persons with a false-negative test attributed to absence of antibody in the early stages of infection is dependent on both the incidence and prevalence of HIV infection in a population (Table 1).

The specificity of the currently licensed EIA tests is approximately 99% when repeatedly reactive tests are considered. Repeat testing of initially reactive specimens by EIA is required to reduce the likelihood of laboratory error. To increase further the specificity of serologic tests, laboratories must use a supplemental test, most often the Western blot, to validate repeatedly reactive EIA results. Under optimal laboratory conditions, the sensitivity of the Western blot test is comparable to or greater than that of a repeatedly reactive EIA, and the Western blot is highly specific when strict criteria are used to interpret the test results. The testing sequence of a repeatedly reactive EIA and a positive Western blot test is highly predictive of HIV infection, even in a population with a low prevalence of infection (Table 2). If the Western blot test result is indeterminant, the testing sequence is considered equivocal for HIV infection.

TABLE 1. Estimated annual number of patients infected with HIV not detected by HIV-antibody testing in a hypothetical hospital with 10,000 admissions/year*

Beginning prevalence of HIV infection	Annual incidence of HIV infection	Approximate number of HIV-infected patients	Approximate number of HIV-infected patients not detected
5.0%	1.0%	550	17-18
5.0%	0.5%	525	11-12
1.0%	0.2%	110	3-4
1.0%	0.1%	105	2-3
0.1%	0.02%	11	0-1
0.1%	0.01%	11	0-1

*The estimates are based on the following assumptions: 1) the sensitivity of the screening test is 99% (i.e., 99% of HIV-infected persons with antibody will be detected); 2) persons infected with HIV will not develop detectable antibody (seroconvert) until 6 weeks (1.5 months) after infection; 3) new infections occur at an equal rate throughout the year; 4) calculations of the number of HIV-infected persons in the patient population are based on the mid-year prevalence, which is the beginning prevalence plus half the annual incidence of infections.

When this occurs, the Western blot test should be repeated on the same serum sample, and, if still indeterminant, the testing sequence should be repeated on a sample collected 3-6 months later. Use of other supplemental tests may aid in interpreting of results on samples that are persistently indeterminant by Western blot.

Testing of Patients

Previous CDC recommendations have emphasized the value of HIV serologic testing of patients for: 1) management of parenteral or mucous-membrane exposures of health-care workers, 2) patient diagnosis and management, and 3) counseling and serologic testing to prevent and control HIV transmission in the community. In addition, more recent recommendations have stated that hospitals, in conjunction with state and local health departments, should periodically determine the prevalence of HIV infection among patients from age groups at highest risk of infection (32).

Adherence to universal blood and body-fluid precautions recommended for the care of all patients will minimize the risk of transmission of HIV and other blood-borne pathogens from patients to health-care workers. The utility of routine HIV serologic testing of patients as an adjunct to universal precautions is unknown. Results of such testing may not be available in emergency or outpatient settings. In addition, some recently infected patients will not have detectable antibody to HIV (Table 1).

Personnel in some hospitals have advocated serologic testing of patients in settings in which exposure of health-care workers to large amounts of patients' blood may be anticipated. Specific patients for whom serologic testing has been advocated include those undergoing major operative procedures and those undergoing treatment in critical-care units, especially if they have conditions involving uncontrolled bleeding. Decisions regarding the need to establish testing programs for patients should be made by physicians or individual institutions. In addition, when deemed appropriate, testing of individual patients may be performed on agreement between the patient and the physician providing care.

In addition to the universal precautions recommended for all patients, certain additional precautions for the care of HIV-infected patients undergoing major surgical operations have been proposed by personnel in some hospitals. For example, surgical procedures on an HIV-infected patient might be altered so that hand-to-hand passing of sharp instruments would be eliminated; stapling instruments rather than

TABLE 2. Predictive value of positive HIV-antibody tests in hypothetical populations with different prevalences of infection

	Prevalence of infection	Predictive value of positive test[*]
Repeatedly reactive enzyme immunoassay (EIA)[†]	0.2%	28.41%
	2.0%	80.16%
	20.0%	98.02%
Repeatedly reactive EIA followed by positive Western blot (WB)[§]	0.2%	99.75%
	2.0%	99.97%
	20.0%	99.99%

[*]Proportion of persons with positive test results who are actually infected with HIV.
[†]Assumes EIA sensitivity of 99.0% and specificity of 99.5%.
[§]Assumes WB sensitivity of 99.0% and specificity of 99.9%.

hand-suturing equipment might be used to perform tissue approximation; electrocautery devices rather than scalpels might be used as cutting instruments; and, even though uncomfortable, gowns that totally prevent seepage of blood onto the skin of members of the operative team might be worn. While such modifications might further minimize the risk of HIV infection for members of the operative team, some of these techniques could result in prolongation of operative time and could potentially have an adverse effect on the patient.

Testing programs, if developed, should include the following principles:
- Obtaining consent for testing.
- Informing patients of test results, and providing counseling for seropositive patients by properly trained persons.
- Assuring that confidentiality safeguards are in place to limit knowledge of test results to those directly involved in the care of infected patients or as required by law.
- Assuring that identification of infected patients will not result in denial of needed care or provision of suboptimal care.
- Evaluating prospectively 1) the efficacy of the program in reducing the incidence of parenteral, mucous-membrane, or significant cutaneous exposures of health-care workers to the blood or other body fluids of HIV-infected patients and 2) the effect of modified procedures on patients.

Testing of Health-Care Workers

Although transmission of HIV from infected health-care workers to patients has not been reported, transmission during invasive procedures remains a possibility. Transmission of hepatitis B virus (HBV) — a blood-borne agent with a considerably greater potential for nosocomial spread — from health-care workers to patients has been documented. Such transmission has occurred in situations (e.g., oral and gynecologic surgery) in which health-care workers, when tested, had very high concentrations of HBV in their blood (at least 100 million infectious virus particles per milliliter, a concentration much higher than occurs with HIV infection), and the health-care workers sustained a puncture wound while performing invasive procedures or had exudative or weeping lesions or microlacerations that allowed virus to contaminate instruments or open wounds of patients (*33,34*).

The hepatitis B experience indicates that only those health-care workers who perform certain types of invasive procedures have transmitted HBV to patients. Adherence to recommendations in this document will minimize the risk of transmission of HIV and other blood-borne pathogens from health-care workers to patients during invasive procedures. Since transmission of HIV from infected health-care workers performing invasive procedures to their patients has not been reported and would be expected to occur only very rarely, if at all, the utility of routine testing of such health-care workers to prevent transmission of HIV cannot be assessed. If consideration is given to developing a serologic testing program for health-care workers who perform invasive procedures, the frequency of testing, as well as the issues of consent, confidentiality, and consequences of test results — as previously outlined for testing programs for patients — must be addressed.

Management of Infected Health-Care Workers

Health-care workers with impaired immune systems resulting from HIV infection or other causes are at increased risk of acquiring or experiencing serious complications of infectious disease. Of particular concern is the risk of severe infection following exposure to patients with infectious diseases that are easily transmitted if appropriate precautions are not taken (e.g., measles, varicella). Any health-care worker with an impaired immune system should be counseled about the potential risk associated with taking care of patients with any transmissible infection and should continue to follow existing recommendations for infection control to minimize risk of exposure to other infectious agents (7,35). Recommendations of the Immunization Practices Advisory Committee (ACIP) and institutional policies concerning requirements for vaccinating health-care workers with live-virus vaccines (e.g., measles, rubella) should also be considered.

The question of whether workers infected with HIV — especially those who perform invasive procedures — can adequately and safely be allowed to perform patient-care duties or whether their work assignments should be changed must be determined on an individual basis. These decisions should be made by the health-care worker's personal physician(s) in conjunction with the medical directors and personnel health service staff of the employing institution or hospital.

Management of Exposures

If a health-care worker has a parenteral (e.g., needlestick or cut) or mucous-membrane (e.g., splash to the eye or mouth) exposure to blood or other body fluids or has a cutaneous exposure involving large amounts of blood or prolonged contact with blood — especially when the exposed skin is chapped, abraded, or afflicted with dermatitis — the source patient should be informed of the incident and tested for serologic evidence of HIV infection after consent is obtained. Policies should be developed for testing source patients in situations in which consent cannot be obtained (e.g., an unconscious patient).

If the source patient has AIDS, is positive for HIV antibody, or refuses the test, the health-care worker should be counseled regarding the risk of infection and evaluated clinically and serologically for evidence of HIV infection as soon as possible after the exposure. The health-care worker should be advised to report and seek medical evaluation for any acute febrile illness that occurs within 12 weeks after the exposure. Such an illness — particularly one characterized by fever, rash, or lymphadenopathy — may be indicative of recent HIV infection. Seronegative health-care workers should be retested 6 weeks post-exposure and on a periodic basis thereafter (e.g., 12 weeks and 6 months after exposure) to determine whether transmission has occurred. During this follow-up period — especially the first 6-12 weeks after exposure, when most infected persons are expected to seroconvert — exposed health-care workers should follow U.S. Public Health Service (PHS) recommendations for preventing transmission of HIV (36,37).

No further follow-up of a health-care worker exposed to infection as described above is necessary if the source patient is seronegative unless the source patient is at high risk of HIV infection. In the latter case, a subsequent specimen (e.g., 12 weeks following exposure) may be obtained from the health-care worker for antibody testing. If the source patient cannot be identified, decisions regarding appropriate follow-up should be individualized. Serologic testing should be available to all health-care workers who are concerned that they may have been infected with HIV.

If a patient has a parenteral or mucous-membrane exposure to blood or other body fluid of a health-care worker, the patient should be informed of the incident, and the same procedure outlined above for management of exposures should be followed for both the source health-care worker and the exposed patient.

References
1. CDC. Acquired immunodeficiency syndrome (AIDS): Precautions for clinical and laboratory staffs. MMWR 1982;31:577-80.
2. CDC. Acquired immunodeficiency syndrome (AIDS): Precautions for health-care workers and allied professionals. MMWR 1983;32:450-1.
3. CDC. Recommendations for preventing transmission of infection with human T-lymphotropic virus type III/lymphadenopathy-associated virus in the workplace. MMWR 1985;34:681-6, 691-5.
4. CDC. Recommendations for preventing transmission of infection with human T-lymphotropic virus type III/lymphadenopathy-associated virus during invasive procedures. MMWR 1986;35:221-3.
5. CDC. Recommendations for preventing possible transmission of human T-lymphotropic virus type III/lymphadenopathy-associated virus from tears. MMWR 1985;34:533-4.
6. CDC. Recommendations for providing dialysis treatment to patients infected with human T-lymphotropic virus type III/lymphadenopathy-associated virus infection. MMWR 1986;35:376-8, 383.
7. Garner JS, Simmons BP. Guideline for isolation precautions in hospitals. Infect Control 1983;4 (suppl) :245-325.
8. CDC. Recommended infection control practices for dentistry. MMWR 1986;35:237-42.
9. McCray E, The Cooperative Needlestick Surveillance Group. Occupational risk of the acquired immunodeficiency syndrome among health care workers. N Engl J Med 1986;314:1127-32.
10. Henderson DK, Saah AJ, Zak BJ, et al. Risk of nosocomial infection with human T-cell lymphotropic virus type III/lymphadenopathy-associated virus in a large cohort of intensively exposed health care workers. Ann Intern Med 1986;104:644-7.
11. Gerberding JL, Bryant-LeBlanc CE, Nelson K, et al. Risk of transmitting the human immunodeficiency virus, cytomegalovirus, and hepatitis B virus to health care workers exposed to patients with AIDS and AIDS-related conditions. J Infect Dis 1987;156:1-8.
12. McEvoy M, Porter K, Mortimer P, Simmons N, Shanson D. Prospective study of clinical, laboratory, and ancillary staff with accidental exposures to blood or other body fluids from patients infected with HIV. Br Med J 1987;294:1595-7.
13. Anonymous. Needlestick transmission of HTLV-III from a patient infected in Africa. Lancet 1984;2:1376-7.
14. Oksenhendler E, Harzic M, Le Roux JM, Rabian C, Clauvel JP. HIV infection with seroconversion after a superficial needlestick injury to the finger. N Engl J Med 1986;315:582.
15. Neisson-Vernant C, Arfi S, Mathez D, Leibowitch J, Monplaisir N. Needlestick HIV seroconversion in a nurse. Lancet 1986;2:814.
16. Grint P, McEvoy M. Two associated cases of the acquired immune deficiency syndrome (AIDS). PHLS Commun Dis Rep 1985;42:4.
17. CDC. Apparent transmission of human T-lymphotropic virus type III/lymphadenopathy-associated virus from a child to a mother providing health care. MMWR 1986;35:76-9.
18. CDC. Update: Human immunodeficiency virus infections in health-care workers exposed to blood of infected patients. MMWR 1987;36:285-9.
19. Kline RS, Phelan J, Friedland GH, et al. Low occupational risk for HIV infection for dental professionals [Abstract]. In: Abstracts from the III International Conference on AIDS, 1-5 June 1985. Washington, DC: 155.
20. Baker JL, Kelen GD, Sivertson KT, Quinn TC. Unsuspected human immunodeficiency virus in critically ill emergency patients. JAMA 1987;257:2609-11.
21. Favero MS. Dialysis-associated diseases and their control. In: Bennett JV, Brachman PS, eds. Hospital infections. Boston: Little, Brown and Company, 1985:267-84.

Appendix A.1

22. Richardson JH, Barkley WE, eds. Biosafety in microbiological and biomedical laboratories, 1984. Washington, DC. US Department of Health and Human Services, Public Health Service. HHS publication no. (CDC) 84-8395.
23. CDC. Human T-lymphotropic virus type III/lymphadenopathy-associated virus: Agent summary statement. MMWR 1986;35:540-2, 547-9.
24. Environmental Protection Agency. EPA guide for infectious waste management. Washington, DC :U.S. Environmental Protection Agency, May 1986 (Publication no. EPA/530-SW-86-014).
25. Favero MS. Sterilization, disinfection, and antisepsis in the hospital. In: Manual of clinical microbiology 4th ed Washington. DC: American Society for Microbiology, 1985;129-37.
26. Garner JS, Favero MS. Guideline for handwashing and hospital environmental control, 1985. Atlanta: Public Health Service, Centers for Disease Control, 1985. HHS publication no. 99-1117.
27. Spire B, Montagnier L, Barré-Sinoussi F, Chermann JC. Inactivation of lymphadenopathy associated virus by chemical disinfectants. Lancet 1984;2:899-901.
28. Martin LS, McDougal JS, Loskoski SL. Disinfection and inactivation of the human T lymphotropic virus type III/lymphadenopathy-associated virus. J Infect Dis 1985; 152:400-3.
29. McDougal JS, Martin LS, Cort SP, et al. Thermal inactivation of the acquired immunodeficiency syndrome virus-III/lymphadenopathy-associated virus, with special reference to antihemophilic factor. J Clin Invest 1985;76:875-7.
30. Spire B, Barre-Sinoussi F, Dormont D, Montagnier L, Chermann JC. Inactivation of lymphadenopathy-associated virus by heat, gamma rays, and ultraviolet light. Lancet 1985;1:188-9.
31. Resnik L, Veren K, Salahuddin SZ, Tondreau S, Markham PD. Stability and inactivation of HTLV-III/LAV under clinical and laboratory environments. JAMA 1986;255:1887-91.
32. CDC. Public Health Service (PHS) guidelines for counseling and antibody testing to prevent HIV infection and AIDS. MMWR 1987;3:509-15..
33. Kane MA, Lettau LA. Transmission of HBV from dental personnel to patients. J Am Dent Assoc 1985;110:634-6.
34. Lettau LA, Smith JD, Williams D, et. al. Transmission of hepatitis B with resultant restriction of surgical practice. JAMA 1986;255:934-7.
35. Williams WW. Guideline for infection control in hospital personnel. Infect Control 1983;4 (suppl) :326-49.
36. CDC. Prevention of acquired immune deficiency syndrome (AIDS): Report of inter-agency recommendations. MMWR 1983;32:101-3.
37. CDC. Provisional Public Health Service inter-agency recommendations for screening donated blood and plasma for antibody to the virus causing acquired immunodeficiency syndrome. MMWR 1985;34:1-5.

Copies of the *MMWR* supplement entitled *Recommendations for Prevention of HIV Transmission in Health-Care Settings* published in August 1987 are available through the National Aids Clearinghouse, P.O. Box 6003, Rockville, MD 20850.

Appendix A.2

Update: Universal Precautions for Prevention of Transmission of Human Immunodeficiency Virus, Hepatitis B Virus, and Other Bloodborne Pathogens in Health-Care Settings

Introduction

The purpose of this report is to clarify and supplement the CDC publication entitled "Recommendations for Prevention of HIV Transmission in Health-Care Settings" (1).*

In 1983, CDC published a document entitled "Guideline for Isolation Precautions in Hospitals" (2) that contained a section entitled "Blood and Body Fluid Precautions." The recommendations in this section called for blood and body fluid precautions when a patient was known or suspected to be infected with bloodborne pathogens. In August 1987, CDC published a document entitled "Recommendations for Prevention of HIV Transmission in Health-Care Settings" (1). In contrast to the 1983 document, the 1987 document recommended that blood and body fluid precautions be consistently used for all patients regardless of their bloodborne infection status. This extension of blood and body fluid precautions to all patients is referred to as "Universal Blood and Body Fluid Precautions" or "Universal Precautions." Under universal precautions, blood and certain body fluids of all patients are considered potentially infectious for human immunodeficiency virus (HIV), hepatitis B virus (HBV), and other bloodborne pathogens.

Universal precautions are intended to prevent parenteral, mucous membrane, and nonintact skin exposures of health-care workers to bloodborne pathogens. In addition, immunization with HBV vaccine is recommended as an important adjunct to universal precautions for health-care workers who have exposures to blood (3,4).

Since the recommendations for universal precautions were published in August 1987, CDC and the Food and Drug Administration (FDA) have received requests for clarification of the following issues: 1) body fluids to which universal precautions apply, 2) use of protective barriers, 3) use of gloves for phlebotomy, 4) selection of gloves for use while observing universal precautions, and 5) need for making changes in waste management programs as a result of adopting universal precautions.

---

*The August 1987 publication should be consulted for general information and specific recommendations not addressed in this update.

Centers for Disease Control. Update: Universal precautions for prevention of transmission of human immunodeficiency virus, hepatitis B virus, and other bloodborne pathogens in health-care settings. *MMWR* 1988; 37 :[377-388].

Body Fluids to Which Universal Precautions Apply

Universal precautions apply to blood and to other body fluids containing visible blood. Occupational transmission of HIV and HBV to health-care workers by blood is documented (4,5). **Blood is the single most important source of HIV, HBV, and other bloodborne pathogens in the occupational setting. Infection control efforts for HIV, HBV, and other bloodborne pathogens must focus on preventing exposures to blood as well as on delivery of HBV immunization.**

Universal precautions also apply to semen and vaginal secretions. Although both of these fluids have been implicated in the sexual transmission of HIV and HBV, they have not been implicated in occupational transmission from patient to health-care worker. This observation is not unexpected, since exposure to semen in the usual health-care setting is limited, and the routine practice of wearing gloves for performing vaginal examinations protects health-care workers from exposure to potentially infectious vaginal secretions.

Universal precautions also apply to tissues and to the following fluids: cerebrospinal fluid (CSF), synovial fluid, pleural fluid, peritoneal fluid, pericardial fluid, and amniotic fluid. The risk of transmission of HIV and HBV from these fluids is unknown; epidemiologic studies in the health-care and community setting are currently inadequate to assess the potential risk to health-care workers from occupational exposures to them. However, HIV has been isolated from CSF, synovial, and amniotic fluid (6–8), and HBsAg has been detected in synovial fluid, amniotic fluid, and peritoneal fluid (9–11). One case of HIV transmission was reported after a percutaneous exposure to bloody pleural fluid obtained by needle aspiration (12). Whereas aseptic procedures used to obtain these fluids for diagnostic or therapeutic purposes protect health-care workers from skin exposures, they cannot prevent penetrating injuries due to contaminated needles or other sharp instruments.

Body Fluids to Which Universal Precautions Do Not Apply

Universal precautions do not apply to feces, nasal secretions, sputum, sweat, tears, urine, and vomitus unless they contain visible blood. The risk of transmission of HIV and HBV from these fluids and materials is extremely low or nonexistent. HIV has been isolated and HBsAg has been demonstrated in some of these fluids; however, epidemiologic studies in the health-care and community setting have not implicated these fluids or materials in the transmission of HIV and HBV infections (13,14). Some of the above fluids and excretions represent a potential source for nosocomial and community-acquired infections with other pathogens, and recommendations for preventing the transmission of nonbloodborne pathogens have been published (2).

Precautions for Other Body Fluids in Special Settings

Human breast milk has been implicated in perinatal transmission of HIV, and HBsAg has been found in the milk of mothers infected with HBV (10,13). However, occupational exposure to human breast milk has not been implicated in the transmission of HIV nor HBV infection to health-care workers. Moreover, the health-care worker will not have the same type of intensive exposure to breast milk as the nursing neonate. Whereas universal precautions do not apply to human breast milk, gloves may be worn by health-care workers in situations where exposures to breast milk might be frequent, for example, in breast milk banking.

Saliva of some persons infected with HBV has been shown to contain HBV-DNA at concentrations 1/1,000 to 1/10,000 of that found in the infected person's serum (15). HBsAg-positive saliva has been shown to be infectious when injected into experimental animals and in human bite exposures (16-18). However, HBsAg-positive saliva has not been shown to be infectious when applied to oral mucous membranes in experimental primate studies (18) or through contamination of musical instruments or cardiopulmonary resuscitation dummies used by HBV carriers (19,20). Epidemiologic studies of nonsexual household contacts of HIV-infected patients, including several small series in which HIV transmission failed to occur after bites or after percutaneous inoculation or contamination of cuts and open wounds with saliva from HIV-infected patients, suggest that the potential for salivary transmission of HIV is remote (5,13,14,21,22). One case report from Germany has suggested the possibility of transmission of HIV in a household setting from an infected child to a sibling through a human bite (23). The bite did not break the skin or result in bleeding. Since the date of seroconversion to HIV was not known for either child in this case, evidence for the role of saliva in the transmission of virus is unclear (23). Another case report suggested the possibility of transmission of HIV from husband to wife by contact with saliva during kissing (24). However, follow-up studies did not confirm HIV infection in the wife (21).

Universal precautions do not apply to saliva. General infection control practices already in existence — including the use of gloves for digital examination of mucous membranes and endotracheal suctioning, and handwashing after exposure to saliva — should further minimize the minute risk, if any, for salivary transmission of HIV and HBV (1,25). Gloves need not be worn when feeding patients and when wiping saliva from skin.

Special precautions, however, are recommended for dentistry (1). Occupationally acquired infection with HBV in dental workers has been documented (4), and two possible cases of occupationally acquired HIV infection involving dentists have been reported (5,26). During dental procedures, contamination of saliva with blood is predictable, trauma to health-care workers' hands is common, and blood spattering may occur. Infection control precautions for dentistry minimize the potential for nonintact skin and mucous membrane contact of dental health-care workers to blood-contaminated saliva of patients. In addition, the use of gloves for oral examinations and treatment in the dental setting may also protect the patient's oral mucous membranes from exposures to blood, which may occur from breaks in the skin of dental workers' hands.

Use of Protective Barriers

Protective barriers reduce the risk of exposure of the health-care worker's skin or mucous membranes to potentially infective materials. For universal precautions, protective barriers reduce the risk of exposure to blood, body fluids containing visible blood, and other fluids to which universal precautions apply. Examples of protective barriers include gloves, gowns, masks, and protective eyewear. Gloves should reduce the incidence of contamination of hands, but they cannot prevent penetrating injuries due to needles or other sharp instruments. Masks and protective eyewear or face shields should reduce the incidence of contamination of mucous membranes of the mouth, nose, and eyes.

Universal precautions are intended to supplement rather than replace recommendations for routine infection control, such as handwashing and using gloves to prevent gross microbial contamination of hands (27). Because specifying the types of barriers needed for every possible clinical situation is impractical, some judgment must be exercised.

The risk of nosocomial transmission of HIV, HBV, and other bloodborne pathogens can be minimized if health-care workers use the following general guidelines:[†]

1. Take care to prevent injuries when using needles, scalpels, and other sharp instruments or devices; when handling sharp instruments after procedures; when cleaning used instruments; and when disposing of used needles. Do not recap used needles by hand; do not remove used needles from disposable syringes by hand; and do not bend, break, or otherwise manipulate used needles by hand. Place used disposable syringes and needles, scalpel blades, and other sharp items in puncture-resistant containers for disposal. Locate the puncture-resistant containers as close to the use area as is practical.
2. Use protective barriers to prevent exposure to blood, body fluids containing visible blood, and other fluids to which universal precautions apply. The type of protective barrier(s) should be appropriate for the procedure being performed and the type of exposure anticipated.
3. Immediately and thoroughly wash hands and other skin surfaces that are contaminated with blood, body fluids containing visible blood, or other body fluids to which universal precautions apply.

Glove Use for Phlebotomy

Gloves should reduce the incidence of blood contamination of hands during phlebotomy (drawing blood samples), but they cannot prevent penetrating injuries caused by needles or other sharp instruments. The likelihood of hand contamination with blood containing HIV, HBV, or other bloodborne pathogens during phlebotomy depends on several factors: 1) the skill and technique of the health-care worker, 2) the frequency with which the health-care worker performs the procedure (other factors being equal, the cumulative risk of blood exposure is higher for a health-care worker who performs more procedures), 3) whether the procedure occurs in a routine or emergency situation (where blood contact may be more likely), and 4) the prevalence of infection with bloodborne pathogens in the patient population. The likelihood of infection after skin exposure to blood containing HIV or HBV will depend on the concentration of virus (viral concentration is much higher for hepatitis B than for HIV), the duration of contact, the presence of skin lesions on the hands of the health-care worker, and — for HBV — the immune status of the health-care worker. Although not accurately quantified, the risk of HIV infection following intact skin contact with infective blood is certainly much less than the 0.5% risk following percutaneous needlestick exposures (5). In universal precautions, *all* blood is assumed to be potentially infective for bloodborne pathogens, but in certain settings (e.g., volunteer blood-donation centers) the prevalence of infection with some bloodborne pathogens (e.g., HIV, HBV) is known to be very low. Some institutions have relaxed recommendations for using gloves for phlebotomy procedures by skilled phlebotomists in settings where the prevalence of bloodborne pathogens is known to be very low.

[†]The August 1987 publication should be consulted for general information and specific recommendations not addressed in this update.

Institutions that judge that routine gloving for *all* phlebotomies is not necessary should periodically reevaluate their policy. Gloves should always be available to health-care workers who wish to use them for phlebotomy. In addition, the following general guidelines apply:
1. Use gloves for performing phlebotomy when the health-care worker has cuts, scratches, or other breaks in his/her skin.
2. Use gloves in situations where the health-care worker judges that hand contamination with blood may occur, for example, when performing phlebotomy on an uncooperative patient.
3. Use gloves for performing finger and/or heel sticks on infants and children.
4. Use gloves when persons are receiving training in phlebotomy.

Selection of Gloves

The Center for Devices and Radiological Health, FDA, has responsibility for regulating the medical glove industry. Medical gloves include those marketed as sterile surgical or nonsterile examination gloves made of vinyl or latex. General purpose utility ("rubber") gloves are also used in the health-care setting, but they are not regulated by FDA since they are not promoted for medical use. There are no reported differences in barrier effectiveness between intact latex and intact vinyl used to manufacture gloves. Thus, the type of gloves selected should be appropriate for the task being performed.

The following general guidelines are recommended:
1. Use sterile gloves for procedures involving contact with normally sterile areas of the body.
2. Use examination gloves for procedures involving contact with mucous membranes, unless otherwise indicated, and for other patient care or diagnostic procedures that do not require the use of sterile gloves.
3. Change gloves between patient contacts.
4. Do not wash or disinfect surgical or examination gloves for reuse. Washing with surfactants may cause "wicking," i.e., the enhanced penetration of liquids through undetected holes in the glove. Disinfecting agents may cause deterioration.
5. Use general-purpose utility gloves (e.g., rubber household gloves) for housekeeping chores involving potential blood contact and for instrument cleaning and decontamination procedures. Utility gloves may be decontaminated and reused but should be discarded if they are peeling, cracked, or discolored, or if they have punctures, tears, or other evidence of deterioration.

Waste Management

Universal precautions are not intended to change waste management programs previously recommended by CDC for health-care settings (*1*). Policies for defining, collecting, storing, decontaminating, and disposing of infective waste are generally determined by institutions in accordance with state and local regulations. Information regarding waste management regulations in health-care settings may be obtained from state or local health departments or agencies responsible for waste management.

Reported by: Center for Devices and Radiological Health, Food and Drug Administration. Hospital Infections Program, AIDS Program, and Hepatitis Br, Div of Viral Diseases, Center for Infectious Diseases, National Institute for Occupational Safety and Health, CDC.

Editorial Note: Implementation of universal precautions does not eliminate the need for other category- or disease-specific isolation precautions, such as enteric precautions for infectious diarrhea or isolation for pulmonary tuberculosis (*1,2*). In addition to universal precautions, detailed precautions have been developed for the following procedures and/or settings in which prolonged or intensive exposures to blood occur: invasive procedures, dentistry, autopsies or morticians' services, dialysis, and the clinical laboratory. These detailed precautions are found in the August 21, 1987, "Recommendations for Prevention of HIV Transmission in Health-Care Settings" (*1*). In addition, specific precautions have been developed for research laboratories (*28*).

References
1. Centers for Disease Control. Recommendations for prevention of HIV transmission in health-care settings. MMWR 1987;36(suppl no. 2S).
2. Garner JS, Simmons BP. Guideline for isolation precautions in hospitals. Infect Control 1983:4;245–325.
3. Immunization Practices Advisory Committee. Recommendations for protection against viral hepatitis. MMWR 1985;34:313-24,329–35.
4. Department of Labor, Department of Health and Human Services. Joint advisory notice: protection against occupational exposure to hepatitis B virus (HBV) and human immunodeficiency virus (HIV). Washington, DC:US Department of Labor, US Department of Health and Human Services, 1987.
5. Centers for Disease Control. Update: Acquired immunodeficiency syndrome and human immunodeficiency virus infection among health-care workers. MMWR 1988;37:229–34,239.
6. Hollander H, Levy JA. Neurologic abnormalities and recovery of human immunodeficiency virus from cerebrospinal fluid. Ann Intern Med 1987;106:692–5.
7. Wirthrington RH, Cornes P, Harris JRW, et al. Isolation of human immunodeficiency virus from synovial fluid of a patient with reactive arthritis. Br Med J 1987;294:484.
8. Mundy DC, Schinazi RF, Gerber AR, Nahmias AJ, Randall HW. Human immunodeficiency virus isolated from amniotic fluid. Lancet 1987;2:459–60.
9. Onion DK, Crumpacker CS, Gilliland BC. Arthritis of hepatitis associated with Australia antigen. Ann Intern Med 1971;75:29–33.
10. Lee AKY, Ip HMH, Wong VCW. Mechanisms of maternal-fetal transmission of hepatitis B virus. J Infect Dis 1978;138:668–71.
11. Bond WW, Petersen NJ, Gravelle CR, Favero MS. Hepatitis B virus in peritoneal dialysis fluid: A potential hazard. Dialysis and Transplantation 1982;11:592–600.
12. Oskenhendler E, Harzic M, Le Roux J-M, Rabian C, Clauvel JP. HIV infection with seroconversion after a superficial needlestick injury to the finger [Letter]. N Engl J Med 1986;315:582.
13. Lifson AR. Do alternate modes for transmission of human immunodeficiency virus exist? A review. JAMA 1988;259:1353–6.
14. Friedland GH, Saltzman BR, Rogers MF, et al. Lack of transmission of HTLV-III/LAV infection to household contacts of patients with AIDS or AIDS-related complex with oral candidiasis. N Engl J Med 1986;314:344–9.
15. Jenison SA, Lemon SM, Baker LN, Newbold JE. Quantitative analysis of hepatitis B virus DNA in saliva and semen of chronically infected homosexual men. J Infect Dis 1987;156:299–306.
16. Cancio-Bello TP, de Medina M, Shorey J, Valledor MD, Schiff ER. An institutional outbreak of hepatitis B related to a human biting carrier. J Infect Dis 1982;146:652–6.
17. MacQuarrie MB, Forghani B, Wolochow DA. Hepatitis B transmitted by a human bite. JAMA 1974;230:723–4.
18. Scott RM, Snitbhan R, Bancroft WH, Alter HJ, Tingpalapong M. Experimental transmission of hepatitis B virus by semen and saliva. J Infect Dis 1980;142:67–71.

19. Glaser JB, Nadler JP. Hepatitis B virus in a cardiopulmonary resuscitation training course: Risk of transmission from a surface antigen-positive participant. Arch Intern Med 1985;145:1653–5.
20. Osterholm MT, Bravo ER, Crosson JT, et al. Lack of transmission of viral hepatitis type B after oral exposure to HBsAg-positive saliva. Br Med J 1979;2:1263–4.
21. Curran JW, Jaffe HW, Hardy AM, et al. Epidemiology of HIV infection and AIDS in the United States. Science 1988;239:610–6.
22. Jason JM, McDougal JS, Dixon G, et al. HTLV-III/LAV antibody and immune status of household contacts and sexual partners of persons with hemophilia. JAMA 1986;255:212–5.
23. Wahn V, Kramer HH, Voit T, Brüster HT, Scrampical B, Scheid A. Horizontal transmission of HIV infection between two siblings [Letter]. Lancet 1986;2:694.
24. Salahuddin SZ, Groopman JE, Markham PD, et al. HTLV-III in symptom-free seronegative persons. Lancet 1984;2:1418–20.
25. Simmons BP, Wong ES. Guideline for prevention of nosocomial pneumonia. Atlanta: US Department of Health and Human Services, Public Health Service, Centers for Disease Control, 1982.
26. Klein RS, Phelan JA, Freeman K, et al. Low occupational risk of human immunodeficiency virus infection among dental professionals. N Engl J Med 1988;318:86–90.
27. Garner JS, Favero MS. Guideline for handwashing and hospital environmental control, 1985. Atlanta: US Department of Health and Human Services, Public Health Service, Centers for Disease Control, 1985; HHS publication no. 99-1117.
28. Centers for Disease Control. 1988 Agent summary statement for human immunodeficiency virus and report on laboratory-acquired infection with human immunodeficiency virus. MMWR 1988;37(suppl no. S4:1S-22S).

☆U.S. GOVERNMENT PRINTING OFFICE: 1988-530-009/84718

Copies of this report are available through the National AIDS Information Clearinghouse, P.O. Box 6003, Rockville, MD 20850.

Appendix B

Revision of the CDC Surveillance Case Definition for Acquired Immunodeficiency Syndrome

Reported by
Council of State and Territorial Epidemiologists;
AIDS Program, Center for Infectious Diseases, CDC

INTRODUCTION

The following revised case definition for surveillance of acquired immunodeficiency syndrome (AIDS) was developed by CDC in collaboration with public health and clinical specialists. The Council of State and Territorial Epidemiologists (CSTE) has officially recommended adoption of the revised definition for national reporting of AIDS. The objectives of the revision are a) to track more effectively the severe disabling morbidity associated with infection with human immunodeficiency virus (HIV) (including HIV-1 and HIV-2); b) to simplify reporting of AIDS cases; c) to increase the sensitivity and specificity of the definition through greater diagnostic application of laboratory evidence for HIV infection; and d) to be consistent with current diagnostic practice, which in some cases includes presumptive, i.e., without confirmatory laboratory evidence, diagnosis of AIDS-indicative diseases (e.g., *Pneumocystis carinii* pneumonia, Kaposi's sarcoma).

The definition is organized into three sections that depend on the status of laboratory evidence of HIV infection (e.g., HIV antibody) (Figure 1). The major proposed changes apply to patients with laboratory evidence for HIV infection: a) inclusion of HIV encephalopathy, HIV wasting syndrome, and a broader range of specific AIDS-indicative diseases (Section II.A); b) inclusion of AIDS patients whose indicator diseases are diagnosed presumptively (Section II.B); and c) elimination of exclusions due to other causes of immunodeficiency (Section I.A).

Application of the definition for children differs from that for adults in two ways. First, multiple or recurrent serious bacterial infections and lymphoid interstitial pneumonia/pulmonary lymphoid hyperplasia are accepted as indicative of AIDS among children but not among adults. Second, for children<15 months of age whose mothers are thought to have had HIV infection during the child's perinatal period, the laboratory criteria for HIV infection are more stringent, since the presence of HIV antibody in the child is, by itself, insufficient evidence for HIV infection because of the persistence of passively acquired maternal antibodies < 15 months after birth.

The new definition is effective immediately. State and local health departments are requested to apply the new definition henceforth to patients reported to them. The initiation of the actual reporting of cases that meet the new definition is targeted for September 1, 1987, when modified computer software and report forms should be in place to accommodate the changes. CSTE has recommended retrospective application of the revised definition to patients already reported to health departments. The new definition follows:

Centers for Disease Control. Revision of the CDC Surveillance case definition for acquired immunodeficiency syndrome. *MMWR* 1987; 36 (suppl no. 1S) :[3S-15S].

1987 REVISION OF CASE DEFINITION FOR AIDS FOR SURVEILLANCE PURPOSES

For national reporting, a case of AIDS is defined as an illness characterized by one or more of the following "indicator" diseases, depending on the status of laboratory evidence of HIV infection, as shown below.

I. Without Laboratory Evidence Regarding HIV Infection

If laboratory tests for HIV were not performed or gave inconclusive results (*See* Appendix I) and the patient had no other cause of immunodeficiency listed in Section I.A below, then any disease listed in Section I.B indicates AIDS if it was diagnosed by a definitive method (*See* Appendix II).

A. **Causes of immunodeficiency that disqualify diseases as indicators of AIDS in the absence of laboratory evidence for HIV infection**
   1. high-dose or long-term systemic corticosteroid therapy or other immunosuppressive/cytotoxic therapy ≤3 months before the onset of the indicator disease
   2. any of the following diseases diagnosed ≤3 months after diagnosis of the indicator disease: Hodgkin's disease, non-Hodgkin's lymphoma (other than primary brain lymphoma), lymphocytic leukemia, multiple myeloma, any other cancer of lymphoreticular or histiocytic tissue, or angioimmunoblastic lymphadenopathy
   3. a genetic (congenital) immunodeficiency syndrome or an acquired immunodeficiency syndrome atypical of HIV infection, such as one involving hypogammaglobulinemia

B. **Indicator diseases diagnosed definitively (*See* Appendix II)**
   1. candidiasis of the esophagus, trachea, bronchi, or lungs
   2. cryptococcosis, extrapulmonary
   3. cryptosporidiosis with diarrhea persisting >1 month
   4. cytomegalovirus disease of an organ other than liver, spleen, or lymph nodes in a patient >1 month of age
   5. herpes simplex virus infection causing a mucocutaneous ulcer that persists longer than 1 month; or bronchitis, pneumonitis, or esophagitis for any duration affecting a patient >1 month of age
   6. Kaposi's sarcoma affecting a patient < 60 years of age
   7. lymphoma of the brain (primary) affecting a patient < 60 years of age
   8. lymphoid interstitial pneumonia and/or pulmonary lymphoid hyperplasia (LIP/PLH complex) affecting a child <13 years of age
   9. *Mycobacterium avium* complex or *M. kansasii* disease, disseminated (at a site other than or in addition to lungs, skin, or cervical or hilar lymph nodes)
   10. *Pneumocystis carinii* pneumonia
   11. progressive multifocal leukoencephalopathy
   12. toxoplasmosis of the brain affecting a patient >1 month of age

II. With Laboratory Evidence for HIV Infection

Regardless of the presence of other causes of immunodeficiency (I.A), in the presence of laboratory evidence for HIV infection (*See* Appendix I), any disease listed above (I.B) or below (II.A or II.B) indicates a diagnosis of AIDS.

A. **Indicator diseases diagnosed definitively (See Appendix II)**
   1. bacterial infections, multiple or recurrent (any combination of at least two within a 2-year period), of the following types affecting a child < 13 years of age:
      septicemia, pneumonia, meningitis, bone or joint infection, or abscess of an internal organ or body cavity (excluding otitis media or superficial skin or mucosal abscesses), caused by *Haemophilus*, *Streptococcus* (including pneumococcus), or other pyogenic bacteria
   2. coccidioidomycosis, disseminated (at a site other than or in addition to lungs or cervical or hilar lymph nodes)
   3. HIV encephalopathy (also called "HIV dementia," "AIDS dementia," or "subacute encephalitis due to HIV") (*See* Appendix II for description)
   4. histoplasmosis, disseminated (at a site other than or in addition to lungs or cervical or hilar lymph nodes)
   5. isosporiasis with diarrhea persisting >1 month
   6. Kaposi's sarcoma at any age
   7. lymphoma of the brain (primary) at any age
   8. other non-Hodgkin's lymphoma of B-cell or unknown immunologic phenotype and the following histologic types:
      a. small noncleaved lymphoma (either Burkitt or non-Burkitt type) (*See* Appendix IV for equivalent terms and numeric codes used in the *International Classification of Diseases*, Ninth Revision, Clinical Modification)
      b. immunoblastic sarcoma (equivalent to any of the following, although not necessarily all in combination: immunoblastic lymphoma, large-cell lymphoma, diffuse histiocytic lymphoma, diffuse undifferentiated lymphoma, or high-grade lymphoma) (*See* Appendix IV for equivalent terms and numeric codes used in the *International Classification of Diseases*, Ninth Revision, Clinical Modification)

      Note: Lymphomas are not included here if they are of T-cell immunologic phenotype or their histologic type is not described or is described as "lymphocytic," "lymphoblastic," "small cleaved," or "plasmacytoid lymphocytic"

   9. any mycobacterial disease caused by mycobacteria other than *M. tuberculosis*, disseminated (at a site other than or in addition to lungs, skin, or cervical or hilar lymph nodes)
   10. disease caused by *M. tuberculosis*, extrapulmonary (involving at least one site outside the lungs, regardless of whether there is concurrent pulmonary involvement)
   11. *Salmonella* (nontyphoid) septicemia, recurrent
   12. HIV wasting syndrome (emaciation, "slim disease") (*See* Appendix II for description)

B. **Indicator diseases diagnosed presumptively (by a method other than those in Appendix II)**
   Note: Given the seriousness of diseases indicative of AIDS, it is generally important to diagnose them definitively, especially when therapy that would be used may have serious side effects or when definitive diagnosis is needed

for eligibility for antiretroviral therapy. Nonetheless, in some situations, a patient's condition will not permit the performance of definitive tests. In other situations, accepted clinical practice may be to diagnose presumptively based on the presence of characteristic clinical and laboratory abnormalities. Guidelines for presumptive diagnoses are suggested in Appendix III.

1. candidiasis of the esophagus
2. cytomegalovirus retinitis with loss of vision
3. Kaposi's sarcoma
4. lymphoid interstitial pneumonia and/or pulmonary lymphoid hyperplasia (LIP/PLH complex) affecting a child <13 years of age
5. mycobacterial disease (acid-fast bacilli with species not identified by culture), disseminated (involving at least one site other than or in addition to lungs, skin, or cervical or hilar lymph nodes)
6. *Pneumocystis carinii* pneumonia
7. toxoplasmosis of the brain affecting a patient >1 month of age

III. With Laboratory Evidence Against HIV Infection

With laboratory test results negative for HIV infection (*See* Appendix I), a diagnosis of AIDS for surveillance purposes is ruled out *unless*:
- A. all the other causes of immunodeficiency listed above in Section I.A are excluded; **AND**
- B. the patient has had either:
    1. *Pneumocystis carinii* pneumonia diagnosed by a definitive method (*See* Appendix II); **OR**
    2. a. any of the other diseases indicative of AIDS listed above in Section I.B diagnosed by a definitive method (*See* Appendix II); **AND**
       b. a T-helper/inducer (CD4) lymphocyte count <400/mm^3.

COMMENTARY

The surveillance of severe disease associated with HIV infection remains an essential, though not the only, indicator of the course of the HIV epidemic. The number of AIDS cases and the relative distribution of cases by demographic, geographic, and behavioral risk variables are the oldest indices of the epidemic, which began in 1981 and for which data are available retrospectively back to 1978. The original surveillance case definition, based on then-available knowledge, provided useful epidemiologic data on severe HIV disease (*1*). To ensure a reasonable predictive value for underlying immunodeficiency caused by what was then an unknown agent, the indicators of AIDS in the old case definition were restricted to particular opportunistic diseases diagnosed by reliable methods in patients without specific known causes of immunodeficiency. After HIV was discovered to be the cause of AIDS, however, and highly sensitive and specific HIV-antibody tests became available, the spectrum of manifestations of HIV infection became better defined, and classification systems for HIV infection were developed (*2-5*). It became apparent that some progressive, seriously disabling, and even fatal conditions (e.g., encephalopathy, wasting syndrome) affecting a substantial number of HIV-infected patients were not subject to epidemiologic surveillance, as they were not included in the AIDS case definition. For reporting purposes, the revision adds to the definition most of those severe non-infectious, non-cancerous HIV-associated conditions that are categorized in the CDC clinical classification systems for HIV infection among adults and children (4,5).

Another limitation of the old definition was that AIDS-indicative diseases are diagnosed presumptively (i.e., without confirmation by methods required by the old definition) in 10%-15% of patients diagnosed with such diseases; thus, an appreciable proportion of AIDS cases were missed for reporting purposes (6,7). This proportion may be increasing, which would compromise the old case definition's usefulness as a tool for monitoring trends. The revised case definition permits the reporting of these clinically diagnosed cases as long as there is laboratory evidence of HIV infection.

The effectiveness of the revision will depend on how extensively HIV-antibody tests are used. Approximately one third of AIDS patients in the United States have been from New York City and San Francisco, where, since 1985, < 7% have been reported with HIV-antibody test results, compared with > 60% in other areas. The impact of the revision on the reported numbers of AIDS cases will also depend on the proportion of AIDS patients in whom indicator diseases are diagnosed presumptively rather than definitively. The use of presumptive diagnostic criteria varies geographically, being more common in certain rural areas and in urban areas with many indigent AIDS patients.

To avoid confusion about what should be reported to health departments, the term "AIDS" should refer only to conditions meeting the surveillance definition. This definition is intended only to provide consistent statistical data for public health purposes. Clinicians will not rely on this definition alone to diagnose serious disease caused by HIV infection in individual patients because there may be additional information that would lead to a more accurate diagnosis. For example, patients who are not reportable under the definition because they have either a negative HIV-antibody test or, in the presence of HIV antibody, an opportunistic disease not listed in the definition as an indicator of AIDS nonetheless may be diagnosed as having serious HIV disease on consideration of other clinical or laboratory characteristics of HIV infection or a history of exposure to HIV.

Conversely, the AIDS surveillance definition may rarely misclassify other patients as having serious HIV disease if they have no HIV-antibody test but have an AIDS-indicative disease with a background incidence unrelated to HIV infection, such as cryptococcal meningitis.

The diagnostic criteria accepted by the AIDS surveillance case definition should not be interpreted as the standard of good medical practice. Presumptive diagnoses are accepted in the definition because not to count them would be to ignore substantial morbidity resulting from HIV infection. Likewise, the definition accepts a reactive screening test for HIV antibody without confirmation by a supplemental test because a repeatedly reactive screening test result, in combination with an indicator disease, is highly indicative of true HIV disease. For national surveillance purposes, the tiny proportion of possibly false-positive screening tests in persons with AIDS-indicative diseases is of little consequence. For the individual patient, however, a correct diagnosis is critically important. The use of supplemental tests is, therefore, strongly endorsed. An increase in the diagnostic use of HIV-antibody tests could improve both the quality of medical care and the function of the new case definition, as well as assist in providing counselling to prevent transmission of HIV.

FIGURE I. Flow diagram for revised CDC case definition of AIDS, September 1, 1987

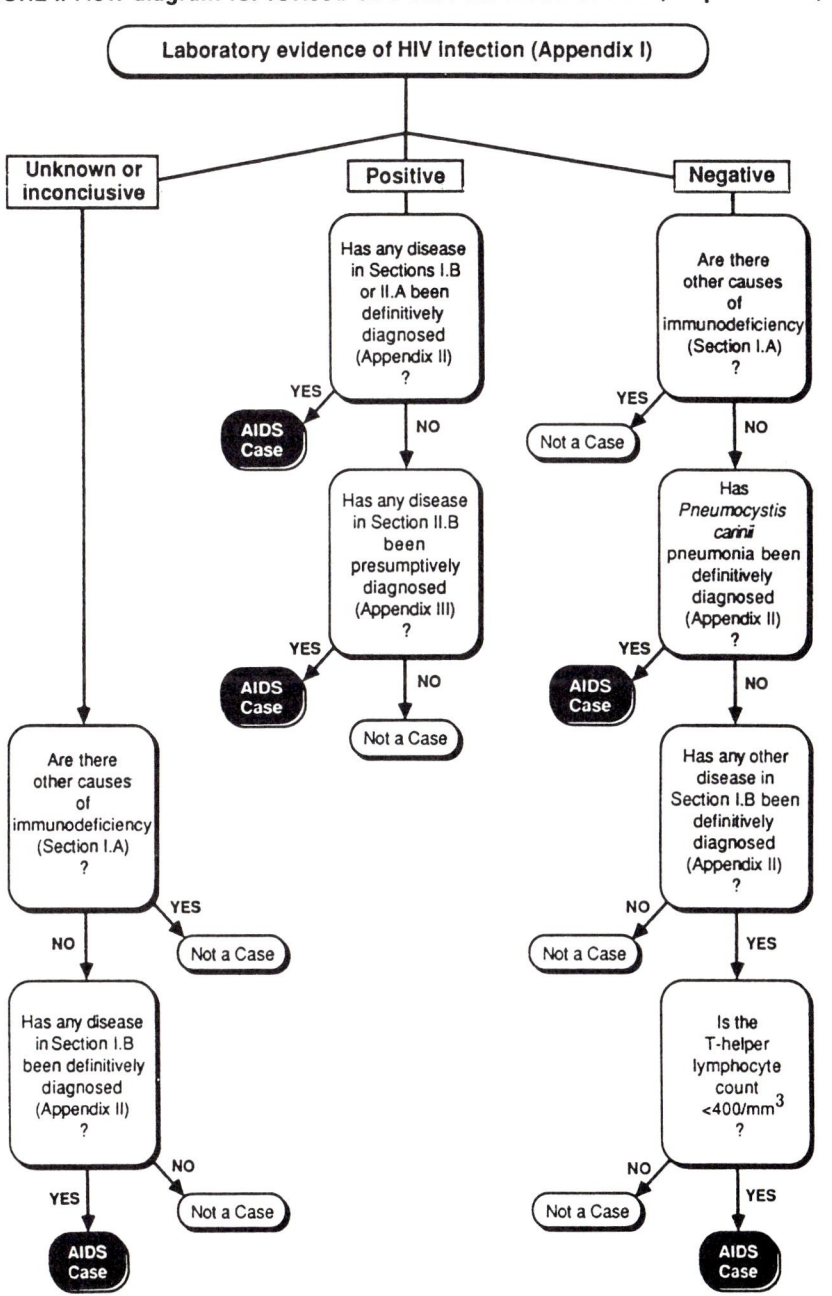

References
1. World Health Organization. Acquired immunodeficiency syndrome (AIDS): WHO/CDC case definition for AIDS. WHO Wkly Epidemiol Rec 1986;61:69-72.
2. Haverkos HW, Gottlieb MS, Killen JY, Edelman R. Classification of HTLV-III/LAV-related diseases [Letter]. J Infect Dis 1985;152:1095.
3. Redfield RR, Wright DC, Tramont EC. The Walter Reed staging classification of HTLV-III infection. N Engl J Med 1986;314:131-2.
4. CDC. Classification system for human T-lymphotropic virus type III/lymphadenopathy-associated virus infections. MMWR 1986;35:334-9.
5. CDC. Classification system for human immunodeficiency virus (HIV) infection in children under 13 years of age. MMWR 1987;36:225-30,235.
6. Hardy AM, Starcher ET, Morgan WM, et al. Review of death certificates to assess completeness of AIDS case reporting. Pub Hlth Rep 1987;102(4):386-91.
7. Starcher ET, Biel JK, Rivera-Castano R, Day JM, Hopkins SG, Miller JW. The impact of presumptively diagnosed opportunistic infections and cancers on national reporting of AIDS [Abstract]. Washington, DC : III International Conference on AIDS, June 1-5, 1987.

APPENDIX I

Laboratory Evidence For or Against HIV Infection

1. **For Infection**:
   When a patient has disease consistent with AIDS:
   a. a serum specimen from a patient ≥15 months of age, or from a child <15 months of age whose mother is not thought to have had HIV infection during the child's perinatal period, that is repeatedly reactive for HIV antibody by a screening test (e.g., enzyme-linked immunosorbent assay [ELISA]), as long as subsequent HIV-antibody tests (e.g., Western blot, immunofluorescence assay), if done, are positive; **OR**
   b. a serum specimen from a child < 15 months of age, whose mother is thought to have had HIV infection during the child's perinatal period, that is repeatedly reactive for HIV antibody by a screening test (e.g., ELISA), plus increased serum immunoglobulin levels and at least one of the following abnormal immunologic test results: reduced absolute lymphocyte count, depressed CD4 (T-helper) lymphocyte count, or decreased CD4/CD8 (helper/suppressor) ratio, as long as subsequent antibody tests (e.g., Western blot, immunofluorescence assay), if done, are positive; **OR**
   c. a positive test for HIV serum antigen; **OR**
   d. a positive HIV culture confirmed by both reverse transcriptase detection and a specific HIV-antigen test or in situ hybridization using a nucleic acid probe; **OR**
   e. a positive result on any other highly specific test for HIV (e.g., nucleic acid probe of peripheral blood lymphocytes).

2. **Against Infection**:
   A nonreactive screening test for serum antibody to HIV (e.g., ELISA) without a reactive or positive result on any other test for HIV infection (e.g., antibody, antigen, culture), if done.

3. **Inconclusive (Neither For nor Against Infection)**:
   a. a repeatedly reactive screening test for serum antibody to HIV (e.g., ELISA) followed by a negative or inconclusive supplemental test (e.g., Western blot, immunofluorescence assay) without a positive HIV culture or serum antigen test, if done; **OR**
   b. a serum specimen from a child < 15 months of age, whose mother is thought to have had HIV infection during the child's perinatal period, that is repeatedly reactive for HIV antibody by a screening test, even if positive by a supplemental test, without additional evidence for immunodeficiency as described above (in 1.b) and without a positive HIV culture or serum antigen test, if done.

APPENDIX II

Definitive Diagnostic Methods for Diseases Indicative of AIDS

Diseases	Definitive Diagnostic Methods
cryptosporidiosis cytomegalovirus isosporiasis Kaposi's sarcoma lymphoma lymphoid pneumonia or hyperplasia *Pneumocystis carinii* pneumonia progressive multifocal leukoencephalopathy toxoplasmosis	microscopy (histology or cytology).
candidiasis	gross inspection by endoscopy or autopsy or by microscopy (histology or cytology) on a specimen obtained directly from the tissues affected (including scrapings from the mucosal surface), not from a culture.
coccidioidomycosis cryptococcosis herpes simplex virus histoplasmosis	microscopy (histology or cytology), culture, or detection of antigen in a specimen obtained directly from the tissues affected or a fluid from those tissues.
tuberculosis other mycobacteriosis salmonellosis other bacterial infection	culture.

HIV encephalopathy* (dementia)	clinical findings of disabling cognitive and/or motor dysfunction interfering with occupation or activities of daily living, or loss of behavioral developmental milestones affecting a child, progressing over weeks to months, in the absence of a concurrent illness or condition other than HIV infection that could explain the findings. Methods to rule out such concurrent illnesses and conditions must include cerebrospinal fluid examination and either brain imaging (computed tomography or magnetic resonance) or autopsy.
HIV wasting syndrome*	findings of profound involuntary weight loss >10% of baseline body weight plus either chronic diarrhea (at least two loose stools per day for ≥ 30 days) or chronic weakness and documented fever (for ≥ 30 days, intermittent or constant) in the absence of a concurrent illness or condition other than HIV infection that could explain the findings (e.g., cancer, tuberculosis, cryptosporidiosis, or other specific enteritis).

*For HIV encephalopathy and HIV wasting syndrome, the methods of diagnosis described here are not truly definitive, but are sufficiently rigorous for surveillance purposes.

APPENDIX III

Suggested Guidelines for Presumptive Diagnosis of Diseases Indicative of AIDS

Diseases	Presumptive Diagnostic Criteria
candidiasis of esophagus	a. recent onset of retrosternal pain on swallowing; **AND** b. oral candidiasis diagnosed by the gross appearance of white patches or plaques on an erythematous base or by the microscopic appearance of fungal mycelial filaments in an uncultured specimen scraped from the oral mucosa.
cytomegalovirus retinitis	a characteristic appearance on serial ophthalmoscopic examinations (e.g., discrete patches of retinal whitening with distinct borders, spreading in a centrifugal manner, following blood vessels, progressing over several months, frequently associated with retinal vasculitis, hemorrhage, and necrosis). Resolution of active disease leaves retinal scarring and atrophy with retinal pigment epithelial mottling.
mycobacteriosis	microscopy of a specimen from stool or normally sterile body fluids or tissue from a site other than lungs, skin, or cervical or hilar lymph nodes, showing acid-fast bacilli of a species not identified by culture.
Kaposi's sarcoma	a characteristic gross appearance of an erythematous or violaceous plaque-like lesion on skin or mucous membrane. (**Note:** Presumptive diagnosis of Kaposi's sarcoma should not be made by clinicians who have seen few cases of it.)
lymphoid interstitial pneumonia	bilateral reticulonodular interstitial pulmonary infiltrates present on chest X ray for ≥2 months with no pathogen identified and no response to antibiotic treatment.
Pneumocystis carinii pneumonia	a. a history of dyspnea on exertion or nonproductive cough of recent onset (within the past 3 months); **AND** b. chest X-ray evidence of diffuse bilateral interstitial infiltrates or gallium scan evidence of diffuse bilateral pulmonary disease; **AND** c. arterial blood gas analysis showing an arterial pO_2 of <70 mm Hg or a low respiratory diffusing capacity (<80% of predicted values) or an increase in the alveolar-arterial oxygen tension gradient; **AND** d. no evidence of a bacterial pneumonia.

toxoplasmosis of the brain	a. recent onset of a focal neurologic abnormality consistent with intracranial disease or a reduced level of consciousness; **AND** b. brain imaging evidence of a lesion having a mass effect (on computed tomography or nuclear magnetic resonance) or the radiographic appearance of which is enhanced by injection of contrast medium; **AND** c. serum antibody to toxoplasmosis or successful response to therapy for toxoplasmosis.

APPENDIX IV

Equivalent Terms and International Classification of Disease (ICD) Codes for AIDS-Indicative Lymphomas

The following terms and codes describe lymphomas indicative of AIDS in patients with antibody evidence for HIV infection (Section II.A.8 of the AIDS case definition). Many of these terms are obsolete or equivalent to one another.

ICD-9-CM (1978)

Codes	Terms
200.0	**Reticulosarcoma** lymphoma (malignant): histiocytic (diffuse) reticulum cell sarcoma: pleomorphic cell type or not otherwise specified
200.2	**Burkitt's tumor or lymphoma** malignant lymphoma, Burkitt's type

ICD-O (Oncologic Histologic Types 1976)

Codes	Terms
9600/3	**Malignant lymphoma, undifferentiated cell type** non-Burkitt's or not otherwise specified
9601/3	**Malignant lymphoma, stem cell type** stem cell lymphoma
9612/3	**Malignant lymphoma, immunoblastic type** immunoblastic sarcoma, immunoblastic lymphoma, or immunoblastic lymphosarcoma
9632/3	**Malignant lymphoma, centroblastic type** diffuse or not otherwise specified, or germinoblastic sarcoma: diffuse or not otherwise specified
9633/3	**Malignant lymphoma, follicular center cell, non-cleaved** diffuse or not otherwise specified
9640/3	**Reticulosarcoma, not otherwise specified** malignant lymphoma, histiocytic: diffuse or not otherwise specified reticulum cell sarcoma, not otherwise specified malignant lymphoma, reticulum cell type
9641/3	**Reticulosarcoma, pleomorphic cell type** malignant lymphoma, histiocytic, pleomorphic cell type reticulum cell sarcoma, pleomorphic cell type
9750/3	**Burkitt's lymphoma or Burkitt's tumor** malignant lymphoma, undifferentiated, Burkitt's type malignant lymphoma, lymphoblastic, Burkitt's type

Copies of this report are available through the National AIDS Information Clearinghouse, P.O. Box 6003, Rockville, MD 20850.

Glossary

acquired immunodeficiency syndrome (AIDS)—an acquired defect in immune system function caused by infection with HIV that reduces the affected person's resistance to certain types of opportunistic infections and cancers.

addiction—compulsive, uncontrollable dependence on a substance, habit, or practice to such a degree that cessation causes severe emotional, mental, or physiologic reactions, as with intravenous drug abuse.

AIDS dementia complex (HIV encephalopathy)—the most common neurologic disorder in persons with AIDS, characterized by its effects on cognition, behavior, and motor function. The dementia may progress from memory loss to intellectual dysfunction, generalized profound weakness, hypokinesia, incontinence, mutism, or death.

AIDS-related complex (ARC)—a manifestation of HIV infection wherein a number of signs, symptoms, or diseases may occur, indicating immune suppression. These include fever, night sweats, oral thrush, weight loss, and persistent diarrhea, among others.

amoebiasis—infection by amoebas, especially *Entamoeba histolytica*. Usually causes severe diarrhea and/or cramping.

antibody (Ab)—a protein belonging to a class of proteins known as immunoglobulins. Antibodies are produced by plasma cells to counteract specific antigens (Ag)—infectious agents such as viruses, bacteria, etc. The antibodies then combine with the antigen they are made to fight and may cause the death of the infectious agent.

antibody negative for HIV–a blood test result showing that a person has not developed antibodies to HIV, although this may show a false result.

antibody positive for HIV—a blood test result showing that a person has been infected with HIV at some time and has developed antibodies to HIV, also termed seropositive. Although people who are antibody positive are presumed to be both infected and infectious, they may be free of symptoms of AIDS or ARC.

antibody test for HIV—blood testing conducted in two stages: 1. ELISA (enzyme-linked immunoabsorbent assay test for antibodies)—a test developed to screen the nation's blood supply; 2. Western Blot—confirmatory test for antibodies.

antigen (Ag)—a substance (often a protein or carbohydrate on the surface of an infectious agent) foreign to the body, which stimulates the formation of antibodies to combat its presence.

asymptomatic infection—an infection in which certain organisms, such as viruses, penetrate a person's cells without resulting in clinical signs or symptoms to indicate that the person is infected.

AZT, Azidothymidine, Retrovir (zidovudine)—the only federally approved antiviral treatment for HIV infection. In persons with AIDS and ARC, short-term studies have shown that it increases life span, decreases the frequency of opportunistic infections, improves functional status, and promotes weight gain. The most significant side effects are anemia, neutropenia, nausea, vomiting, and headache. Long-term side effects are yet undetermined.

bacterium—a microscopic organism composed of a single cell. Many bacteria can cause disease in humans.

basophil—a special white blood cell, called a granulocyte, the normal functions of which are unknown. It has been most commonly identified with allergic reactions.

B-cells—see *lymphocytes*.

B-lymphocytes—B-cells (see *lymphocytes*).

bone marrow—soft tissue located in the cavities of the bones; responsible for producing blood cells.

buying club a group of individuals who purchase non-FDA-approved medication from foreign countries for their personal use.

candidiasis—a yeastlike infection caused by *Candida albicans*. In persons with HIV infection, it is commonly found in the mouth and esophagus. Oral infections are called thrush and exhibit creamy white patches of exudate on inflamed and painful mucosa. Common sites may also include the nail beds, axilla, umbilicus, and around the anus. It may occur systematically and affect the heart, the lining around the brain, and the spinal cord. This infection has become a standard problem seen in immunosuppressed people. It also occurs frequently in the vaginal area in cases that are not associated with HIV.

carcinogenic—any substance that may induce the cancerous transformation of cells.

case manager—the person responsible for daily assessment and coordination of a client's home care services.

cell-mediated immunity—the reaction to antigenic materials by specific defensive cells (macrophages) rather than antibodies.
colitis—inflammation of the colon (the part of the large intestine that terminates at the rectum).
community of color—a term used to describe neighborhoods of primarily black or Latino people; may also include other racial minorities.
complementary therapies or alternative therapies—nontraditional approaches to health care treatment with the goal of restoring clients' equilibrium so that their own healing processes can take over. Some complementary therapies include biofeedback, pain control, massage, visualization, and Chinese acupuncture.
cryptococcus—a fungal infection of the meninges commonly found in persons with AIDS. It is caused by the fungus *Cryptococcus neoformans*. Meningitis with headache, blurred vision, confusion, depression, agitation, or inappropriate speech is the most common form.
cryptosporidiosis—an infection caused by a protozoan parasite found in the intestines that causes severe diarrhea.
cytomegalovirus (CMV)—a virus related to the herpes family. CMV infections may occur without any symptoms, or may result in mild flulike symptoms of aching, fever, mild sore throat, weakness, and enlarged lymph nodes. Severe CMV infections can result in hepatitis, mononucleosis, or pneumonia, even in nonimmunosuppressed persons. CMV is "shed" in body fluids and substances—urine, semen, saliva, feces, sweat.
depression—a mental illness characterized by dejected mood, apathy, insomnia, weight loss, and physical inactivity.
diffuse, undifferentiated non-Hodgkins lymphoma (DUNHL)—a rare B-cell lymphoma that is difficult to distinguish from Burkitt's lymphoma. DUNHL patients exhibit generalized lymphadenopathy and enlarged spleens. The disease is usually fatal in persons with HIV infection.
dissemination—spread of a disease internally throughout the body.
dysentery—infection of the intestines, especially the colon, that produces abdominal pain and diarrhea containing blood and mucus.
enteric infections—infections of the intestine.
epidemic—spreading rapidly and extensively through a significant number of people at the same time; a disease that spreads rapidly through a demographic segment of the human population.
epidemiology—the study of relationships among various factors thought to determine the frequency and distribution of health/illness in humans; the study of epidemics and epidemic diseases.
Epstein-Barr virus (EBV)—a herpeslike virus that causes one of the two kinds of mononucleosis (the other is caused by CMV). It affects the nose and throat and is transmitted by kissing. EBV lies dormant in the lymph glands. This is the clearest link to date between virus and cancer.

exposure—the act or condition of coming in contact with, but not necessarily being infected by, a pathogenic agent.
family of choice—the person(s) selected as family members in adulthood; the family that one creates as an adult.
family of origin—the family into which one is born, usually including biological parents and siblings.
fungus—member of a class of relatively primitive vegetable organisms, including mushrooms, yeasts, rusts, molds, and smuts.
gay family—a family of choice, whose members are predominantly gay or lesbian, though it frequently includes heterosexual members as well.
giardiasis—infection of the intestinal tract by *Giardia lambila* (a protozoan) that may cause intermittent diarrhea of lengthy duration or that may be asymptomatic.
granulocytes—white blood cells of the immune system filled with granules of toxic chemicals that enable them to digest microorganisms. Basophils, neutrophils, eosinophils, and mast cells are examples of granulocytes.
guerrilla clinics—places where HIV-infected clients may go to receive drug treatment they cannot administer themselves, such as dinitrochlorobenzene (DNCB).
helper cells—T-4 cells (see *lymphocytes*).
herpes simplex II (HSV II)—a viral infection that causes painful sores on the anus or genitals, but can also be transmitted to the face or mouth.
herpes varicella (zoster virus [HZV])—the varicella virus that causes chicken pox in children. It may reappear in adulthood as herpes zoster, also called shingles. It is characterized by very painful blisters on the skin and follows nerve pathways.
HIV antibody screening—a test for the purpose of revealing the presence of antibodies to HIV. It is used on all donated blood and organs and in all medical and clinical testing programs. If antibodies are detected, it is assumed that the individual or organ is infected.
human immunodeficiency virus (HIV)—the retrovirus that causes AIDS. Formerly referred to as LAV or HTLV-III.
human T-lymphotropic virus (HTLV-III)—the former name of the virus associated with AIDS development in humans (now called HIV).
immune complex—large molecules formed when an antigen and antibody bind together.
immune response—the activity of the immune system against foreign substances.
immune status—the ability of the body's natural defense to fight diseases. It is influenced by heredity, age, past illness history, diet, and physical and mental health. It includes production of circulating and local antibodies and their mechanics of action.
immune system—the system within the body that helps to resist disease-causing organisms such as germs, viruses, or other infectious agents.
immunostimulant—any agent that triggers the body's defenses.

immunosuppression—a condition in which the body's immune system defenses do not work normally. This may be the result of illness or the administration of certain drugs (ones commonly used to fight cancer).

incubation period—the interval between infection and the appearance of the first symptoms.

infection—the invasion of a part or parts of the body by a pathogenic agent that ordinarily multiplies and causes harmful effects.

interferon—an antiviral chemical secreted by an infected cell that strengthens the defenses of nearby cells not yet attacked.

intravenous drugs—drugs injected by needle directly into a vein.

Kaposi's sarcoma (KS)—a tumor of the walls of the blood vessels. It usually appears as painless, pink to purple spots on the skin, but may also occur internally in addition to, or independent of, the skin lesions. Death occurs from major organ involvement. Originally seen in elderly men or in equatorial Africa as a slow-growing, benign lesion, it is now occurring in young people with HIV infection.

latency—the period when the virus is still in the body but resting in an inactive state.

leukocyte—a white blood cell.

leukopenia—a decrease in the white blood cell count.

lymph—a transparent, slightly yellow fluid containing primarily lymphocytes. Lymph is composed of tissue fluids collected from all parts of the body and returned to the blood via the lymphatic vessels.

lymphadenopathy—enlargement of lymph nodes.

lymph nodes—small bean-sized organs of the immune system distributed widely throughout the body; an outpost for B-lymphocytes.

lymphoblast—a T-lymphocyte that has changed (e.g., during a viral attack) to release a variety of chemicals that encourage greater defensive activity by the immune system.

lymphocytes—small white cells, normally present in the blood and lymphoid tissues, that bear the major responsibility for carrying out the functions of the immune system. Different types of lymphocytes include:

T-lymphocytes (T-cells)—processed in the thymus, they produce *lymphokines*, powerful substances that stimulate other cells in the immune system.

T_4 *lymphocytes (T-4 cells, helper cells)*—stimulate the B-lymphocytes to produce antibodies.

T_8 *lymphocytes (suppressor cells)*—shut down antibody production by the B-cells.

Helper (T_4)-Suppressor (T_8) Ratio—the normal ratio of helper T-cells to suppressor T-cells is about 2:1. This becomes inverted in AIDS clients by the dramatic reduction in the number of helper (T-4) cells.

B-lymphocytes (B-cells)—derived from bone marrow, they detect the presence of a foreign agent. Once exposed to an antigen on the agent, these cells differentiate into plasma cells to produce antibodies.

lymphocytosis—a decrease in the total number of lymphocytes.

lymphokines—powerful substances produced and released into the blood stream by T-lymphocytes and capable of stimulating other cells in the immune system.

macrophage—a scavenger cell found in the tissues, able to destroy invading bacteria or other foreign material.

malaise—a generalized feeling of bodily discomfort.

methadone—a semisynthetic, long-acting narcotic used to treat heroin addiction.

monocyte—a large white blood cell that acts as a scavenger, capable of destroying invading bacteria or other foreign material.

morbidity—the degree of symptomatic illness associated with an infectious organism.

mycobacteria avium complex (MAC)—a common opportunistic bacterial infection in persons with AIDS. Sites of infection include the lungs, blood, lymph nodes, and other areas throughout the body. Occurs widely in nature, but does not often cause disease except in immunosuppressed individuals.

Mycobacterium tuberculosis (MTB)—the bacterium that causes tuberculosis. In persons with AIDS, tuberculosis is commonly found in areas other than the lung, such as lymph nodes and the pericardium.

natural killer cells—large granular lymphocytes that attack and destroy other cells such as tumor cells and those infected by viruses or other microbes.

neutropenia—an abnormal decrease in the number of neutrophils in the blood. Neutropenia is noted as a major side effect of AZT treatment as well as a common disorder in HIV infection.

neutrophil—a special white blood cell, called a granulocyte, that can digest microorganisms.

nonpathogenic organisms—microorganisms that are not disease-producing.

oncogenic—any substance that may produce tumors, especially malignant ones.

opportunistic infections—those diseases caused by agents that are frequently present in our bodies or environment, but that cause disease only when there is an alteration from normal health conditions, such as when the immune system becomes depressed.

parasite—a plant or animal that lives, grows, and feeds on or within another organism.

pathogen—any disease-producing microorganism or substance.

perinatal—occurring in the period during, just before, or just after birth.

persistent generalized lymphadenopathy (PGL)—a persistent swelling of the lymph nodes, frequently associated with HIV infection.

pneumocystis carinii pneumonia (PCP)—a lung infection seen in immunosuppressed people. It is caused by the protozoan *Pneumocystis carinii*, which is present almost everywhere but normally is destroyed by healthy immune systems. Once individuals contract PCP, they are susceptible to recurrence of the disease.

power packing—maintaining a high-calorie, high-protein diet.

prevalence—the total number of persons with a disease in a given population at a given point in time—usually expressed as a percentage.
proctitis—inflammation of the rectum.
prodrome—a period of vague or minor symptoms that precedes the characteristic signs or symptoms at the onset of a disease.
psychoneuroimmunology (PNI)—a new field of research that explores the correlation of consciousness and the central nervous system to immune function, targeting stress, grief, and depression as causes of immunosuppression and the onset of various diseases.
PWA—person with AIDS.
remission—the lessening of the severity or duration of disease, or the abatement of symptoms altogether over a period of time.
retrovirus—a genus of viruses that contain the enzyme reverse transcriptase, and that require the synthesis of proviral DNA for their replication.
safer sex—sexual practices that deter the transmission of potentially infectious body fluids from one person to another.
salmonella—a microorganism that may cause diarrhea with cramps and, sometimes, fever; usually self-limiting.
sensitivity—in reference to a blood test, the degree of accuracy for detection; the probability that the test will be positive when infection is present.
seroconversion—the point at which antibodies to specific antigens are produced by B-lymphocytes and become detectable in the blood; the point of changing from antibody negative to antibody positive.
seronegative—see *antibody negative*.
seropositive—see *antibody positive*.
shigella—a microorganism that may cause dysentery.
"slims"—the progressive weight loss resulting from HIV infection.
specificity—in reference to a blood test, the degree of accuracy in identifying a particular entity; the probability that the test will be negative when the infection is not present.
subclinical infections—infections with minimal or no apparent symptoms.
suppressor cell (T_8)—(see *lymphocytes*.)
syndrome—a set of signs and symptoms that occur together.
T-cells—T-lymphocytes (see *lymphocytes*).
thymus—a central lymphoid organ important in the development of immune capability.
toxoplasmosis—an opportunistic infection of the brain caused by the protozoan *Toxoplasma gondii*.
transmission of HIV—HIV is a fragile virus that needs direct blood-to-blood or parenteral contact to be transmitted. There must be mucous membrane contact or breaks in the skin to allow the virus to reach the bloodstream. There must also be sufficient virus in the body fluid to infect. HIV infection spreads by

infusion of contaminated blood, semen, or vaginal secretions through sexual activity and from mother to fetus or newborn.

universal precautions—practices employed to protect health workers to the fullest extent from occupational exposure to HIV or hepatitis B. The most effective means of protection is through consistent use of protective barriers, i.e., gloves, face protection (goggles, mask), and impervious gowns.

vaccine—a substance containing the antigen of an organism that stimulates active immunity and future protection against infection by the organism.

virus—a submicroscopic microbe causing infectious disease that can reproduce only in living cells.

Sources

AIDS Action Committee (1988). *AIDS glossary.* Boston: AIDS Action Committee.

Dorland's illustrated medical dictionary (26th ed.) (1985). Philadelphia: W.B. Saunders Company.

List of terms. (Winter/Spring, 1988). *New England Journal of Public Policy, 4,* 1.

Mosby's medical and nursing dictionary (2nd ed.) (1986). St. Louis: The C.V. Mosby Company.

Index

Abandonment, 204, 206, 221
Abdominal cramping, 142
Acquired immunodeficiency syndrome. *See* AIDS
Actinomycin D, 98
Activity/exercise, assessment of, 113
Acupressure, 186
Acupuncture, 186
Acyclovir, 240
Addiction and addicts
    attitudes toward, 54
    psychosocial profile, 54-55
    referral for, 63
    See also Intravenous drug abuse; specific drugs
Adriamycin, 98
AIDS, 231
    cancer as rehearsal for, 184
    in children, 157-164
    and communities of color, 70-71
    diagnosis of, 91
    education about. *See* Education about AIDS
    emotional issues and, 46-49
    ethical dilemmas about, 23
    family response to, 115, 158-159, 221-223
    infection control guidelines, 246-250
    and intravenous drug abuse, 5, 14, 63-65, 76-77, 80
    and mothering, 84
    nursing care plan for persons with, 119-128
    and pregnancy, 78
    psychological interventions (table), 214-215
    relationships, effect on, 45-46
    spiritual questions about, 207-211
    symptoms, early (table), 232
    terminology related to (table), 231
    and tuberculosis, 19-20, 94
    See also ARC; HIV
AIDS Dementia Complex, 94-96
    See also Dementia
AIDS related complex. *See* ARC
AIDS virus. *See* HIV
AL-721, 134, 190
Algae therapy, 189

Anger, 217-218
    among family members, 222-223
    See also Rage
Anorexia, 130
Antibodies, 231
    retention of mother's by newborn, 159-160
    tests for, 91-92
    time lag in formation, in response to HIV infection, 4, 90
Anti-yeast diet, 134
ARC, 91, 231, 246-250
Arthritis, 113
Aseptic meningitis, 94, 96
Attitudinal healing, 185
AZT. See Zidovudine

Bach flower remedies, 189
Bactrim, 238
Bactrim DS, 238
B-cells, 89, 94
Blacks. See Communities of color
Bladder elimination. See Elimination - bowels and bladder
Bleomycin, 98
Blood transfusions, in transmission of HIV, 14-15, 206-207
Body fluids, HIV found in, 14
Bodywork therapies, 186-189
Bowel elimination. See Elimination - bowels and bladder
Breast feeding, 80
Burnout, 35-36
Butylated-hydroxytoluene (BHT), 134
"Buying clubs" for unapproved or experimental drugs, 190

Calories, increasing intake, 136
Cancer
    as rehearsal for AIDS, 184
    See also Kaposi's sarcoma
Candida, 18, 103, 239, 241
Centers for Disease Control (CDC), 16-18
Central nervous system, effect of HIV on, 94-96
    See also Dementia

Change, dealing with, 199-204
Chemotherapy, 97-98
Children with AIDS, 157-164
    clinical symptoms of, 159-160
    community response to, 163-164
    diagnosis of, 160-161
    family response to, 158-159
    foster care and residential programs for, 164
    nursing role for, 161-163
    and public schools, 163-164
    sibling involvement in caring, 159
    support to families of, 162-163
Chiropractic, 187
CMV. See Cytomegalovirus infection
Cocaine, 58-59
    effects of, 59
    treatment for addiction, 62-63
Coccidiomyocosis, 94
Coenzyme Q, 134
Cognition/perception, assessment of, 114
Communities of color
    AIDS and, 70-71
    barriers against, 68-70
    cultural diversity in, 71
    and the health care system, 71-73
    homophobia in, 71
    and poverty, 69
Complementary therapies
    kinds of, 184-186
    and long-term survivors, 183-184
    mind-body connections, 182-183
    nursing response to, 191-194
    overview, 181-182
    resources for, 194
    See also specific therapy
Condoms, 81-82, 174, 175
Confidentiality, 25-26, 92
Constipation, 140-141
Coping, assessment of, 116
Cramps, abdominal, 142
Creative visualization, 187
Cryptococcal meningitis, 104
Cryptospordium, 105
Crystal therapy, 187
Cytomegalovirus infection (CMV), 105

and activity assessment, 113

Dehydration, 141
Dementia, 94-96, 114, 216
Denial, 200-201, 215-217
Depression, 202, 219-221
  assessment of, 221
Dextran sulfate, 190
Diarrhea, 140
  and self-image, 115
Diet therapies, 185
  See also Nutrition/metabolism
Dinitrochlorobenzene (DNCB), 190
Discharge planning, 150-155
DNA, production by HIV, 4, 89-90
Doxyrubicin, 98
Drug abuse. See Addiction and addicts; Intravenous drug abuse
DTIC, 98
Duty to care, 27-28
Duty to warn, 25-26
Dysphagia, 130

Education about AIDS
  additional learning tools for, 234
  disease process, 228
  follow-up care, 230
  individualizing, 225-226
  infection control, 230
  medications, 229-230
  reportable signs and symptoms, 229
  symptom management, 228-229
  timing of, 226-227
Elimination - bowel and bladder, assessment of, 112-113
  See also Diarrhea, Urinary tract infections
ELISA test, 92, 231
Encephalitis, 94
Enzyme-Linked Immunoabsorbent Assay. See ELISA
Etoposide, 98
Exercise, assessment of, 113

Family, 115, 158-159, 221-223
  biological, 45, 221-222
  gay, 43-46, 221-222
  response to children with AIDS, 158-159
Fatigue, and eating, 136-137
Fear
  of abandonment, 202, 204
  building community despite, 204-207
  of contagion, 6-7
  of dying, 203, 208-209, 213-215
  overcoming, 8-9
  of pain, 203
  roots of, 7-8
  spiritual dimension of, 32-34, 203-204
  of transmission, 203-204
Flower essences, 189
Food supplements, 148
Functional health patterns assessment, 111-117
Fungus infections, 94, 239, 241

Gastrointestinal disorders, 130-131
Gay families
  and biological families, 221-222
  emotional issues in, 46-49
  nurse's interaction with, 49-51
  understanding, 43-46
Grief, 35-36, 201-202
  among family members, 223
"Guerrilla clinics," 190
Guided imagery, 187
Guilt, feelings of, 207-208, 218
  among family members, 222
  survivor response, 222

Hatha yoga, 187
Healing groups, 185
Health perception/health management assessment of, 111-112
Heartburn, 140
Helplessness, feelings of, 36-37
Hepatitis B, transmission of, 14
Herbal remedies, 190
Heroin, 57-58
  effects of, 57
  and pregnancy, 58
  treatment for addiction, 59-62

withdrawal symptoms of, 58
Herpes viruses, 19
   genital herpes, 240
   herpes simplex, 106, 240
   herpes zoster, 94
Heterosexual transmission of HIV, 77
Histoplasmosis, 94
HIV, 231
   asymptomatic infection, 93
   barrier techniques against infection by, 18
   and central nervous system, 94-96
   classification system for infection by, 90-91
   dormancy period of, 90
   effects on body, 93
   and immune system, 93-94
   and lymphocytes and platelets, 97
   and peripheral nervous system, 96
   exposure risk, 4-6, 15-17
   incubation period, 4
   infection control guidelines, 246-250
   infectious mechanism of, 89-90, 228
   malignancies associated with, 97-98
   mutation of, 4
   transition to illness, 90
   transmission of, 5, 13, 14-15, 76-78
   See also AIDS, ARC
HIV encephalopathy, 94-96
HIV testing. *See* Testing
Holistic remedies, 186-191
   See also specific remedy
Home care
   education/information needs, 225-235
   evaluation of home for, 151-152
   evaluation of patient's needs, 152-153
   implementing of, 154-155
   and intravenous equipment, 153-154
   need for, 149-150
   packaging of, 153-154
   reimbursement for, 153
Homeopathy, 190
Homophobia, 71
Homosexuality and homosexual relationships
   attitudes towards, 49-50, 71

   biological family reaction to, 45
   See also Gay families
Hope
   burnout and, 35-36
   grief and, 35-36
   and helplessness, 36-37
   meaning of and need for, 31
   sources of, 38-40
HTLV-III. *See* HIV
Human immunodeficiency virus. *See* HIV

Immune system, effect of HIV on, 93-94
Infection control guidelines, 246-250
Informed consent, 23-25
Interferon, 97
Intravenous drug abuse
   and AIDS, 5, 14, 63-65
   among women, 82-83
   gender and, 82-83
   needle use, prevention education for, 64-65
   and persons with HIV infection, 65
   referral for, 14, 63-65
   self-esteem and, 82-83
   by sexual partner, 80
   among women, 58, 76-77, 80
   See also Addiction and addicts
Isolation, 218-219

Kaposi's sarcoma (KS), 18, 97-98
   definition and treatment, 237
   pulmonary lesions of, 113
   and self-image, 115
   skin lesions from, 112, 237
Ketoconazole, 239
Kubler-Ross, Elizabeth, 34-35

Lactose intolerance, 141-142
Loss, dealing with, 199-204
Lymphocytes, effect of HIV on, 97
Lymphoid interstitial pneumonitis (LIP)
   mortality rate in children, 161

MAC. *See* Mycobacterium avium complex
Macrobiotic diet, 134
Macrophaghes, 89

Magnetic resonance imaging, 186
MAI (mycobacterium avium-intracellulare).
    See Mycobacterium Avium Complex
Manna, blue green, therapy, 189
Mandatory testing, 23-25
Massage, 188
Meal
    plans, 135, 143-147
    supplements, 148
Megadosing of vitamins, 134
Methadone maintenance, 60-62
    drug interactions with, 61, 62
    pain management and, 60, 62
    side effects of, 61
Mind-body connections, 182-183
Mistletoe extract, 134
Mortality, feelings of, 34-35
Mothering and AIDS, 84
Mouth care, 137-138
Mucositis, 130
Mycobacterium tuberculosis (MTB), 19
Mycobacterium avium complex (MAC), 19, 107
Mycobacterium avium-intracellulare (MAI). See Mycobacterium Avium Complex
Mycostatin. See Nystatin suspension

Nadostine. See Nystatin suspension
Nalbuphine, 62
Naltrexone, 59, 62
Narcotic antagonist therapy, 59, 62
Nausea, 130, 139-140
Needlestick injury, 14, 17
    precautions against, 18
Needs assessment, 109-111
    functional health patterns, 111-117
    physical, 117-118
NHL. See Non-Hodgkin's Lymphoma
Nilstat. See Nystatin suspension
Nizoral. See Ketoconazole
Non-Hodgkin's Lymphoma (NHL), 98
Nubain, 62
Nursing and nursing care, 119-128, (table), 214-215
    for children with AIDS, 161-163
    and complementary therapies, 191-194
    diagnosis, role in, 118-119
    disease-oriented vs. people-oriented, 182
    with gay families, 49-51
    precautions, 17-19
    self-care issues for, 31-32, 37-38
    support groups for, 32, 50
Nursing care plan, 120-128
Nursing diagnosis, 118-119
    See also Needs assessment
Nutrition/metabolism, 249
    assessment of, 112, 131-133
    for children with AIDS, 161
    effect of AIDS on, 129-131
    food supplements, 148
    meal plans, 135, 143-147
    requirements, 136-142
    solutions for common problems, 136-142
    supplements, 148
    unproven regimes, 133-134
    vitamin/mineral therapy, 134
Nutritional risk, measurement (table), 133
Nystatin suspension, 241

Odynophagia, 130
Opportunistic infections, 18-19, 89, 90
    list of, 102-108
Oral lesions, 130
Overinvolvement, 50

Pain, 60, 62, 203, 216
Parasite infections, 94
Parenteral exposure, 14
PCP. See Pneumocystis carinii pneumonia
Pediatric AIDS. See Children with AIDS
Pentam 300. See Pentamidine isethionate
Pentamidine isethionate, 190, 242-243
Pentazocine, 62
Perinatal transmission of HIV, 15, 78-79, 158
Peripheral nervous system, effect of HIV on, 96, 113
Persistent generalized lymphadenopathy (PGL), 130-131

Personal hygiene, 246-248
Personal risk taking, 27-28
Pets, 249
PGL. *See* Persistent generalized lymphadenopathy
Phenytoin, 61
Physical examination
   guidelines for, 117
Platelets
   effect of HIV on, 97
Pneumocystis carinii pneumonia (PCP), 18, 108, 236, 242
   and activity assessment, 113
   definition and treatment, 236
   mortality rate in children, 161
Polarity therapy, 188
Prayer, 210-211
Pregnancy
   and AIDS, 78
   and drug abuse, 58, 79
Progressive relaxation, 188
Project Inform, 191
Prostitution, 78
Protein, increasing intake, 138
Psychoneuroimmunology, 182-183
Psychosocial interventions (table)
   general, 214-215
   for physical problems, 216

Race. *See* Communities of color
Radiation therapy, 98
Rage, 201-202
   See also Anger
Rashes, 112
Reiki therapy, 188
Relationships
   assessment of, 115-116
   gay families, 44-45
   nurses and, 49
   reenvisioning, 205-206
   support groups, 50
Retrovir. *See* Zidovudine
Retrovirus, 4, 13, 89
Ribavarian, 190
Rifampin, 61
Right to die, 26-27
Right to treatment, 26-27

Roles, assessment of, 115-116

Safer sex. *See* Sex and sexuality
Salmonellosis, 94
Sanitation in household chores, 248-249
Self-care diary, 233
Self-care issues for nurses, 37-38
   changes with increased involvement with HIV-infected people, 31-32
   hope and, 31
   support groups, 32, 50
Self-care issues for patients, 228-230
   guidelines, 246-250
   items to have on hand, 251
   "to do list," 252-253
Self-perception/self-concept
   assessment of, 115
   and depression, 219-220
   weight loss and, 115
Septra. *See* Bactrim
Sex and sexuality
   assessment of, 116, 168-172
   barriers to safer practices, 176-177
   choosing partners, 81
   comfort in talking about, 168
   and drug abuse by partner, 80
   risk factors (table), 173
   safer practices, 167-177
   slang expressions (table), 171
   stages of behavior change (table), 175
   teaching safer practices, 172-176
Skin disorders, 112
Sleep/rest, assessment of, 114
Spiritual matters, 207-211
   and fear, 32-34, 203-204
   values and beliefs, 116-117
Spirulima therapy, 189
Stress tolerance, assessment of, 116
Strongyloidosis, 94
Suicide, 209, 220-221
Sulfamethoxazole. *See* Bactrim

T4 lymphocytes, 93
   See also T-helper cells
Talwin, 62
Taste disorders, 138-139
Testing, 91-92, 231

importance of counseling and education, 92
interpreting results, 92
mandatory, 23-25
for women, 82
T-helper cells, 89, 184
Therapeutic massage, 188
Therapeutic touch, 189
Thrombocytopenia, 112
Thrush. *See* Candida
Thymus gland stimulation, 185-186
Touch, therapeutic, 189
Toxoplasma gondii, 18
Toxoplasmosis, 102
Trexan. *See* Naltrexone
Trimethoprim. *See* Bactrim
Trust, 206-207
Tuberculosis, and AIDS, 19-20, 94

Universal Precautions (Centers for Disease Control), 17-18, Appendix A.1, Appendix A.2
Urinary tract infections, 238

Vacuolar myelopathy, 94, 96
Values/beliefs, assessment of, 116-117
  See also Spiritual matters
Vinblastine, 98
Vincristine, 98
Visualization and imagery, 184

Vitamin/mineral therapy, 134
Vomiting, 130
  See also Nausea

WARN. *See* Women's AIDS Risk Network
Weight loss, 129
  and self-image, 115
  See also Nutrition/metabolism
Western blot test, 92, 231
Women, 68, 72
  and children, 67, 157
  epidemiology of AIDS in, 76
  HIV testing for, 82
  HIV transmission in, 76-78
  risk-reduction strategies for, 80-82
  self-esteem and drug abuse, 82-83
  sexual transmission of HIV between, 78
  social networks for, 83-84
Women's AIDS Risk Network (WARN), 70

Yeast infections, 239, 241
  See also Candida

Zidovudine (AZT), 96, 98-99, 162, 190, 244-245
  cost of, 245
  dosage of, 99, 245
  side effects of, 98-99, 244
Zovirax. *See* Acyclovir